The Complete Diabetes Guide

FOR TYPE 2 DIABETES

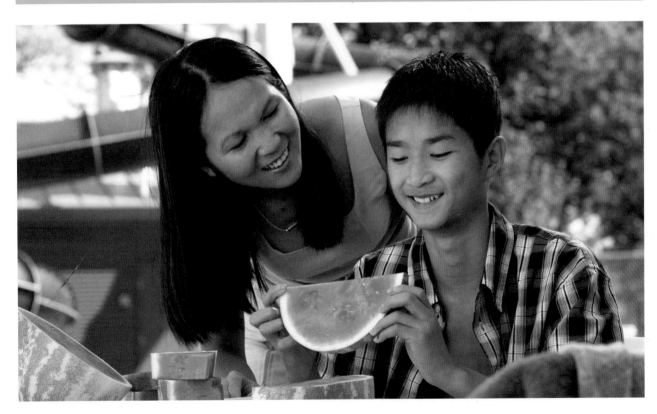

Karen Graham, RD, CDE
Certified Diabetes Educator

Robert ROSE

The Complete Diabetes Guide for Type 2 Diabetes

Disclaimer

The recipes in this book have been carefully tested by our kitchen and our tasters. To the best of our knowledge, they are safe and nutritious for ordinary use and users. For those people with food or other allergies, or who have special food requirements or health issues, please read the suggested contents of each recipe carefully and determine whether or not they may create a problem for you. All recipes are used at the risk of the consumer. We cannot be responsible for any hazards, loss or damage that may occur as a result of any recipe use. For those with special needs, allergies, requirements or health problems (such as kidney disease), in the event of any doubt, please contact your medical adviser prior to the use of any recipe.

The suggestions and information contained in this publication are based on a thorough assessment of all the latest research and information. Reasonable steps have been taken to ensure the accuracy of the information presented. However, we cannot ensure the safety or efficacy of any product or service described in this publication. Individuals are advised to consult a physician or other appropriate health care professional before undertaking any diet, exercise, activity or treatment program or taking any herb or medication referred to in this publication. Professionals must use and apply their own professional judgment, experience, and training and should not rely solely on the information contained in this publication before prescribing any diet, exercise, treatment or medication. While we thank the professional expertise of the reviewers of this publication, neither they nor the author or publisher assumes any responsibility or liability for personal or other injury, loss, or damage that may result from the suggestions or information in this publication.

This book is not intended as a substitute for professional medical care. Only your doctor can diagnose and treat a medical problem.

Design & Production: Durand and Graham, Ltd., with assistance from Tom Powell Design Studio and Fine Line Design
Additional Production: PageWave Graphics Inc.
Editors: Joanne Seiff (primary editor), Janice Madill and Roslyn Graham
Photographer: Brian Gould, Brian Gould Photography Inc.
Food Stylist: Judy Fowler
Photograph on page 43 credit to Casey Hein, on page 266 to Rick Durand, on page 313 to Scott Grant, and on page 359 to Roslyn Graham
Graphic Artwork: Sandi Storen
Water image on cover: ©iStockphoto.com/roman_sh

We acknowledge the financial support of the Government of Canada through the Book Publishing Industry Development Program (BPIDP) for our publishing activities.

Published by Robert Rose Inc.
120 Eglinton Avenue East, Suite 800, Toronto, Ontario, Canada M4P 1E2
Tel: (416) 322-6552 Fax: (416) 322-6936
www.robertrose.ca

Printed and bound in Canada

1 2 3 4 5 6 7 8 9 TCP 21 20 19 18 17 16 15 14 13

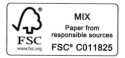

Thank you to:

Robert Rose Inc.
Over the past twenty years, Robert Rose has built a high standard in the promotion of wellness through the publication of cookbooks and lifestyle books that have been extensively researched to address diabetes and chronic disease.

Therefore, I am exceptionally pleased that this book is now included in Robert Rose's collection. I am also proud to note that my first book, *Diabetes Meals for Good Health*, was published by Robert Rose in 2010.

Several years ago, Bob Dees, President of Robert Rose, encouraged me to write a complete diabetes guide. Bob shares my vision and commitment to bringing you – the person with diabetes – a practical and easy-to-read book to help you better understand diabetes, and the health complications that can arise. This book was written to provide you with the answers on how to be as healthy as you can be.

Editors
I am appreciative and grateful for the collective expertise and guidance of my editors; thank you to Joanne Seiff (primary editor), Janice Madill and Roslyn Graham.

Photographer, food stylist, models and graphic artist
Thank you to Brian Gould, photographer, and Judy Fowler, food stylist, for your consistently amazing photography work! Your work shines throughout the book.

Thank you to the models; each one of you brought your enthusiasm, patience and joy that have enhanced the pages of this book.

Thank you, Sandy Storen, your artistic talent has created meaningful and beautiful drawings.

Recipe creators and tasters
I develop my own recipes found in the book, and appreciate recipe ideas of family and friends; thanks to Carol Fraize, France Marcoux, Maize Regular, Mary Vivian, Carl Durand, Marg Graham and Sharon Maciejko for each contributing a recipe idea. Also, many thanks to Rick Durand and others who tested recipes.

Nutrient Analysis
Barbara Selley, RD, and Cathie Martin of Food Intelligence reviewed the nutrient calculations of the meals, snacks and recipes.

Thank you to the National Aboriginal Diabetes Association, especially Anita Ducharme and Dina Bruyere, for their review of the book and their partnership in the fight against diabetes.

Thanks to those who shared your diabetes stories
I learned from you that many of you have overcome challenges, prevented complications and made significant changes in your lives. I wanted everyone to learn from your experience and wisdom. This book includes your real stories. To protect contributors' privacy, I did not include your full names or your name was changed. For most stories, my photographer used models to illustrate your experiences.

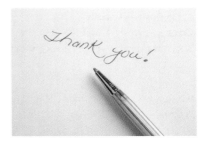

To be sure that this book contained accurate and up-to-date information, health professionals reviewed it on a volunteer basis. These professionals are experts in their particular diabetes or medical specialties. Thank you for taking time out of your busy schedules and providing such essential contributions.

Professional reviewers

- Full book review by: Dr. Jim Price, MB, ChB, CCFP, family physician in Portage la Prairie, Manitoba; Teresa Bodin, RN, CDE, diabetes nurse educator in The Pas, Manitoba; Wilma J. Koersen, BSc, secondary school math and science teacher, Grand Prairie, Alberta; and Diane Unruh, RD, CDE, diabetes educator in Carman, Manitoba.

- Partial book review by: The Riverside-San Bernardino County Diabetes Project in California: Dr Kendall Shumway, DPM (podiatrist and Diabetes Program Director), Marcia Ruhl, RD, CDE (dietitian), Antonia Roots, ACSM, HFS (fitness specialist) and Kristopher Hamlin, BS (fitness assistant).

- Dr. Sheldon Tobe, MD, FRCPC, FACP, Associate Scientist, Sunnybrook Health Sciences Centre, Toronto, reviewed the *Heart attack and stroke, kidney damage* and *urinary tract infection* sections.

- Dr. Blair Lonsberry, MS, OD, Med., FAAO, Clinic Director at Portland Vision Clinic and Associate Professor of Optometry at Pacific University College of Optometry, reviewed the *Eye problems* section and consulted on eye questions throughout the book.

- Casey Hein, BSDH, MBA, Interprofessional Education and Dentistry at the University of Manitoba, Winnipeg, and the President of Casey Hein & Associates in Evergreen, Colorado, reviewed the dental sections.

- Gina Sunderland, MSc, RD, a dietitian who practices in Winnipeg, reviewed sections 1, 2, 3, 6 and 10 of *Top ten nutrition topics*.

- Joan Rew, RD, nutrition educator at Red River College, Winnipeg, reviewed section 4 of *Top ten nutrition topics*.

- Shannon Roode, RD, CDE, at the Collingwood General and Marine Hospital Diabetes Program, reviewed sections 7, 8 and 9 of *Top ten nutrition topics*.

- Pan Am Clinic, Sports Physiotherapy Centre, Winnipeg: Physiotherapists Sam Steinfeld, BSc, BMR (PT), Tim Thiessen, BMR (PT) and Shanna Semler, BSc, BMR (PT) reviewed *Step 2. Being Active*. Dr. Brian Lukie, MD from the Pan Am Clinic reviewed the precautions section in Step 2.

- Murray Gibson, Executive Director, Manitoba Tobacco Reduction Alliance (MANTRA) in Winnipeg, reviewed *Step 3. Becoming a Non-Smoker*.

- Canadian Association of Wound Care, Toronto: Kimberly Stevenson, RN, BN, IIWCC; Heather Orsted, RD, BN, ET, BSc.; Mariam Botros, DcH (Chiropody) reviewed *Foot and lower leg infections* and *Step 4. Preventing Infections, Ten steps to keep your feet healthy.* Also thanks to Dr. Karen Philp, Chief Executive Officer.

- Mary Bertone, RDH, Centre for Community Oral Health, University of Manitoba, Winnipeg, and Roxena Trembath, BSc, RDH (Dental Hygienists) reviewed *Gum disease* and *Step 4, Ten tips for mouth care.*

- Dr. J. Robin Conway, MD, Diabetes Clinic, Smith Falls, Ontario, and Dr. Sora Ludwig, MD, FRCPC, Section of Endocrinology and Metabolism, University of Manitoba, Winnipeg, reviewed *Step 5, Taking Medications and Tests* (2011 edition), and in 2013, Dr. Maureen Clement, MD, CCFP, Vernon, British Columbia, reviewed key sections of *Step 5.*

- Pharmacists Scott McGibney, BSc (Pharm) of Portage la Prairie, Manitoba, and Travis Petrisor, BSc, BSP, of Penticton, British Columbia, reviewed section 7 of *Top ten nutrition topics* and *Step 5, Taking Medications and Tests.*

- Stephanie Staples, LPN, Certified Life Coach and Motivational Speaker, Winnipeg, reviewed *Step 6, Staying Upbeat.*

- The Diabetes Education Resource for Children team, Winnipeg, reviewed *Step 7, Preschoolers to teenagers.* The team included Phyllis Mooney, MSW, RSW; Julie Dexter, BN, CDE and Pam Matson, BN, CDE; Nicole Aylward, RD, CDE and Norma Van Walleghem, RD, CDE; and Dr. Heather Dean, MD, FRCPC, Dr. E. Sellers, MD, FRCPC and Dr. B. Wicklow, MD, FRCPC.

- Holliday Tyson, RM, RN, MHSc (Registered Midwife), Director, International Midwifery Pre-registration Program, Ryerson University, Toronto, reviewed *Step 7. Pregnancy and gestational diabetes.*

- Dr. Stacy Elliott, MD, Director for the BC Centre for Sexual Medicine, and Clinical Professor, Departments of Psychiatry and Urologic Sciences, University of British Columbia, Vancouver; and Dr Richard J. Wassersug, Department of Urologic Sciences, University of British Columbia, Vancouver, reviewed *Step 7. Sexuality and diabetes.*

- Barb Komar, RN, MC, RCC (Masters in Counselling and Registered Clinical Counsellor), St. Paul's Hospital, Vancouver, and private practice counselor, reviewed *Step 7. Pregnancy and gestational diabetes,* and *Sexuality and diabetes.*

My family

My children, Carl Durand and Roslyn Graham, and my parents, Marg and Bill Graham have provided important ideas and nourishment. My husband Rick Durand, as the one closest to me in every way – contributed regular and important inspiration and feedback. This book required many hours of my life, and Rick gave me flexibility and time to support its writing. Thank you, Rick.

Contents

Introduction   *9*
    Straight answers to common diabetes questions   10

Learning About Diabetes   *13*
    Types of diabetes   14
    What is type 2 diabetes?   16
    Symptoms of type 2 diabetes   18
    Risks for type 2 diabetes   19

Diabetes Complications   *21*
    How high blood sugar harms blood vessels   24
    How high blood sugar harms nerves   26
    Heart attack and stroke   27
    Foot and lower leg infections   29
    Kidney damage   33
    Eye problems   38
    Other complications   42

7 STEPS TO PREVENT OR REDUCE DIABETES COMPLICATIONS

    1. Eating Well   *54*
    Karen Graham's Hands-on Food Guide   55
    Top ten nutrition topics   60
      1. How to lose weight and keep it off   61
      2. Carbohydrates and your blood sugar   85
      3. Food labels   94
      4. Light desserts and sweeteners   100
      5. Reducing sodium   109
      6. Lowering cholesterol levels   118
      7. Herbs and vitamins   122
      8. Alcohol   134
      9. What to eat when ill   138
    10. How to gain weight   143

    Seven Day Meal Plan with Recipes   149
    4 Breakfasts   152
    4 Lunches   160
    7 Dinners   168
    Snacks   196
    Eat This – Not That   201

2. Being Active — 217

A prescription for exercise — 218
Getting started — 219
Ten benefits of regular exercise — 221
Low-impact aerobic exercise — 223
Staying flexible — 238
Strengthening exercises — 240
A fitness plan for you — 246
Precautions — 255

3. Becoming a Non-Smoker — 263

Why you should stop smoking — 264
Ten steps to stop smoking — 267

4. Preventing Infections — 281

Keeping your feet healthy — 282
Good skin care — 296
Ten tips for mouth care — 297
Avoiding urinary tract infections (UTIs) — 301
Preventing a flu, cold or food poisoning — 306

5. Taking Medications and Tests — 309

Appointments with health care providers — 310
Pills and insulin — 315
Low blood sugar — 331
Regular laboratory tests — 339
Testing your own blood sugar — 345

6. Staying Upbeat — 351

Coping with stress — 352
Coping with depression — 365

7. Managing at Other Life Stages — 367

Preschoolers to teenagers — 368
Pregnancy and gestational diabetes — 381
Sexuality and diabetes — 392

Diabetes Glossary — 412
Index — 413

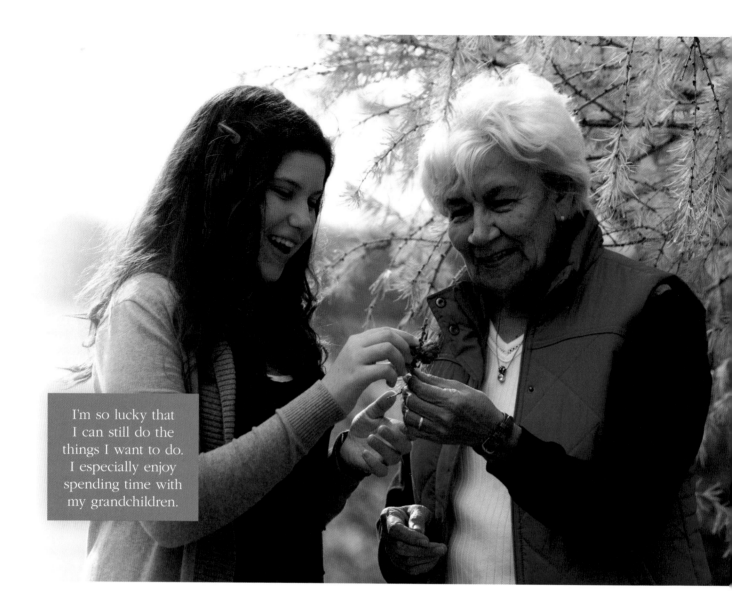

I'm so lucky that I can still do the things I want to do. I especially enjoy spending time with my grandchildren.

Lena's Story

When I was first diagnosed with diabetes I was in terrible shock. I thought my life would change for the worst. However, what I discovered is that with small changes my life actually got richer in an unexpected way. I think you do appreciate life more and in a different way when you have a crisis in your life or you have to deal with a chronic disease. I don't do things the same way I did in the past, but I've adjusted to a new way of living. You reflect and enjoy those things and the people you have around you. I still have wonderful foods to eat, I just don't eat as much. I still watch my favorite TV shows, but I turn the TV off in between. I use this time to go for a walk and exercise, and to organize all my pills and medical appointments. I'm so lucky that I can still do the things I want to do. I especially enjoy spending time with my grandchildren.

Introduction

A journey of a thousand miles begins with a single step.

The Chinese philosopher Lao-tzu said these words more than 2,500 years ago. He understood that our difficult journeys in life start with small changes.

From your diabetes diagnosis, you are starting on a new lifetime journey with one small change at a time. As with all journeys, you might need to ask for directions. You may lose a favorite possession, like giving up a favorite food. You may meet new people, learn new skills, try new foods and learn new ways of cooking. You may feel like a stranger in a foreign land at first, but after a while your new experiences can become routine.

Over the past thirty years as a diabetes educator, I've learned that people have many similar concerns and questions about diabetes. The next three pages outline some common questions that people have asked when first diagnosed. I've provided some straightforward answers to these questions. After you've had diabetes for a while, you may have more questions. This book will help. There are suggestions here about which sections of the book you can read for additional information.

This book also includes stories from everyday people with diabetes – stories to inspire you to manage your diabetes.

The book is for you if you're:

- at risk of type 2 diabetes
- newly diagnosed with type 2 diabetes
- you have had type 2 diabetes for many years.

In this book "diabetes" refers to "type 2 diabetes" unless specified otherwise. A definition of the different types of diabetes is outlined on pages 14–15.

Diabetes Meals for Good Health

Consider obtaining a copy of my first book, *Diabetes Meals for Good Health,* for a full guide to meal planning, portion sizes and healthy eating. I'll refer to this cookbook in order to build on its valuable nutritional information.

What isn't in this book?

Talk to your doctor, pharmacist, or diabetes educator for your individual medical and technical information about diabetes, such as:

- *what medications to take*
- *how to take or adjust insulin*
- *how to operate a blood sugar machine and other changing technology*
- *special needs of people with type 1 diabetes.*

Straight Answers to Common Diabetes Questions

Do I really have diabetes?
You may not feel any different, which makes you wonder whether you really do have diabetes. Many people do not have any symptoms, but blood tests will confirm if you have diabetes. To learn more, read: *What is diabetes,* pages 16–17; *Risks for type 2 diabetes,* pages 19–20; *Symptoms of type 2 diabetes,* page 18 and *Regular laboratory tests,* pages 339–344.

Do I have to stop eating chocolate bars and desserts?
No, you don't have to stop. You can have all your favorite foods, but in moderation. It's a good idea to limit how often you eat chocolate bars, so if you eat them daily, you'll need to start cutting back. There are many wonderful lighter diabetic desserts that you can enjoy. Save the rich dessert for special times. To learn more, read: *Light desserts and sweeteners,* pages 100–108 and *A plan for special occasions,* pages 75–77.

What can I eat?
You can mostly eat the same things you have always eaten, but eat less. If you eat a lot of fatty and sugary foods you'll need to replace some of these with fruits and vegetables and other healthy choices. To learn more, read: *1. Eating Well,* pages 54–216.

Will I go blind?
Having diabetes does not mean you will go blind. However, poorly controlled diabetes makes you more likely to have eye problems. With good blood sugar control and regular visits to your eye doctor, you can do things that will help you have healthy eyes for life. To learn more about keeping your eyes healthy, read pages: 38–41, 313 and 342.

Will I need to go on dialysis?
Having diabetes does not mean you will need kidney dialysis. You can protect your kidneys with good levels of blood sugar, blood pressure and cholesterol, and by not smoking. To learn more, read: *Kidney Damage,* page 33–37.

Will I need to take insulin?
Not everyone that has diabetes needs to take insulin. If your blood sugar levels are high, insulin can be a good way to help bring down your blood sugar. Some people never need insulin. Some start insulin the day they are diagnosed. Others, take insulin five, ten or twenty years after their diagnosis. To learn more, read: *Pills and insulin,* pages 315–330.

Will I lose my leg like my grandpa did?

The good news is that the vast majority of amputations in people with diabetes are preventable. Daily foot care helps prevent infections from happening in the first place. Having good blood sugar control is also important to help reduce the risk of infection. With care, you can keep your feet for life. To learn more about keeping your feet healthy, read pages 29–32 and 282–295.

Do I have to stop smoking?

This is a very good question. Please seriously think about quitting. When you have diabetes and you smoke you are more likely to get complications than if you didn't smoke. This would include gum disease, a foot amputation, heart attack, kidney problems or blindness. To learn more, read: *Becoming a Non-Smoker*, pages 263–280.

Can I eat in restaurants?

Yes. Restaurant meals tend to be higher in fat, sugar and salt, so try to order less and choose healthier meal choices. Limiting how often you eat in restaurants and switching to more home made meals is also a positive step. To learn more, read: *How to lose weight and keep it off, Dine out sensibly*, pages 70–74.

Can I still drink alcohol?

Yes. There may be some benefits to drinking, in moderation. There are also reasons to not drink or to drink less. Alcohol has unwanted calories, so it can make weight loss difficult. Also, if you take insulin or diabetes pills, you will need to take some precautions so you can drink safely. To learn more, read: *Alcohol*, pages 134–137 and *Low blood sugar*, pages 331–338.

How will diabetes affect the cooking I do for my family?

Diabetes tends to run in families, so you are all at a greater risk for diabetes. It's good if you all eat the same healthy way: smaller portions, and less fatty and sugary foods. If you gradually make small changes to your cooking, your family may not even notice any difference. Experiment with new recipes, new flavors (herbs and spices), and new desserts. To learn more, read: *Risks for type 2 diabetes*, pages 19–20; *Light desserts and sweeteners*, pages 100–108, *Seven Day Meal Plan with Recipes*, pages 149–200 and *Eat this – Not that*, pages 201–216.

There are tips to prevent and manage diabetes in preschoolers and children (pages 368–380), and during pregnancy (pages 381–391).

Is diabetes going to make me feel sick?

When your blood sugar is high, you can feel tired and unwell. When your blood sugar improves and you begin to exercise and eat better, you may feel better than you have ever felt. Diabetes may be your reason to quit smoking – after this, you'll start feeling younger. To learn more, read: *Symptoms of type 2 diabetes*, page 18; *Being Active*, pages 217–262 and *Becoming a Non-Smoker*, pages 263–280.

Research proves that you are responsible to make a difference in your health. The earlier a doctor diagnoses your diabetes, and you learn to manage it, the better your chance to live a long and healthy life.

Is diabetes going to shorten my life?

Statistics show that people with diabetes overall have a shorter life. But you can change your lifestyle with moderate daily exercise and weight loss – and live a longer, healthier life. To learn more, read: *7 Steps to Prevent or Reduce Diabetes Complications*, pages 54–411.

Will I have to prick my finger for blood every day?

No, not necessarily. Talk to your doctor or diabetes educator. You may do fine with little or no blood sugar testing at home, and rely on regular blood tests recommended by your doctor. For others, daily blood sugar testing is helpful in managing their blood sugar, especially if they are on insulin or at risk for low blood sugar. To learn more about testing your blood sugar, read pages 309–350.

How am I going to cope with one more thing?

Your doctor may diagnose your diabetes at a time when you have other stress too. This makes things difficult, but not impossible. Going to see a diabetes education team or your doctor is an important first step. You can tell them how you feel, and work out ways to cope better. Take just one step at a time. To learn more, read: *Staying Upbeat*, pages 351–366.

Is this going to stop me from being active?

If you are an active person, that is great. Continue activities, sports and hobbies that you love. Walking and exercise are an essential part of diabetes management. There will be things to do to reduce your risk for injury during exercise, such as wearing supportive shoes. To learn more, read: *Being Active,* including *Precautions*, pages 255–262 and *Footwear*, see pages 290–293.

Will diabetes affect my sex life?

As you make lifestyle changes and bring your blood sugar down, you will find more energy for everything, including sex. Good health and good sex go together. After a number of years of diabetes, some people find sexual changes may happen, but today there are prevention and treatment options. To learn more, read: *Sexuality and diabetes*, pages 392–411.

How do I get rid of diabetes?

There is no cure for type 2 diabetes. Taking medication and making lifestyle changes help many people bring their blood sugar very close to, or within, the normal range. Your risk for problems will then be low. When you are ready, read through the *7 Steps to Prevent or Reduce Diabetes Complications* on pages 54–411. This will give you the tools to make gradual, small changes so you control the diabetes, and it isn't controlling you.

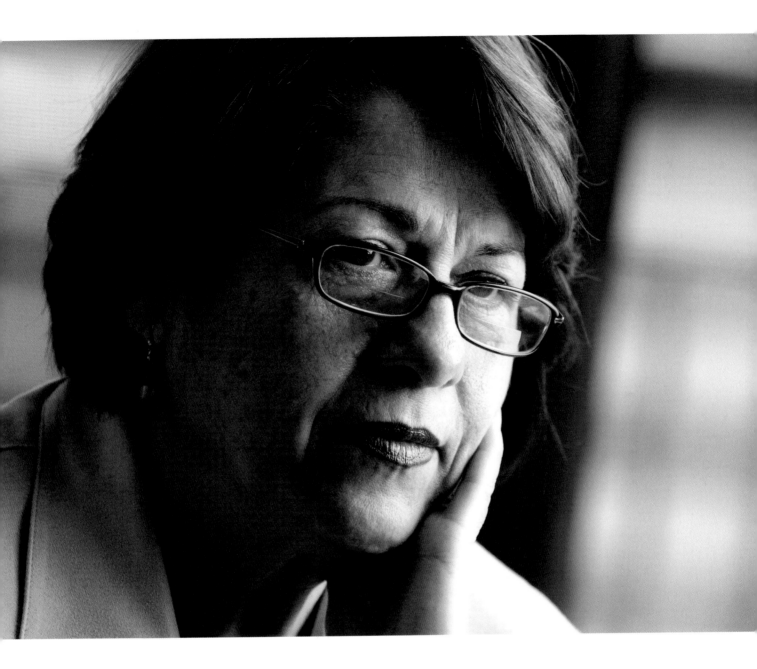

Learning about Diabetes

Types of Diabetes

Diabetes means there is too much sugar in your blood.

Pre-diabetes

Pre-diabetes means your blood sugar levels are higher than normal but lower than what is diagnosed as type 2 diabetes. You may hear this condition called:

- borderline diabetes
- Impaired fasting glucose, or
- Impaired glucose tolerance

If your doctor discovers you have pre-diabetes, you have a great chance to prevent type 2 diabetes by making healthy changes to your lifestyle. Also, your doctor may recommend that you take a diabetes pill to try to reduce your chance of getting type 2 diabetes.

Type 2 diabetes

The most common type of diabetes
Type 2 diabetes is on the rise around the world. This is because many people are less physically active and are overweight.

Caused by genetics and how we live
Type 2 diabetes runs in families. If one or both parents, or a brother or sister has diabetes, you have a higher risk of getting diabetes. In addition to the genes we inherit, we also learn how to eat and exercise from our families. People in the same household tend to eat similar foods and to be either active or inactive. Children who learn from their parents how to eat healthy foods and to be active, will have a decreased risk for diabetes, even if diabetes runs in their family.

What happens in type 2 diabetes?
In type 2 diabetes, the pancreas continues to make some insulin. Therefore, some people will need no medication, and can manage their diabetes with their diet and exercise. Others will benefit from taking diabetes pills and/or insulin. Early use of diabetes pills or insulin can often help improve blood sugars and delay diabetes complications.

Lab tests help to diagnose diabetes

Your doctor may order a fasting blood sugar, random blood sugar or A1C (see page 340). Generally, an A1C of 6–6.4% means pre-diabetes, and an A1C of 6.5% or more means diabetes. To make sure you really have diabetes, the tests are often done twice.

An A1C is not used to diagnose diabetes if you are pregnant, a child or have type 1 diabetes.

Type 2 diabetes is on the rise.

It generally develops after age 40, but now also occurs in some children, teenagers, and young adults. This is because people of all ages are gaining too much weight and are less physically active. Only about 10% of people with type 2 diabetes are lean or underweight when they get diabetes.

Gestational Diabetes

This is a type of diabetes that develops during pregnancy.

There are two things that happen during pregnancy that can increase a woman's blood sugar:

1) The weight gained during pregnancy means the woman's pancreas needs to make more insulin. The pancreas becomes overworked. It cannot make enough insulin, and blood sugar rises.

2) The hormones produced during pregnancy can result in the woman's insulin not working as well. After the baby is born, weight loss reduces the workload on the mother's pancreas. Then her blood sugar goes down.

To learn more about gestational diabetes, see pages 381–386.

Type 1 diabetes

In type 1 diabetes, the pancreas makes less insulin, and eventually makes no insulin at all. Without insulin, sugar isn't removed from the blood and it builds up quickly. Doctors generally diagnose type 1 diabetes in children over the age of 5 and teenagers. It is diagnosed less often in children under age 5 or adults.

Typical symptoms of type 1 diabetes may look like a severe flu:

- extreme thirst
- frequent urination
- stomach pains
- weight loss
- fruity-smelling breath caused by a production of unhealthy acids called ketones.
- see page 18 for a list of other symptoms of diabetes.

Usually within days or several weeks, the pancreas stops making insulin and symptoms rapidly worsen. In order to survive, the young person must take insulin every day.

Type 1 diabetes also runs in families. Caucasians (whites) have the highest risk of developing type 1 diabetes. Studies show that having diabetes genes and exposure to certain viruses are important factors. The viruses may have been contracted up to two years prior to the diabetes onset. These viruses can cause the body's immune system to attack the once-healthy part of the pancreas that makes the insulin.

Lab tests to diagnose gestational diabetes

When you are 24–28 weeks pregnant, your doctor may order a glucose tolerance test. You will be asked to drink a glassful of sweet liquid, then your blood sugar is tested over 1–3 hours.

Gestational diabetes increases the chance that both the mother and her child may develop type 2 diabetes later in life.

People with type 1 diabetes make no insulin at all.

People with type 2 diabetes still make some of their own insulin.

Studies show there is some protection against type 1 diabetes for those who have been breastfed. The protection against type 1 diabetes is greatest when the infant has been exclusively breastfed (no formula, and table foods delayed until 4–6 months). Another protection may be higher levels of vitamin D through sun exposure or diet.

What Is Type 2 Diabetes?

Here is what happens in a person without diabetes

Blood sugar levels before you eat.
Normal blood sugar is about 4–7 mmol/L (70–130 mg/dL).

Blood sugar levels after you eat.
For a person without diabetes, blood sugar will rise a few points after eating a meal, perhaps up to 8 mmol/L (150 mg/dL), but it quickly returns to normal as insulin removes the extra blood sugar to your tissues and organs.

Your blood sugar goes up because much of the food digested changes into a special kind of sugar called glucose. The glucose moves into your bloodstream and is called blood glucose, or blood sugar.

Insulin quickly brings down blood sugar.
Insulin is a hormone made by your pancreas. Insulin is extremely important because it enters the bloodstream after you eat and removes extra sugar. Insulin stimulates "receptors" on your body cells (especially in your muscles and liver) to take up the extra sugar.

When the extra sugar is removed from your blood and stored in your body cells and liver, it can be used later for fast energy.

Normal blood sugar levels

Before eating:
4-7 mmol/L
(70-130 mg/dL).

After eating:
8 mmol/L or less
(150 mg/dL).

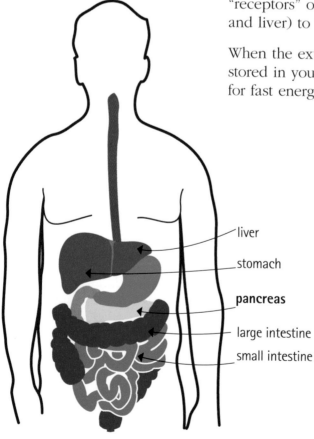

liver

stomach

pancreas

large intestine

small intestine

Insulin is a hormone made by your pancreas.

Here is what happens when you have diabetes

Blood sugar levels before you eat.
Blood sugar is often high in the morning before eating, above 7 mmol/L (130 mg/dL).

Blood sugar levels after you eat.
After eating a meal the blood sugar can go up quickly, for example up to 10 mmol/L (180 mg/dL) or more. Blood sugar levels take longer to come back down.

Extra body fat causes insulin resistance.
Insulin resistance means that the "receptors" on your body cells are blocked, most often because of extra body fat, and extra sugar is not being removed from your bloodstream. Your pancreas then makes more insulin to try to remove the extra sugar. Unfortunately, now the extra insulin in your bloodstream can make you feel hungry and overeat.

Extra sugar builds in your bloodstream, and can worsen over time because of changes in how your organs work:

- **Your pancreas** works overtime to make extra insulin and this organ gets worn down. Then it cannot make enough insulin. Too much sugar remains in your bloodstream. Therefore, your muscles do not have an adequate source of energy and you feel tired.

- **Your liver** releases extra stored sugar, even when you don't need it.

- **Your stomach** makes less of certain hormones that would help insulin work better.

These three things happen in diabetes:

1) *Extra sugar builds up in your blood.*

2) *Your muscles are short of sugar for energy, so you feel tired.*

3) *Over time, the extra sugar in your blood causes premature damage to your blood vessels, heart, nerves, eyes and kidneys.*

Symptoms of Type 2 Diabetes

Symptoms are what you feel. Some people go to their doctor because they have a symptom of diabetes such as extreme thirst, see 1) below. However, because blood sugar can build up gradually in your bloodstream, you may have no recognizable symptoms of diabetes, see 2) below.

1) Symptoms of high blood sugar

- extreme thirst or hunger
- frequent urination
- unexplained weight loss
- extreme fatigue
- blurred vision
- a urinary tract infection
- a cut that is slow to heal

You or your doctor will recognize one or two of these symptoms. Blood tests will confirm the diagnosis.

2) No symptoms

Diabetes diagnosed at annual check-up at doctor's office
If you go to your doctor once a year for a complete check-up, routine blood tests include a blood sugar test. If your blood sugar test is high, your doctor will assess further for diabetes, even if you have no symptoms of diabetes.

Diabetes diagnosed after diabetes complications
If you don't go to a doctor for check-ups, diabetes could go undiagnosed for many years. You may have adapted to high blood sugar so may be unaware of the symptoms. However, during this time your pancreas has been overworked, making more insulin to try and remove the extra blood sugar. The extra sugar will have been building up in your blood vessels, nerves, eyes and kidneys. Eventually, you go to the doctor because you notice symptoms of diabetes complications:

- nerve tingling or pain in your hands, feet or legs

- an infection or ulcer on your foot or leg

- men may experience some erectile dysfunction (difficulty getting hard or maintaining an erection)

- a change or loss of some vision

- shortness of breath, swelling in your legs, or pain in the back of your lower leg (your calf) – these could mean circulation or heart problems.

In some cases, it is after a heart attack or stroke that diabetes is diagnosed.

Risks for Type 2 Diabetes

It is important to know the risks for getting type 2 diabetes because the symptoms may not show up for many years. If you have one or more of the risks below, see your doctor once a year for a complete check-up.

- Being overweight, especially when you carry the extra weight around your waist or upper body.

- You don't exercise regularly.

- You are more at risk of diabetes if your heritage is:
  - Aboriginal (in Canada, including Indian, Inuit and Métis)
  - Native American
  - Hispanic, African, or Asian.

- Having a parent, sister or brother with type 2 diabetes.

- Being 40 or older; your risk increases with age.

- High blood pressure and/or high blood cholesterol.

- If you developed gestational diabetes during pregnancy, or gave birth to a large baby that weighed 9 lbs (4 kg) or more.

Smoking

New evidence is suggesting that smoking may be a risk for diabetes.

When you are at risk for diabetes, have an annual check-up with your doctor

Your doctor will do routine blood tests that include a blood sugar test. See pages 339–344 for more information about different lab tests.

19

Other risks for type 2 diabetes

- A major life stress, such as death of a spouse.

- A physical stress, such as a heart attack, stroke or infection.

- Pancreas surgery or infection of the pancreas.

- Hemochromatosis (a genetic condition where excess iron damages the pancreas).

- Some medications increase blood sugar or interfere with how your insulin works. For example, some blood pressure pills and steroids.

- Medications with a side-effect of unwanted weight gain, such as drugs given for depression or schizophrenia.

- Medical conditions that cause an unwanted weight gain, such as hypothyroidism.

- Other conditions that are related to insulin resistance, such as polycystic ovary syndrome (a hormonal disorder in women) or acanthosis nigricans (darkening of the skin at the back of the neck and armpits).

- Being born to a mother with gestational diabetes.

- Being overweight as an infant, child or teenager.

- Being formula-fed rather than breastfed, as a baby. The current research shows that exclusive and extended breastfeeding reduces the risk of type 2 diabetes.

- Poor sleeping habits such as not enough sleep, sleeping too much or sleep apnea (a condition where you briefly stop breathing while sleeping).

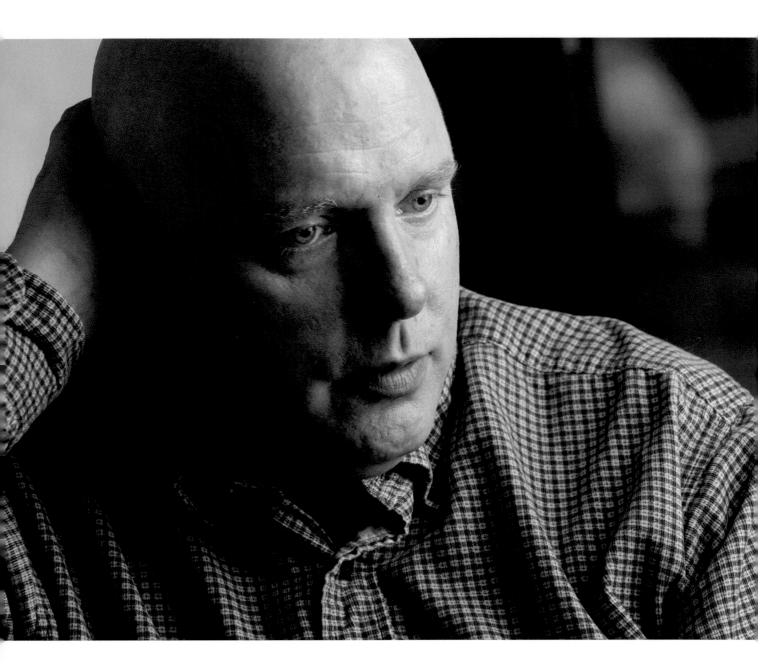

Diabetes Complications

This Diabetes Complications chapter will help you understand why diabetes affects all parts of your body. Taking steps early to prevent these complications is so important.

Many years of having high blood sugar will harm blood vessels and nerves. Blood vessels and nerves work together and are everywhere throughout your body. This is why diabetes complications can occur to almost all parts of the body.

Diabetes can lead to kidney disease and blindness. Controlling blood sugar and blood pressure can reduce these problems. After a heart attack, some people have said that if they had known that diabetes is the leading cause of heart attacks, they might have made some changes earlier. Knowledge is power. Knowing why a problem can occur is the first step in preventing or solving it.

Foot infections and amputations are a serious, yet preventable, complication of diabetes. If you understand how diabetes affects your feet and why it can cause foot infections, I hope you'll be motivated to check your feet everyday. This small change could mean you will have your feet for life, and never have an amputation.

This chapter includes the following topics:

Talking about diabetes complications   23
How high blood sugar harms blood vessels   24
How high blood sugar harms nerves   26
Heart attack and stroke   27
Foot and lower leg infections   29
Kidney damage   33
Eye problems   38
Other complications   42
    Skin problems   42
    Gum disease   43
    Urinary tract infections   46
    Genital problems and sexuality   49
    Stomach and bowel problems   51
    Stress, depression and sleeping problems   52

Talking about Diabetes Complications

Mary's story

When I first found out I had diabetes my doctor sent me to classes at a diabetes education center. In the first class the nurse talked about all the things that could go wrong when you have diabetes. She told us I could lose my vision or I could have my foot amputated. This really scared me. I have an uncle who lost his foot to diabetes. Then she said diabetes is the main cause of stroke and heart attack. I didn't know that. I definitely do not want to have a stroke.

After I got home from this class, I so felt alone that I just sat down and cried. I was upset and worried and didn't understand why this happened to me. What scared me the most was that I didn't want to lose my vision. If I lost my vision I wouldn't be able to drive. And if I couldn't drive I'd be helpless and have to depend on other people to get me around. Back then I had so many family issues to worry about and looking after my grandkids was like a full-time job, so I didn't have time to think about me. I just kept doing what I was doing and pretended to myself that I didn't have diabetes that bad, that I was okay. After all, I could see and drive fine.

And I didn't go back to any more of those classes.

Three months later I had to go back to my doctor for an appointment, and she told me my blood sugar was still high. She asked me if I had gone to the diabetes classes, and I told her what happened and how scared I was really feeling.

She told me that it was important to know the diabetes complications that the nurse talked about. But she told me not to focus on those complications and instead to think about one change I could make right now. I decided I could start that day with a 15-minute walk, and try every day. My doctor said this small change could make a big difference in my day-to-day blood sugars, and that would reduce my chance of getting diabetes complications later. She asked me to write down my plan and reward myself with a coin in a jar every day that I walked. She gave me an appointment to see her in one month and I had to bring in my record of when I went for a walk.

This is how I began my diabetes plan to better health. I added in more changes over time, like drinking more water, especially after I had gone for a walk. My blood sugars slowly got better. I eventually went back to the diabetes education center and met with the nurse and dietitian; this time I didn't feel so upset and overwhelmed and was able to listen to their other suggestions.

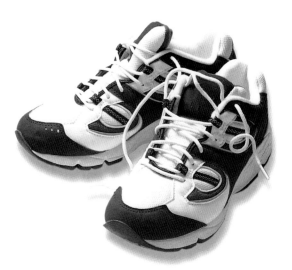

How High Blood Sugar Harms Blood Vessels

Our lifestyles and the genes that we inherit can speed up the narrowing of our blood vessels. Things that cause this problem are diabetes (high blood sugar), high blood pressure, and high blood cholesterol. Smoking, stress, eating a high fat diet, lack of fruits and vegetables, drinking too much alcohol, and being overweight and inactive also contribute.

Over many years, high blood sugar can:

- Cause the inside lining of the blood vessels to absorb more blood sugar than normal. This causes thickening and weakening of the blood vessel walls.
- Increase the build up in your blood of cholesterol and triglycerides (blood fat).
- Make the blood thicker (due to the extra sugar and fat) and more likely to clot.

As a result of these changes, blood vessels become narrow and blocked. This decreases blood circulation. Every part of your body that has less blood flowing to it will suffer. As a result, high blood sugar can cause: a heart attack or stroke, foot problems, vision loss, kidney failure, erectile dysfunction, poor digestion, and gum and tooth decay.

1) Healthy young blood vessels
When we are young, our blood vessels are clean inside and the blood flows freely. Our blood vessels are elastic and can easily stretch to pump more blood quickly when we exercise.

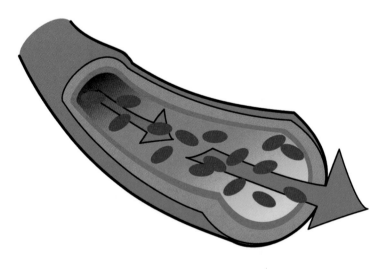

Looking inside a healthy blood vessel.

2) Blood vessels narrow

As we get older, the walls of our blood vessels thicken, harden and become less elastic. Fatty deposits, cholesterol and cells build up under the inner lining of the blood vessel wall. The medical term for these areas of thickening is plaques. We call "hardening of the arteries" atherosclerosis. The blood vessel channel narrows from this thickening (causing decreased circulation). The heart must over-work to pump the blood through. Blood pressure often goes up. This high blood pressure places extra stress on the inner blood vessel walls.

With decreased circulation, you will now have:

- *less oxygen, nutrients and hormones such as insulin circulating to your muscles, tissues and organs*
- *waste materials building up*

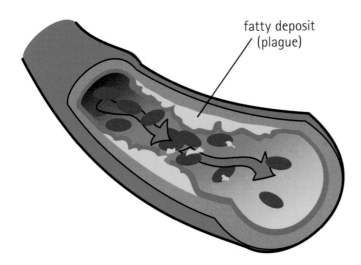

fatty deposit (plague)

The inner blood vessel wall becomes inflamed, rough and weakened from many years of high blood sugar and high blood pressure. Sometimes a plaque can rupture, and the contents will spill out. When this happens, a blood clot can form.

3) A blood vessel is blocked

This is now very serious. A blood clot or blob of fat can totally block a blood vessel. If the blocked blood vessel is in your leg, you could lose blood flow to your lower leg and foot. Then an infection can't heal and you could need an amputation. If the blocked blood vessel goes to your heart, you could have a heart attack. If a blocked blood vessel goes to your brain, you could have a stroke.

Another serious problem, called an embolism, is when a blood clot breaks away, and travels in the blood. It can block a blood vessel somewhere else. For example, it could move from a blood vessel in the leg up to the lung.

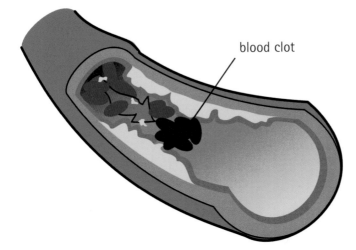

blood clot

How High Blood Sugar Harms Nerves

Healthy Nerve

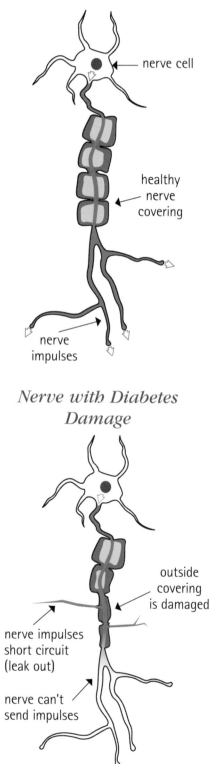

nerve cell

healthy nerve covering

nerve impulses

Nerve with Diabetes Damage

outside covering is damaged

nerve impulses short circuit (leak out)

nerve can't send impulses

Over many years, high blood sugar harms nerves in two main ways:

1) **Less blood flows to nerves.** The nerve and blood systems are very closely connected. To work properly, blood vessels need healthy nerves. Nerves need healthy blood vessels for a supply of oxygen and nutrients. Therefore, damage to the blood vessels also results in damage to the nerves. As blood vessels narrow, there is nerve damage, especially in the small blood vessels of your the hands, feet and eyes.

2) **Direct nerve damage.** Excess blood sugar moves into nerve cells. The sugar is changed into unhealthy proteins and other types of sugars that then damage the nerves. The part of the nerve that is most damaged is the outside cover (this can be compared to when the plastic around a covered wire becomes frayed).

Some of the effects of nerve damage are:
- pain in your legs or feet
- numbness or loss of feeling in your hands or feet
- a sore on your foot that you can't feel that then becomes infected
- some vision loss
- Poor digestion, constipation or diarrhea
- bladder control problems
- Sexual changes such as erectile dysfunction in men, and decreased lubrication and sensation in women

Other factors that increase your risk for nerve damage:
- smoking
- drinking too much alcohol
- having high blood pressure
- having high blood triglycerides (a type of blood fat that is increased when blood sugars are high)
- being overweight
- malnutrition

Heart Attack and Stroke

Visit your doctor for blood cholesterol and blood pressure tests, to make sure any hardening and narrowing of your blood vessels is found early (see pages 339–344 and 350). Tell your doctor if you have any unusual symptoms that may indicate a blocked large blood vessel, such as:

- **Swelling to your fingers or feet**
  With a weaker heart and narrowed blood vessels, the circulation to your kidneys is reduced. Your kidneys hold extra sodium and water. After a long day on your feet, this sodium and water becomes trapped in the tissues of your feet causing swelling.

- **Loss of protein in your urine**
  If you are losing protein in your urine you may be at a greater risk of a heart attack or stroke. This is also a sign of kidney problems, see page 33. Tiny blood vessels in your kidneys filter your blood. If these are damaged, protein leaks into your urine. When blood vessels in your kidneys are damaged, other blood vessels in your body may also be damaged.

- **Shortness of breath**
  This can happen even with small amounts of exercise. This could mean the heart muscle is not able to pump enough oxygen throughout your body.

- **Chest pain**
  Decreased blood flow to your heart could cause chest pain, especially when exercising. Nerve damage to the heart can result in irregular heartbeats.

- **Difficulty concentrating or headaches**
  This could be due to decreased blood flow of oxygen and nutrients to your brain.

- **Calf pain or cramps**
  Decreased blood flow to your legs may cause pain in your calves (back of your legs) when walking and even when you are resting.

If you've had diabetes for many years you may have nerve damage to the heart. That means you may not feel all the usual heart pain of a heart attack. Therefore, it is very important to have regular check-ups with your doctor.

> **See next page for the signs and symptoms of a heart attack or stroke.**

Call 911 or your local hospital emergency right away if you have any signs of a heart attack or stroke. Minutes can make a difference.

Warning Signs of a Heart Attack
Immediately seek medical help if you have

- Sudden pain, heaviness or discomfort in your chest, neck, jaw, shoulder, arms or back, lasting more than a few minutes
- Chest pain when exerting yourself
- Shortness of breath
- Nausea, indigestion or vomiting
- Sudden sweating
- Unusual fear or anxiety

Warning Signs of a Stroke
Immediately seek medical help if you have

- weakness (even if temporary)
- trouble speaking (even if temporary)
- vision problems (even if temporary)
- headache
- dizziness

Foot and Lower Leg Infections

High blood sugar over the years can cause a variety of changes to your feet that put you at risk for foot and lower leg infections. You'll be at higher risk depending on how long you've had diabetes and how high your blood sugar has been. It is difficult to know exactly how at risk you are, or when your risk increases. Therefore, it's important to look after your feet every day.

Six reasons why you are at risk of foot and lower leg infections

1) Loss of feeling (nerve damage)

Symptoms of nerve damage to the feet:

- feeling of pins and needles, or burning and aching (this may also occur in your legs, fingers or arms)

- extreme sensitivity to touch (for example, when sleeping, the blanket on your feet might be bothersome)

- loss of feeling on the bottoms of your feet

- loss of hair growth on your lower leg and on the tops of your feet and toes (hair needs nerve stimulation to grow)

- dry feet (nerves stimulate oil glands that keep your skin soft)

- loss of balance and feeling unstable when standing or walking

These symptoms can be mild or severe. When blood sugar improves, nerve damage can be reduced.

Feelings of pins and needles and aching is uncomfortable or painful, but the greatest risk is when there is a loss of feeling. With loss of feeling, you may not feel light touch, dangerously hot water or pain. Pain is your body's way of telling you something is wrong. You may not know that your shoes are too tight. You won't feel the shoe rubbing on your skin, causing a corn or an injury to a bunion. You may not feel an infected hangnail or a stone in your shoe. You will not know that you need to treat the injury right away.

After having diabetes for 10 years you have a 50% chance you will develop some nerve damage.

You may not feel an open sore on the bottom or side of your foot.

Do you have pain, weakness and cramping of your calf?

You may have Peripheral Arterial Disease (PAD). This is when a blood vessel to your lower leg is blocked. Talk to your doctor.

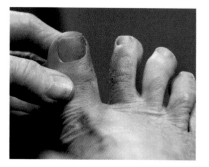

2) Poor blood flow (circulation)

The large blood vessels in your legs and smaller blood vessels in your feet and toes become narrowed and less elastic, causing reduced blood flow. When you are standing, poor circulation affects your feet and toes the most, because of gravity. Nutrients, oxygen and white blood cells that fight infection cannot as easily get to your toes. Your nails may become yellowed, brittle or hard, and your feet are often cold or discolored. Cuts don't heal as well.

Smoking decreases circulation. It is a major contributor to the need for amputations. Don't smoke! See Becoming a Non-Smoker, pages 263–280.

3) High blood sugar feeds germs

Germs (bacteria and fungus) feed on sugar. When you have extra sugar in your blood, germs grow and reproduce fast. Bacterial infections can spread quickly. A serious infection can develop in a short time. Fungus can grow on the foot (athlete's foot) particularly between the toes and under toenails.

High blood sugar can also decrease your body's ability to fight infection (immunity).

4) Dry, cracked skin

Nerves help stimulate oil and sweat glands that moisturize your feet. So, when nerves don't work well, your ability to sweat can be lost and your skin gets dry. Also, if your blood sugar is high, your body pulls fluid out of your tissues (to make extra urine in an attempt to get rid of extra sugar) and this can make dry skin worse. When the skin is dry, you are more likely to get cracks that break open. Once the skin is broken, germs get in and start growing and cause an infection. An infection can cause gangrene and possibly even mean you need an amputation.

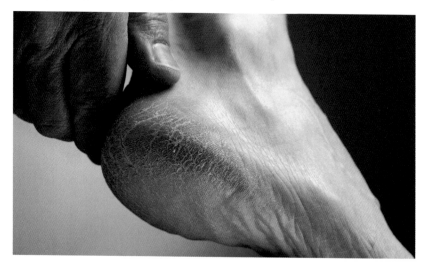

5) Distorted foot shape

Nerves help control the muscles which hold your foot in place and give you balance. The muscles may get weak because diabetes can damage the nerves in your feet. The bones in your feet (and the joints between your bones) may also weaken in some cases.

For example, most people have a natural arch in the soles of their feet. If your muscles weaken, this arch can fall and you will develop a flat foot. Certain bones and parts of your foot that used to be raised will now touch the ground when you walk. This creates pressure and wear on these parts of your foot.

Here are some other problems that can occur when your foot shape changes:

- poor balance
- toes that angle in or out
- corns or calluses
- thinning of the pads on the ball of your foot

6) Extra body weight

The more you weigh, the more weight and burden is on the bottoms of your feet as you stand and move around. Doing high impact exercise (such as running) further increases the weight and pressure on the bottom of your feet.

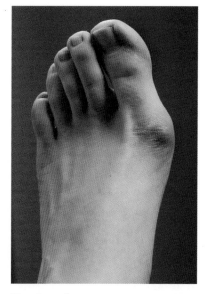

Bunion that creates a pressure point in a shoe that is too tight.

Example of how an infection can happen:

1. You lost some feeling in your foot, due to nerve damage.
2. You get a cut on your toe but you don't feel it.
3. Germs get into your cut and grow quickly because of the extra sugar in your blood.
4. Your cut becomes infected.
5. You notice blood on your sock and see that you have a red and infected sore.

Just a few days later, the sore looks redder. You make an appointment with your doctor, but you don't seek help immediately. Ten days later when you see your doctor, gangrene is developing. Gangrene is dead tissue and needs to be cut out. In order to prevent infection in the rest of your body, you may need to have a toe, foot or part of your leg amputated.

Check your feet daily

Prevent injuries and treat simple injuries immediately.

See pages 282–295.

31

*With proper foot care, up to 85% of amputations
in people with diabetes could be prevented.*

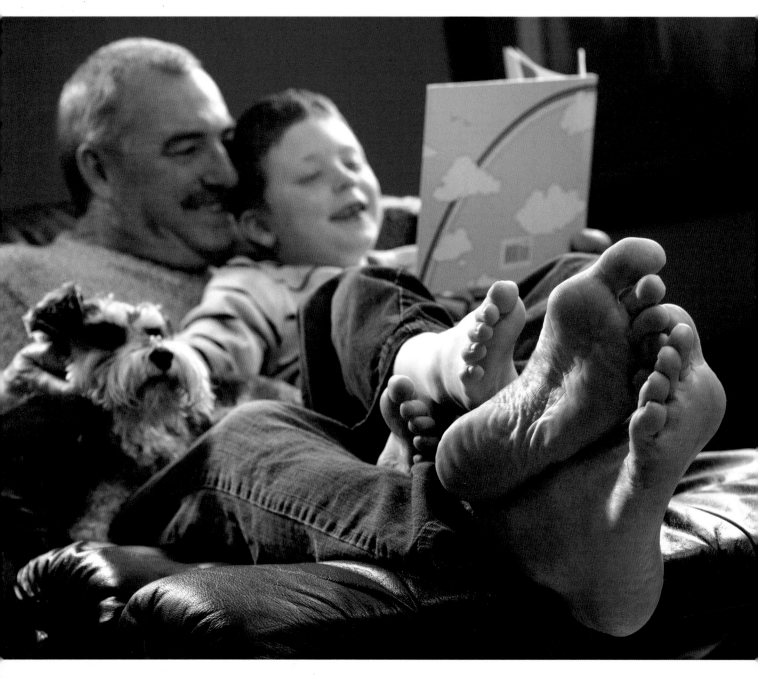

FIGHT AGAINST AMPUTATION – KEEP YOUR FEET FOR LIFE.

Kidney Damage

The kidneys have tiny filtering units surrounded by many tiny blood vessels and nerves. Years of high blood sugar and high blood pressure harms these vessels and nerves. This leads to loss of the filtering units. The kidneys won't work as well. With advanced kidney failure, you will feel unwell, and some people may even need dialysis.

What do healthy kidneys do?

Your two kidneys are like a filter on your furnace or car that removes unwanted compounds and keeps the motor clean. Each kidney has an elaborate network of about a million tiny filters to filter your blood. This keeps fluids and compounds at the right level in your blood and helps control blood pressure.

Your kidneys work to:

- Maintain a healthy balance of water and salts (such as sodium, potassium, calcium and phosphorus) in your body. Extra amounts are filtered out into your urine.

- Maintain normal blood pressure. Damaged kidneys result in extra sodium in your blood and higher blood pressure.

- Filter out waste products from your blood and dispose of them in your urine. This includes compounds that are the result of your body's digestion and metabolism such as urea and creatinine. It also includes excess medications.

- Help make red blood cells. This is why you may be anemic if you have kidney problems.

- Keep these important red blood cells, as well as white blood cells and proteins in the blood. The kidneys don't filter these out.

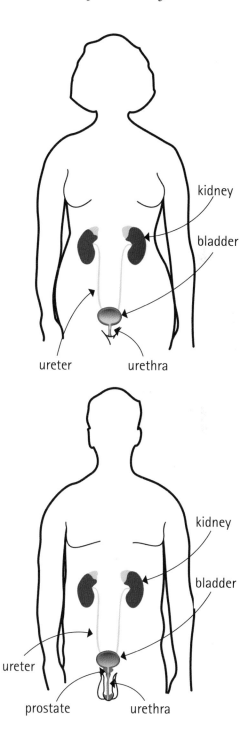

Location of kidneys in your body

kidney

bladder

ureter   urethra

kidney

bladder

ureter

prostate   urethra

33

Healthy Kidney

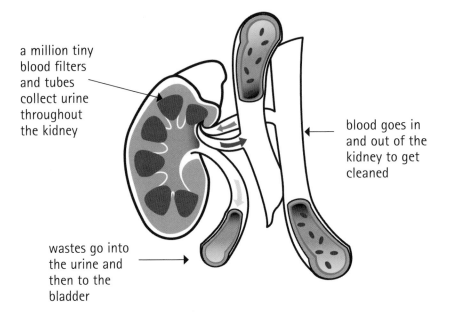

a million tiny blood filters and tubes collect urine throughout the kidney

blood goes in and out of the kidney to get cleaned

wastes go into the urine and then to the bladder

What does a kidney filter look like and how does it work?
There are about one million filters in each of your two kidneys. Each of these million filters includes two connected parts: the glomerulus (the main filter) and the nephron (the second filter).

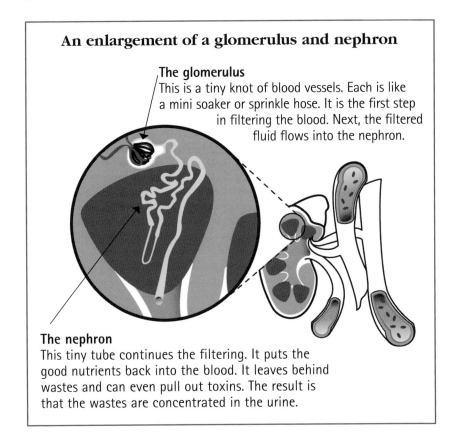

An enlargement of a glomerulus and nephron

The glomerulus
This is a tiny knot of blood vessels. Each is like a mini soaker or sprinkle hose. It is the first step in filtering the blood. Next, the filtered fluid flows into the nephron.

The nephron
This tiny tube continues the filtering. It puts the good nutrients back into the blood. It leaves behind wastes and can even pull out toxins. The result is that the wastes are concentrated in the urine.

Early kidney damage
(microalbuminuria)

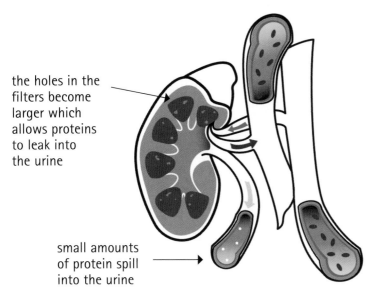

the holes in the filters become larger which allows proteins to leak into the urine

small amounts of protein spill into the urine

The glomeruli (the main filters) become damaged by the excess blood sugar and high blood pressure. They plug up and no longer work. The nephron that is attached to each of them also stops working and becomes useless. This results in fewer filtering units. The rest try to make up the extra work by increasing the pressure inside them. This causes the remaining glomeruli to get bigger holes and wear out faster still. Protein now leaks out into the urine.

If your doctor consistently finds small amounts of protein in your urine, this is an early sign of kidney damage. One type of protein that is measured at the lab is called albumin. "Microalbuminuria" means the loss of small amounts of albumin in the urine.

Page 341 has more information on kidney lab tests.

If you recently have had a kidney or bladder infection, you may have extra protein in your urine. This returns to normal after the infection is gone.

Advanced kidney damage
(macroalbuminuria)

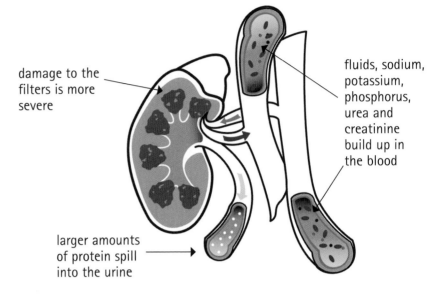

damage to the filters is more severe

fluids, sodium, potassium, phosphorus, urea and creatinine build up in the blood

larger amounts of protein spill into the urine

Special diet when you have advanced kidney damage or are on dialysis

You will need to still follow a diabetes diet but there will be other diet changes needed.

Please talk to a dietitian for individual advice.

More glomeruli and nephrons are damaged. More protein leaks into the urine. This is called "macroalbuminuria."

As the kidney function worsens, the remaining filters can't balance the fluids, salts and wastes. Sodium, potassium, phosphorus, urea and creatinine are normal parts of blood, except when their levels are too high. These now build up to dangerous levels in the blood.

As fluids and compounds build up in blood, some of the symptoms of kidney disease are:
- swollen ankles or legs
- fatigue
- shortness of breath
- nausea and sometimes vomiting
- dry, itchy skin

When your kidneys are so damaged, they can no longer remove enough of the toxins building up in your blood. Your symptoms of kidney damage will get worse. You may require dialysis, or in some cases you may be a candidate for a kidney transplant.

What is hemodialysis?

Dialysis is needed when your kidney damage has advanced to a point that your kidneys are no longer doing their job and you are very unwell. A hemodialysis machine works like a kidney. When you are attached to a dialysis machine, your blood is removed from your body. It is then filtered through the dialysis machine where it is cleaned and returned to your body. Typically, this takes four hours, and needs to be done three times a week, either during the day or at night. Hemodialysis is usually done at a hospital or dialysis centre, but in some cases, people can dialysis themselves at home. In this case, you would use a special hemodialysis home machine.

Peritoneal dialysis

Peritoneal dialysis is a more common form of home dialysis. If this is an option for you, it is simpler than home hemodialysis. Clean dialysis fluid is trickled into the tissues in your belly through a tiny silicone tube. It dwells there and the wastes leave your blood and enter the dialysis fluid. The fluid can be exchanged four times daily or at night using a small machine. This gives you more freedom as you aren't attached to a machine for so many hours, and you can do this at home.

Are you wondering whether you might someday need dialysis?

This depends on your lab results and how you are feeling (your symptoms). Talk to your doctor, kidney specialist (nephrologist) or kidney nurse.

Protecting the kidneys from damage and reducing the need for dialysis

In order to try and protect the kidneys, many doctors now treat blood sugar and blood pressure with medication earlier. You may start taking medication right after you are diagnosed with diabetes. Control of both blood sugar and blood pressure are critical to prevent or slow down kidney damage.

Eye Problems

Like the kidneys, the eyes have many tiny blood vessels and nerves that can be damaged by high blood sugar and high blood pressure.

Three ways diabetes can affect your eyes:

1) Blurring of vision
2) Cataracts or glaucoma
3) Retinopathy (damage to the retina, the back of the eye)

Macular degeneration can affect central vision. It is an eye condition that older adults get, but diabetes has not been found to increase it.

1) Blurring of vision

This happens when blood sugar is high or is swinging from high to low. At the front of your eye is the lens (see diagram on next page). As the level of sugar goes up in your blood, water goes into your lens causing the lens to swell. This change in shape is what causes the blurring. This makes it difficult to see long distances (or in some cases, to read), but it doesn't mean you are going blind. Once you get your blood sugar under control, the lens goes back to its normal shape and your usual vision returns.

2) Cataracts or glaucoma

These eye problems are more likely to develop at an earlier age in people who have diabetes.

- *Cataracts* are when the lens of your eye becomes cloudy (see next page). Signs may include blurred vision or a feeling of having a film over your eyes that doesn't clear up when you blink. Cataracts generally develop slowly. With surgery, doctors remove the cloudy lens and replace it with a new lens.

- *Glaucoma* is damage to the optic nerve that causes a loss of vision. At first, you lose peripheral vision (on the outside part of what you see, see next page). However, you may not notice this damage at this stage. Eventually, you will also lose the middle part of your vision. Because there may not be early warning signs, a regular eye exam is so important. Your optometrist will measure your eye pressure but will also look at the optic nerve for changes, see pages 313 and 342. If you have glaucoma, you may need treatment or surgery.

Retinopathy is the most serious diabetes-related eye problem. If not treated, retinopathy can lead to blindness.

When blood sugar improves, there is less blurring of vision.

Factors that affect the development of eye problems:

- *age*
- *diabetes*
- *smoking*
- *drinking too much alcohol*
- *eating an unhealthy diet*
- *high blood pressure*
- *excess bright sun exposure*
- *pregnancy*

Side view of the eye (enlarged)

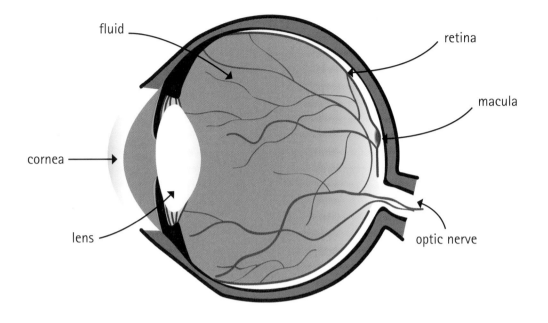

fluid

retina

macula

cornea

lens

optic nerve

What you see with different eye problems

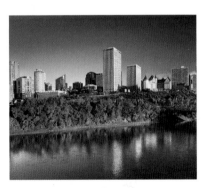

Normal vision

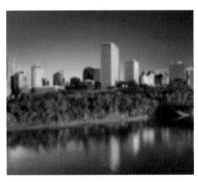

Blurring of vision

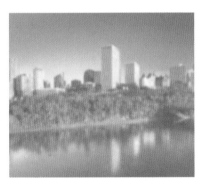

Cataracts

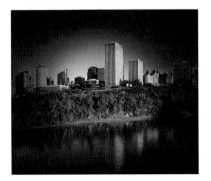

Glaucoma

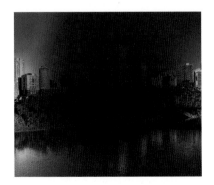

Macular degeneration

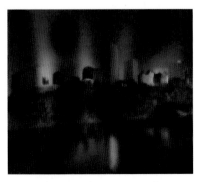

Advanced retinopathy

3) Retinopathy (damage to the back of the eye)

Retinopathy is when high blood sugar over many years causes damage and abnormal growth of the tiny blood vessels at the back of the eye (the retina). See diagrams on page 41.

Early retinopathy (non-proliferative retinopathy)

- Small bulges in blood vessels. This can be a sign of reduced blood flow to the retina. Blood vessels can break (hemorrhage) and leak fluid. This can cause swelling in the retina. This swelling may affect your macula that gives you your detailed vision.

- Small blobs of hard yellow fat. This comes from leaking blood vessels.

- Whitish patches or "cotton wool spots." These are caused by reduced blood flow to nerves in your retina.

Advanced retinopathy (proliferative retinopathy)

- Many new thin and fragile blood vessels on the surface of the retina. These grow because the retina is trying to get more oxygen and nutrients. They grow in response to chemicals that are produced by the retina.

- Blood spots. These indicate that these new tiny blood vessels are weak and tend to break (haemorrhage). Broken blood vessels can leave scar tissue behind. These two things, broken blood vessels and scarring, can threaten your vision.

- Blood in the eye socket. This is due to bursting of the new fragile blood vessels.

If advanced retinopathy is left untreated, several things can lead to loss of vision:

1. Retinal detachment – this is when the retina pulls away from the back wall of the eye (usually as a result of scar tissue).

2. Vitreous hemorrhage – this is when blood leaks into the eye socket.

3. Macular edema – leaking of the blood vessels around the macula.

Treatment

Early detection of retinopathy allows for treatment, if needed. The usual treatment is the use of laser (high powered tiny light beams) which are directed to the outside of the retina. This helps increase blood flow and reduce leakage to the remaining tissues in the inner part of the retina.

There are no warning signs of early retinopathy. See your eye doctor once a year. Only the eye doctor will be able to tell when early changes develop by looking at the back of your eye. See page 342.

Warning Signs Advanced Retinopathy

Immediately seek medical help if you have

- persistent blurring not associated with blood sugar changes

- a sudden decrease, or loss of vision, in one or both eyes

- seeing flashing lights, black spots or spider webs

- shapes or objects look distorted

- red color (meaning bleeding in the eye)

View of the back of the eye

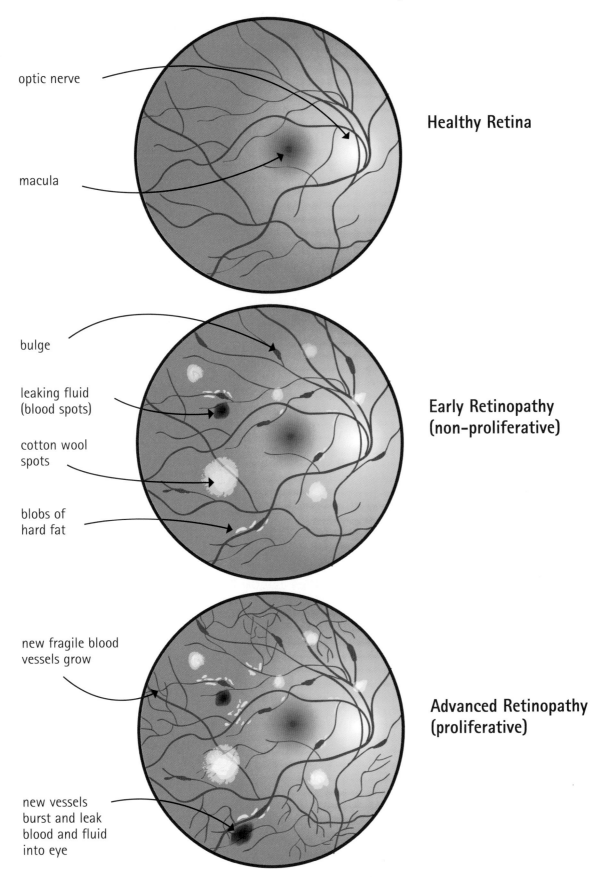

optic nerve

Healthy Retina

macula

bulge

leaking fluid
(blood spots)

Early Retinopathy
(non-proliferative)

cotton wool
spots

blobs of
hard fat

new fragile blood
vessels grow

Advanced Retinopathy
(proliferative)

new vessels
burst and leak
blood and fluid
into eye

Other Complications

Skin Problems

High blood sugar and decreased nerve function affects the skin on your legs and feet, as well as the skin everywhere on your body.

Examples of skin problems in people with diabetes:

- Small sores on your shins or front lower legs.
- A variety of conditions occur with dry, itchy or scaly skin.
- Bacterial infections that can develop into sores.
- Fungus infections develop under the breasts or folds of skin, in armpits, or in the groin area, or on hands.
- Blisters or boils (most often on feet, lower legs or hands).
- Darkened skin on the neck, armpits, hands, elbows or groin.
- If you take insulin, bumps or pits can occur on your skin if you inject in the same spot over and over. It is important to rotate your injection sites (talk to your doctor or nurse).

Report to your doctor any skin condition that doesn't go away. A skin problem can look different on you than someone else. Some skin conditions are uncommon or rare.

Improving your blood sugar and good skin care are essential for preventing and managing skin problems related to diabetes.

Skin care is discussed on page 296.

Painful skin

This is caused by damage to the nerves in your skin because of high blood sugar over many years. This nerve pain is also called neuropathic pain. You may have numbness or tingling, or you may have a burning or deep pain. You are most likely to have pain in your feet or legs. Some people have pain in their hands. The pain can be mild or severe.

There are things that may help:

- Keep active and quit smoking to improve your circulation.
- If your blood sugar is high, bring it down to help reduce your pain.
- Try gentle massage.
- Place warm or cold compresses on your skin.

If pain becomes severe, talk to your doctor. Ask about the cause of your pain and what to do about it. Your doctor may recommend an ointment to put on your skin (to dull the pain), or prescribe a pill. Medications can include pain killers, or anti-depressant pills or other types of pills. If your pain is making it difficult to cope, your doctor may refer you to another doctor who is a pain specialist.

Gum Disease

Gum disease is a serious bacterial infection of your gums and the jaw bone
that supports your teeth.

It is more likely to occur when your blood sugar is high.

Gum disease is one of the most common infections in people with diabetes.
Yet, it is often overlooked.

If gum disease is not treated, it may cause you to lose teeth.

How do I know if I have gum disease?

At first, you may not know you have gum disease.
This is because it doesn't usually hurt in the beginning.

Early warning signs:

- red, puffy gums
- gums that bleed when you brush, floss, or eat hard food

Later signs of gum disease:

- gums that pull away from your teeth; this makes your
  teeth look longer
- bad breath
- your blood sugar may go up
- sores or pain in your mouth
- pus between your gums and teeth
- loose teeth or toothaches
- when you bite, your teeth or dentures may not fit together
  the way they used to
- it's hard to chew raw fruits and vegetables

Early Gum Disease

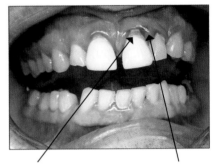

plaque   red, puffy gums
that bleed easily

**Are you having a hard time getting your blood sugar under control?
Gum disease might be part of the cause.**

There are two reasons:

1. If you have a gum infection with inflammation (redness) your insulin may not work as well.

2. A gum infection, like all infections, may cause your body to make stress hormones.
   These, in turn, may increase your blood sugar.

It's very important to see your dentist or dental hygienist at least two times a year
to make sure you don't have gum disease.

Healthy gums and teeth begin in infancy.

As an adult, we can't change how we were fed as an infant. However, here are important things to know to help protect your children and grandchildren's teeth.

- *Breastfeeding is best for an infant's healthy gums and teeth (see pages 387–389).*

- *If you bottle feed, there are steps you can take to protect your baby's gums and teeth:*
  1) don't give babies or toddlers bottles with juice, soft drink or sweetened beverages
  2) don't give a baby a bottle when putting them to bed.

- *Don't put sugar, honey or other sweet liquids on a soother (pacifier). Also, don't give a child a soother after age two.*

- *Gently clean your baby's gums daily with a clean, soft moist cloth. Once your baby's teeth appear, gently brush every day (use an infant toothbrush). Ask your dentist when to start using toothpaste with fluoride.*

Three main causes of gum disease:

1) Plaque

Bacteria (germs) that are a normal part of your mouth attach to your gums and teeth everyday. Gum infections begin when the build up of bacteria turns into a sticky, clear film, called plaque. When you don't brush and floss your teeth, plaque builds up around the gum line. Often the plaque attaches to tartar, a hard deposit that may build up under your gums, around the roots of your teeth. When this happens, your gums and the bone that supports your teeth are covered all the time by the bacteria in the plaque. This causes gum infection. That's why it's so important to clean your teeth everyday, and have your teeth cleaned by a dental hygienist every six months. This removes the plaque.

2) Smoking

Smoking or chewing tobacco reduces blood circulation. This significantly decreases your ability to fight infection, and makes you more likely to get gum disease. Tobacco use also slows healing after gum surgery.

3) High blood sugar

High blood sugar, especially over many years, can damage blood vessels and nerves. High blood sugar, even over a short time, results in more sugar in your saliva.

Damaged blood vessels: You are less able to fight infections.
As with other parts of your body, blood vessels in your mouth can be damaged by high blood sugar. When blood vessels become narrow, less blood can reach the gums. This makes it difficult to fight the infection and heal the gums.

Damaged nerves: Your glands make less saliva.
Nerves stimulate your glands to make saliva, especially when you eat. Saliva helps wash away bits of food. This reduces bacteria and plaque which start gum disease. Saliva also keeps your mouth clean and moist. With high blood sugar, nerves in your glands may be damaged. As a result, less saliva may be produced in your mouth.

More sugar in your blood and saliva: More germs grow.
Extra sugar in your blood can feed the growth of bacteria at the infected area. Also, when your blood sugar is high, some of this extra sugar goes into your saliva. This sweeter saliva around the infected area, is even more sugar for bacteria to grow. Your infection can be difficult to heal or can worsen.

Thrush

Thrush is another type of infection, caused by yeast. A yeast infection can be in the mouth or on the gums, lips or tongue.

It is normal to have some bacteria and yeast in your mouth. However, too much yeast can grow when you take antibiotics, have a poor immune system, or have high blood sugar. You are more likely to get thrush than someone who doesn't have diabetes.

Common signs of a yeast infection:

- white or yellow patches on your mouth and tongue, or sides of your lips
- the corners of your mouth may be dry and crack

Tooth decay

Tooth decay is when the white surface of your teeth (enamel) is broken down leaving cavities (holes) in your teeth.

Tooth decay is caused by acid
When the bacteria in plaque mixes with sugar from the foods that you eat, acid is made. This acid attacks the surface of your teeth (enamel). Eating acidic foods (such as lemons or soft drinks) can also break down enamel. These acid attacks last for twenty minutes or more after eating, and over time can break down the tooth enamel causing cavities. As a person with diabetes you have more sugar in your saliva and are more likely to get tooth decay.

The good news!

Studies show that if you keep your blood sugar at a good level you are less likely to get gum disease, thrush and tooth decay. See targets for blood sugar on page 346. Having good blood sugar is very important. When gum disease is treated, this may reduce how much insulin you need.

See pages 297–300 for specific things that you can do to keep your teeth and gums healthy.

Urinary Tract Infections

If UTIs occur frequently they may damage the kidneys – so prompt treatment is important.

See pages 301–305 for prevention and treatment of UTIs.

Symptoms of a UTI:

- *increased need or urgency to urinate*

- *pain during urination or sex*

- *blood or pus in the urine*

- *abdominal cramps or pain (back pain if kidneys or prostate are infected)*

- *urine may be smelly*

- *women with a vaginal yeast infection, often have vaginal itching or burning, or notice a yeasty smell or thick white discharge.*

Urinary tract infections (UTIs) are infections that affect the kidney, bladder or urethra (the tube that carries the urine from your bladder out of your body). In women, UTIs are often associated with vaginal infections. In men, UTIs can be associated with an enlarged prostate gland or kidney stones. UTIs can occur if your blood sugar is high for even a few days or a week.

When your blood has extra sugar in it, your body feels overwhelmed by the extra sugar. Your kidneys filter it into your urine which goes to your bladder, and you pee it out. When your blood sugar is high, for example, 15 mmol/L (270 mg/dL) or more, some sugar comes out in your urine.

Bacteria and yeast can feed and multiply rapidly when there's extra sugar in your kidneys, bladder and urine. An infection can develop. When your blood sugar is high, your body has reduced immunity (slow-moving white blood cells). This means your body is less able to fight infection.

Two things happen. First, high blood sugars contribute to a UTI. Second, once you have a UTI, the infection increases stress hormones in your body. These make blood sugar go even higher. If left untreated, you can become very sick.

With nerve damage to the bladder, it is more difficult to feel when your bladder is full. Therefore, you don't empty your bladder as often as you should, or as fully. Urine sits in the bladder for a longer time. This gives bacteria more time to grow, so the chance of a UTI increases.

In some cases, nerve damage to the bladder can mean you may experience some opposite symptoms. For example, having to urinate frequently, or some incontinence.

For women:

Women with high blood sugar have more sugar in their urine and in their vaginal secretions.

The biggest source of germs is your stool. A woman's vagina is located so near to her anus, that germs can easily spread. Germs that get in the vagina can then spread up the urethra (the tube between the bladder and opening) and into the bladder and kidneys. A woman's urethra is only about 1½ inches (4 cm) long so germs can easily travel that distance. The extra sugar in the genital area can also cause a yeast infection.

Sexual activity can increase the infection risk because germs get pushed into the vagina and urethra.

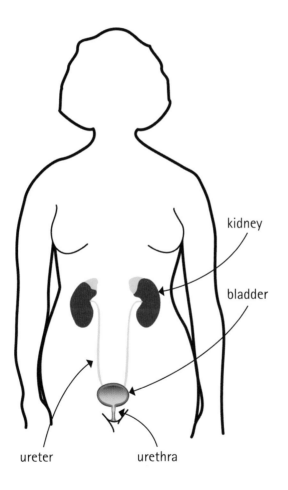

For men:

Men have a significantly lower risk of UTIs compared to women. This is in large part because of a longer urethra (about 8 inches/20 cm) compared to women. A man's urethra extends from the bladder down the length of the penis. Usually, bacteria from the outside cannot travel this distance, so infections are less. Also the urethra opening at the end of the penis is separated from your anus so is less likely to get contaminated by stool.

However, the risk for a UTI does increase if you have an enlarged prostate. An enlarged prostate pushes against your urethra or bladder and makes it hard to fully empty your bladder. Germs then can grow in the urine that is left sitting in the bladder. Having a catheter to drain your bladder also increases your risk for a UTI.

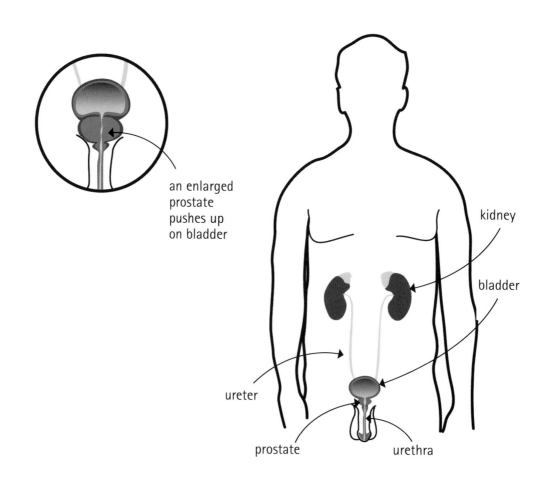

an enlarged
prostate
pushes up
on bladder

kidney

bladder

ureter

prostate   urethra

Genital Problems and Sexuality

Our sexual organs (see diagrams below) are highly sensitive. The reason these areas are so sensitive is because they have a lot of nerves and blood vessels. However, since diabetes can damage nerves and blood vessels, over time, you may lose some sensation or sexual functioning. In some cases, the changes are temporary. Improving your blood sugar and blood pressure can help slow down this damage.

Some people with diabetes experience no changes when it comes to sex.

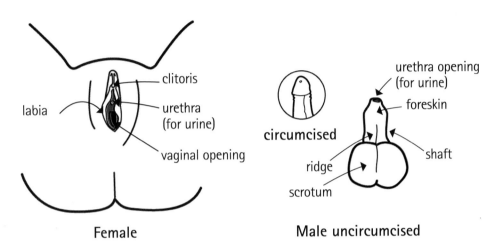

Female   Male uncircumcised

As a man or woman with type 2 diabetes, here are some changes that *might* happen:

- You may have decreased sex drive. Sometimes dealing with a chronic disease like diabetes can be overwhelming and makes it difficult to do things you used to enjoy. If you are feeling tired or depressed, you may feel less interest in all things in life, including sex. For men, a lower level of the hormone testosterone can also affect your drive. As you get older it is natural to have less testosterone, but this is more likely if you have diabetes. For women, estrogen (and even testosterone) decreases after menopause, and the effects of this can affect your sex drive. Also, some medications (such as certain pills for treating depression) might decrease your sex drive.

- You may have aches and pains (such as arthritis in the knees or back) that can make your usual sexual activity uncomfortable, or even painful.

Alternately, you may have an increased sex drive! This can be because you may have more time, especially private time, with your partner (for example, if you have children who have now left home or you are retired). You may like the opportunity to have sex at different times. When the woman is past child-bearing age, you no longer need to worry about pregnancy.

49

**For women, here are some other changes
that *might* happen:**

- You may have less of a sensitive feeling or feel dry while having sex. After you stop having your period (menopause) you also have less estrogen in your body, which causes less lubrication. This can make intercourse less enjoyable, and sometimes even painful.

- As discussed on pages 46–48, diabetes can also cause vaginal tract or urinary tract infections. This can mean itching, pain or odor that may affect a woman's (or a man's) interest in sex for a little while.

- As an older woman, you probably know how to orgasm, but you may need a little more stimulation to get there.

**For men, here are some other changes
that *might* happen:**

- Sometimes you may find it takes longer to reach orgasm. Getting older, and/or a lower level of testosterone, might be the reason for this.

- You may find you have some difficulty getting hard or maintaining an erection (called erectile dysfunction). In some cases, this can be the result of nerve or blood vessel damage. Over time this may get worse if your high blood sugar and high blood pressure continues or worsens.

*These things can
affect erection
hardness:*

- *psychological stress*

- *physical stress (fatigue, pain, illness or surgery)*

- *a side effect of certain medications, such as some pills for blood pressure or depression*

- *smoking or heavy drinking*

*However, the cause
may be diabetes-related
if the problem develops
slowly.*

**Read pages 392–411 for solutions and
approaches to sexual changes to enhance
your sex life.**

Stomach and Bowel Problems

Our stomach, small intestine and large intestine (bowel) are large muscles that digest food with help from:

- a network of nerves
- a healthy flow of blood, and
- digestive enzymes and acids.

As a result, diabetes nerve and blood vessel damage also affects the stomach and intestines.

A couple of changes can happen. A decrease in nerve function may mean that the muscles in our stomach and intestines don't contract as well, or in some cases over-contract. You may feel nausea and bloating because food sits in your stomach too long. Carbohydrates and nutrients may be absorbed at a fluctuating rate because of uneven nerve or blood function. This results in fluctuating blood sugar levels. If there are damaged bowel nerves, you may have either constipation (a slowing down of the bowel) or diarrhea (a speeding up of the bowel).

For constipation prevention, try a high fiber diet along with lots of water and exercise. For information on high fiber foods, see pages 58 and 92–93. For severe gastroparesis with diarrhea, a low fiber, low fat diet that is mostly liquids is often helpful. It is recommended you see a dietitian. You may also need medications, for either constipation or diarrhea.

***Gastroparesis** is the term for stomach and intestine changes caused by diabetes. It can cause an uneven absorption of carbohydrate. This can sometimes explain strange blood sugar fluctuations.*

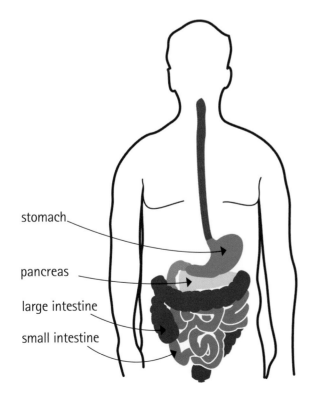

stomach

pancreas

large intestine

small intestine

Stress, Depression and Sleeping Problems

Stress

Having diabetes can make you feel overwhelmed. You may feel denial, fear, frustration, sadness, anger and guilt. This stress can make other diabetes complications worse because it increases both blood pressure and blood sugar.

See pages 351–366 for information on managing stress.

Depression

We don't know why, but depression is more common in people with diabetes. This doesn't mean you will get depressed, but it does mean you should be aware of signs of depression (see page 365). If you feel depressed, you might feel tired and less motivated to look after your diabetes. You may gain weight and your blood sugar would go up. Many pills given for depression can cause some weight gain. To prevent this unhealthy cycle, it is important to diagnose depression early and take steps to manage it.

See pages 365–366 for information on depression.

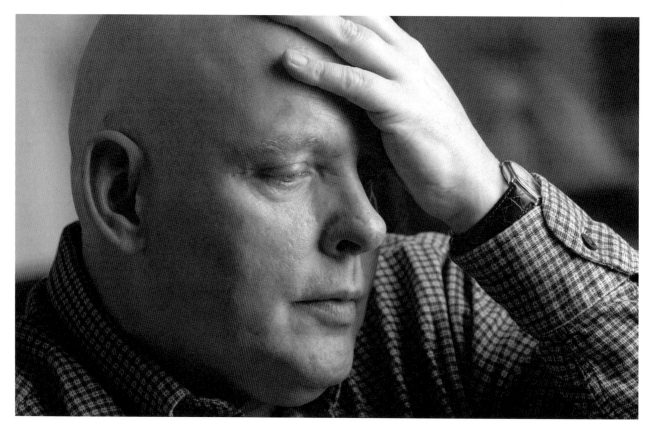

Sleeping problems

Lack of sleep, sleep apnea or too much sleep may contribute to diabetes. High blood sugar can make these problems worse.

Lack of sleep

Worry and stress can cause sleep problems. Diabetes nerve damage can cause your legs to be restless or sore. This can keep you awake. High blood sugar can make you thirsty so you drink more and wake up more during the night needing to pee.

A lack of sleep disrupts the production of your appetite hormones, so when you are awake you eat more. It also increases your stress hormones, which increases your blood sugar.

Sleep apnea

If you have sleep apnea you may be a heavier person that falls asleep quickly and snores a lot. While you are sleeping you briefly stop breathing many times during the night. This can wake you up, or you can sleep through it, but the result is a poor sleep. You wake up not feeling rested. Sleep apnea can contribute to high blood pressure, insulin resistance, lack of energy to exercise, weight gain and erectile dysfunction.

Too much sleep

High blood sugar can cause you to be very tired and sleep too much. This fatigue will likely mean you will be less active. Your metabolism will go down, and your weight and blood sugar go up.

Do you have a problem sleeping?

Early diagnosis and treatment is essential in managing your diabetes.

See pages 362–363 for tips on sleeping better.

7 Steps to Prevent or Reduce Diabetes Complications

1. Eating Well

Karen Graham's Hands-On Food Guide

55

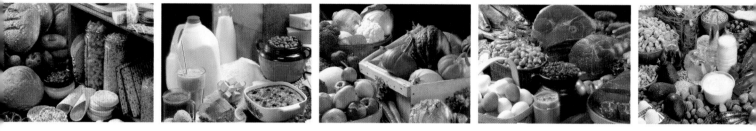

Top Ten Nutrition Topics   **60**

1.	How to lose weight and keep it off	61
2.	Carbohydrate foods and your blood sugar	85
3.	Food labels	94
4.	Light desserts and sweeteners	100
5.	Reducing sodium	109
6.	Lowering cholesterol levels	118
7.	Herbs and vitamins	122
8.	Alcohol	134
9.	What to eat when ill	138
10.	How to gain weight	143

Seven-Day Meal Plan with Recipes   **149**

4 Breakfasts	152
4 Lunches	160
7 Dinners	168
Snacks	196
Eat this – Not that	201

This Eating Well section of the book builds on the meal planning information and meal plans found in my first book *Diabetes Meals for Good Health*, including part of the popular "Eat This – Not That" section. Here you will find my "Hands-On Food Guide," answers to frequently asked nutrition questions in the "Top Ten Nutrition Topics," and an additional one week menu. You will also read about challenges to making diet changes, and practical advice for overcoming these.

Karen Graham's
Hands-On Food Guide

Enjoy a variety of foods from the five food groups. Choose the right portions for a healthy weight. Eat three balanced meals a day. Include snacks if needed. Choose high-fiber foods. Drink lots of water. Keep active everyday.

Use your hands as a guide for your portions.

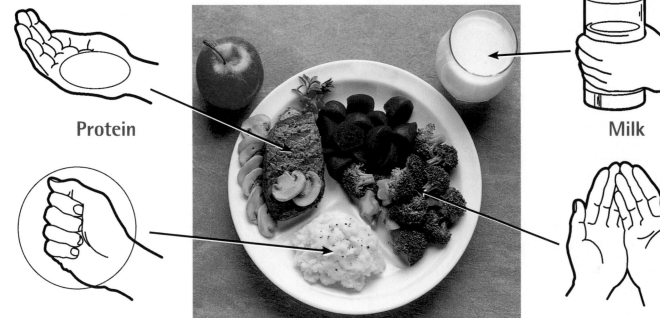

Protein

Milk

Grains & Starches

Vegetables

For Infants

Offer breast milk exclusively for the first six months. Continue with breast milk for one year or more.

At six months, add soft table foods rich in iron and vitamins.

For Children & Teenagers

As children grow, so do their hands — so use their hands as a guide for portions. Larger portions may be needed during growth spurts.

For Adults

Very active adults may need larger portions than shown in this Food Guide. Women during pregnancy and breastfeeding may also need more.

For Older Adults

Eat a variety of colorful and nutrient-rich foods, but smaller portions are needed.

Start with Grains & Starches

How much?

✓ Have a fistful at each of your meals; 3 or 4 fistfuls a day.

✓ Teenagers and young or active adults may need a two-fisted serving at meals; 5 to 8 fistfuls a day.

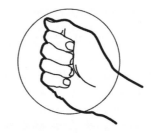

Good choices:

✓ Choose whole grain starches more often; these are an excellent source of fiber.

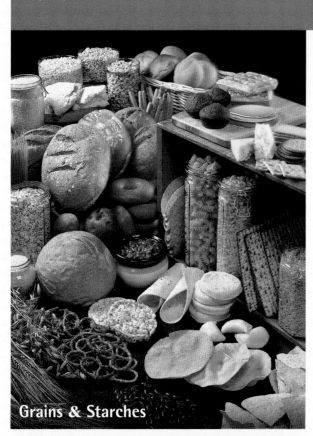

Grains & Starches

Fill Up on Vegetables & Fruits

How many vegetables?

✓ A serving is one fistful size.

✓ Eat one or more servings at lunch, and two or more at dinner.

✓ Fill your hands to overflowing and you have a daily amount of vegetables.

Good choices:

✓ Choose a variety of colors; dark green and orange are especially good for you.

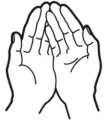

How much fruit?

✓ One serving equals:

- A fresh fruit serving is a fistful size.
- A dried fruit serving is 1 or 2 thumb-size amounts.
- A juice serving is $1/2$ cup (125 mL).

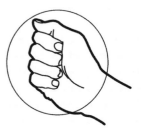

✓ Eat 3 or more fruit servings a day.

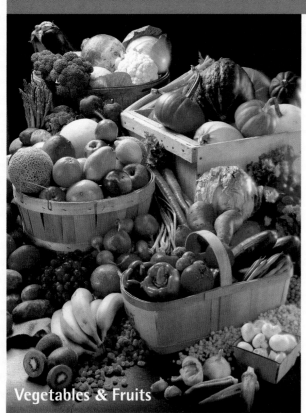

Vegetables & Fruits

Choose Milk & Calcium-Rich Foods

How much?

✓ One serving equals:

- 1 cup (250 mL) of milk or yogurt
- a bowlful of calcium-rich vegetables such as cabbage or broccoli.
- a thumb-size amount of cheese, nuts or tofu.

✓ At each meal, choose at least one calcium-rich food; 3–4 servings a day.

✓ For youths 10–16 years, and pregnant or breastfeeding women, have an extra daily serving.

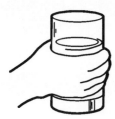 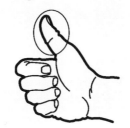

Good choices:

✓ Choose lower-fat choices more often.

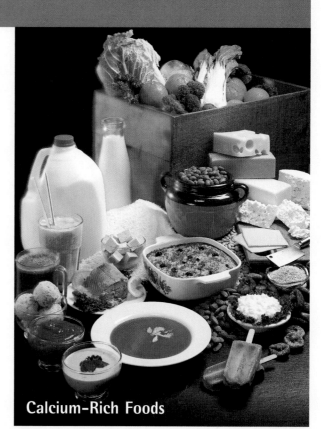

Calcium-Rich Foods

Eat the Right Amount of Protein

How much?

✓ Limit your portion to your palm size at your main meal; half or less at your other two meals.

✓ For children and women this means about 3–5 ounces (90–150 g) of cooked meat or other protein, and for men and active teens 4–7 ounces (125–210 g), at the main meal.

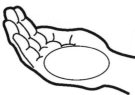

Good choices:

✓ Choose lean meat and poultry.

✓ Trim off visible fat.

✓ Bake and broil rather than fry in fat.

✓ At some meals, instead of meat, choose eggs, cheese, beans and lentils, or nuts and seeds.

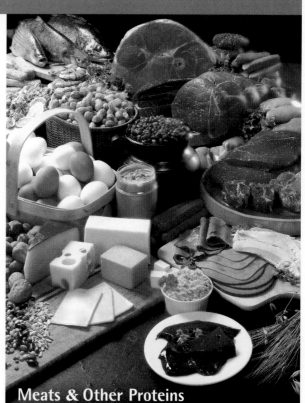

Meats & Other Proteins

Include Some Healthy Fats

How much?

✓ A serving of fish or seafood is about the size of your palm.

✓ A serving of olives, nuts or seeds, avocado or ground flax is the amount that fits in the small part of your palm.

✓ Each day have at least one serving of an omega-enriched food or other healthy fat choice.

✓ A serving of olive oil or vegetable oil or soft margarine is the amount that fits in the tip of one or two of your thumbs.

Good choices:

✓ Fish is the best source of omega-3 fat.

✓ Olives and avocados are excellent sources of monounsaturated fat.

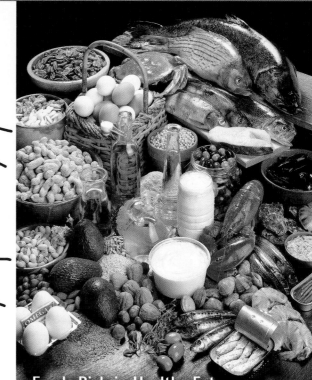

Foods Rich in Healthy Fats

Other Things to Remember

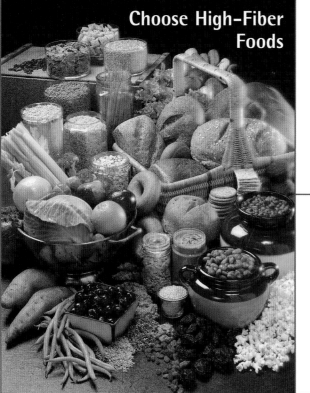

Choose High-Fiber Foods

Keep Active Everyday

Walk, bike or play to keep fit.

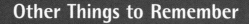
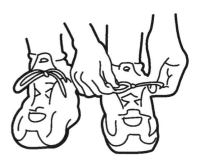

Drink Lots of Water

Drink six or more glasses of water a day. Drink more if the day is hot or you are active. Tap water with fluoride is good for your teeth and bones.

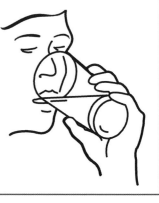

Food and Drinks to Limit

Foods High in Saturated or Trans Fats

Butter, lard, palm oil, some margarines, fried foods, potato chips and French fries, donuts, chocolates and sweet desserts

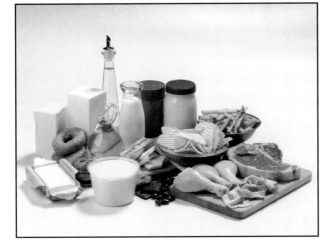

Sugar-Packed Drinks

Cappuccinos, milkshakes, iced drinks, sports drinks, energy drinks, flavored milks, beer, sweet wines, sweetened teas and coffees, juices and sweet drinks

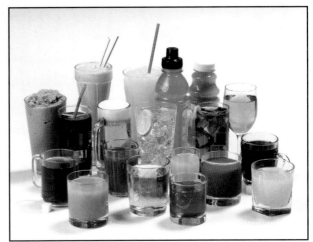

These high-fat, sweet foods and drinks taste good — so they are easy to overeat and overdrink. Enjoy them for special treats, rather than daily.

Restaurant Meals

These are too often large portions and high in fat, salt and sugar. Eat out less often, and enjoy healthy and fast homemade meals.

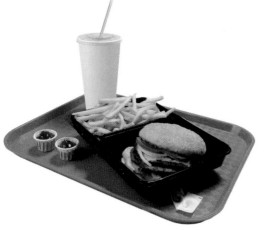

Salty Foods

Most of the salt in your diet comes from processed foods and restaurant meals. Cut back on these as well as table salt.

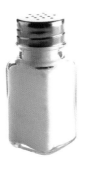

Alcohol

Talk to your doctor about whether small amounts of alcohol are healthy for you. There is no safe limit for children and pregnant women. Doctors generally recommend no alcohol during breastfeeding.

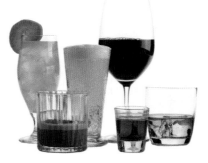

Choosing the right food portions is in your own hands.

Top Ten Nutrition Topics

1 How to lose weight and keep it off   61

2 Carbohydrates and your blood sugar   85

3 Food labels   94

4 Light desserts and sweeteners   100

5 Reducing sodium   109

6 Lowering cholesterol levels   118

7 Herbs and vitamins   122

8 Alcohol   134

9 What to eat when ill   138

10 How to gain weight   143

1. How to lose weight & keep it off

Begin your Journey

Your body is for life; don't go on a short-term diet.

The most important step to eating better and achieving a healthy weight loss is the decision to make health changes for the better. These changes happen in small steps. Looking for more information means that you are on your way to better choices for your health.

If you've been gaining a few pounds or more every year over the last few years, then even halting this continual weight gain is a success. When you are ready, aim for gradual weight loss, perhaps 1 pound (0.5 kg) a month. This will lead to a terrific weight loss of 12 pounds (5.5 kg) over the year. Gradual weight loss is less stressful on you and your body. Studies show that a weight loss of even 5–10 pounds (2 to 5 kg), especially in the pre-diabetes stage or at the time of diagnosis, can significantly improve blood sugar. We all want a quick fix like what we see on TV, but patience does pay off. Anticipate standstills and be realistic about how weight loss works. Slowly, you will see benefits.

Diabetes is for life and so is healthy eating and exercise. All foods can fit in a healthy eating pattern, but small portions are critical. Plan for a small indulgence occasionally. Enjoy it, and don't feel guilty about it. Studies show that including some favorite foods is important for a lifelong commitment to healthy eating.

Success is losing a few pounds and keeping it off for life, not losing a lot of weight and regaining it within the year.

Take it slowly, one step at a time.

Tony's story:

I've lost more than 40 pounds (18 kg) over the last three years, and my blood sugar is now normal!

For years I yo-yo dieted. I would lose and gain, lose and gain, then gain more. When you're dieting, you can say, "Oh, I'll have something extra, just this one time." Now that I have diabetes I know that it's not just the diet that I'm putting at stake, it's my health too. That's why I knew I had to stop my dieting cycle. I didn't just need to lose weight; I needed to change my lifestyle. I knew I could do it. Once I started, it wasn't so hard. I love to bake, so all I had to do was change the recipes a little. These were changes I knew that I could make forever.

I've told family and friends, this probably is the best thing that could have happened to me. Diabetes is a bad thing and I don't wish it on anybody, but it got me under control… and it wasn't that difficult.

Record your Progress

Studies show that keeping a record of what you eat helps you lose weight, and keep the weight off.

No matter how tedious it may seem, writing down what you eat each day works! It helps you see how you are doing – and you feel rewarded for your efforts.

I recommend you do this for a week. Return to record keeping as soon as you are falling off your healthy pattern.

Why keep a record of the food you eat?

- It helps you realize what foods you usually eat, and how much you eat. We tend to minimize the extent of our bad habits. Food records help break this pattern of denial. My clients tell me that one of the best things about keeping a diary of their eating habits is that it shocks them into realizing how much they actually eat.

How to keep a food record?

- **Write down everything you eat and drink (even water).**

- **Write down the amounts of all the foods that you eat.** Instead of saying a glass of juice, record the amount, such as 1 cup (250 mL). Instead of saying a bowl of cereal, measure out how many cups or mL of cereal you put in your bowl. You might be surprised at the amounts. Once you are familiar with the portions you are eating, you don't need to keep measuring.

- **Read food labels.** Different brands can vary.

- **Record all added fats and spreads.** Fat is the highest calorie food in our diet, so it is very important to record all added butter, margarine, vegetable oil, olive oil, shortening, lard, etc. Record even a ½ teaspoon (2 mL) of fat added in cooking or at the table – the calories add up. Also, record added amounts of spreads like jams, ketchup, etc.

- **Estimate the ingredients and portions of homemade recipes.**

Reward your daily efforts:

- *Add a coin to a jar each day you achieve your daily goal. Let the coins add up, and then buy something nice for yourself!*

- *Sometimes a reward can be a small food treat. See Treat Budget on page 68.*

If you eat a meal or snack that matches the portions of one shown on pages 149–200, record the calories as listed. A calorie check is on page 151.

Write down other things in your food record.

- What are your feelings at different times of the day?

- Where and when do you eat?

- When are you exercising? Studies show that at the same time that we underestimate how much we eat, we overestimate how much exercise we do. That's one more reason to write it down (see page 254).

- Write down your blood sugar at different times of the day.

- Record your weight. Weighing yourself once a week can be motivating, but when your weight loss goal is a gradual one, a monthly weigh-in is usually better.

You've got a record of what you ate.
What should you do with it?

First, calculate your daily calories. If you are seeing a dietitian, you could ask her to work this out for you, or use a calorie app on your smart phone or tablet. Otherwise, use the handy Calorie Counter that follows. Figure out which high calorie foods you need to decrease.

Second, review your records to learn what leads you to overeat and what helps you eat better. Ask yourself:

- What times of the day do I tend to overeat?

- What made me overeat?

- Do I eat less when I eat regular meals?

- Was I really hungry – or was I bored, tired, frustrated or angry, or just being sociable?

- What helped make a good day?

- Does drinking water help me eat or drink less?

- Do I eat more in front of the TV or computer, instead of at my kitchen or dining room table?

- Do I eat more in restaurants or in my car than at home?

- Do I eat differently on days that I am busy or active?

- Do I need to allow myself some comfort food and if so how much and how often?

- How can I limit or change situations that lead me to overeat?

Asking these questions will lead you to solutions that will work for you. Try changing one habit at a time.

It's hard to give up favorite foods, but one amazing thing about a food record is that you feel rewarded right away for your good choices.

Calorie apps

There are some great calorie app programs that you can download onto your smart phone or tablet. You will then be linked to a database of information. On the internet search "diabetes apps" or "calorie apps." There are also great "exercise apps" and "quit smoking apps" – you'll find an app for almost everything! Some apps are free and others have a small charge to download.

Internet links:

To find more detailed calorie information search these key words:

- *calorie counter*
- *nutrient value of some common foods*
- *USDA nutrient database*

Mistakes happen.

Don't beat yourself up. These aren't easy changes and sometimes you'll get fed up, feel anxious or even mad. Get back to your healthy pattern as soon as you can. Start another one week food record. Try and understand what led to the slip and see if you can prevent it or manage it better next time. Imagine the situation happening again, and plan ahead how to react and deal with it. If needed, talk to a friend or professional for support.

63

Karen's Calorie Counter

- I rounded portions off to 25, 50, 75, 100 and so on to make it easier to add.

- Unless marked, the calories are for the commercial or usual available product, rather than a light, or lighter homemade version. Commercial products vary depending on brand.

- Short forms used: tablespoon = tbsp; teaspoon = tsp; ounce = oz and grams = g. Most meat portions are shown in 5-ounce portions, which equals 150 grams.

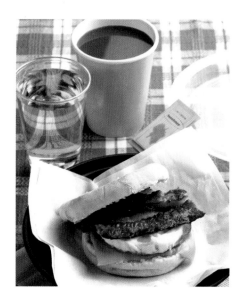

Almonds, 2 tbsp (30 mL)	100
almonds, ½ cup (125 mL)	425
apple, 1 medium	75
applesauce, unsweetened, ½ cup (125 mL)	50
apple juice, unsweetened, 1 cup (250 mL)	125
avocado, ½ medium	100
Bacon, crisp, 2 strips	75
bagel, 6-inch (15 cm)	325
banana, 1 medium	100
bannock, one 3-inch (7.5 cm) piece	200
barley, cooked, ½ cup (125 mL)	100
beans or lentils, cooked, 1 cup (250 mL)	125
beans, canned, baked with tomato sauce, 1 cup (250 mL)	125
beans, kidney, canned, 1 cup (250 mL)	125
beer, regular, Canadian, one 12-oz (341 mL) bottle	175
beer, regular, American, one 12-oz (341 mL) bottle	150
biscuit, tea, 1 medium	250
blueberries, 1 cup (250 mL)	75
bologna, 1 slice (21 g)	50
bread, whole wheat, 1 slice (28 g)	75
bread, white, 1 slice (25 g)	75

bread, 1 thick slice (48 g)	125
bun, hamburger or hotdog bun, 1	125
butter, 1½ tsp (7 mL)	50
Cake, angel food, 1/12 of cake	75
cake, chocolate with icing, 1/12 of cake	200
cake, cheesecake, cherry, 1/12 of a cake	325
cappuccino, with whole milk, medium (12 oz/375 mL)	100
carrot, raw, 1 medium	25
cereal, dry, unsweetened, 1 cup (250 mL)	100
cereal, dry, sweetened, 1 cup (250 mL)	150
cereal, granola, commercial, 1 cup (250 mL)	500
cereal, hot, cooked, 1 cup (250 mL)	150
Cheez Whiz, 1 tbsp (15 mL)	50
cheese, cheddar, 1 oz (30 g)	125
cheese, cheddar, low fat, 1 oz (30 g)	75
cheese, cottage, 2%, ½ cup (125 mL)	100
cheese, processed, 1 slice (thick)	75
chicken wings, roasted, with skin, 4 wings	400
chicken, baked, breast, no skin, 5 oz (150 g)	225
chicken, deep fried, drumstick and thigh	500
chili con carne, restaurant, 1¼ cups (300 mL)	300

chocolate bar, standard size, 1 bar (65 g)	275
cinnamon bun, 1 large	500
coffee or tea, black, large	0
coffee, double cream and sugar, large	75
cola, regular, 12-oz (355 mL) can	150
coleslaw, commercial, ½ cup (125 mL)	150
cookies, 2 digestive or 3 graham wafers	75
cookies, chocolate chip, 2 (2½-inch/6 cm)	100
corn on the cob, 1 medium	125
corn, kernel, ½ cup (125 mL)	75
crackers, 4 soda, 2 Breton or 2 melba toast	50
cranberry juice cocktail, regular, 1 cup (250 mL)	125
cranberry juice cocktail, light, 1 cup (250 mL)	50
cream, half and half (cereal cream), 1½ tbsp (22 mL)	25
cream, whipping, whipped, ½ cup (125 mL)	200
croissant, 1 medium	225
Crystal Light beverage, 1 cup (250 mL)	0
Danish pastry, 1	275
donut, cake, 1	200
donut, cream or jelly filled, 1	300
Egg, 1 large	75
English muffin, 1	125
Fish, canned salmon or tuna, ½ can (3½ oz/105 g)	175
fish, fresh, cooked, salmon, 5 oz (150 g)	250
fish, fresh, cooked, white, 5 oz (150 g)	175
French fries, small, with 1 package ketchup	225
French fries, supersize, with 2 packages ketchup	650
fruit, 1 fist-sized	75
fruit, canned in juice, ½ cup (125 mL)	75
Granola bar, single bar	150
grapefruit, half	50
grapes or cherries, 10	50
Ham, cooked, 5 oz (150 g)	250
hamburger with bun, fast food, plain	300
hamburger, equal to a Big Mac size with cheese	700
hash browns, frozen, fried, ½ cup (125 mL)	175
honey, 1 tsp (5 mL)	25
hot chocolate light, 1 cup (250 mL)	50
Ice cream, 1 scoop	125
iced tea, regular, 12-oz (355 mL) bottle	150
Jam, 1½ tsp (7 mL) regular or 1–2 tbsp (15–30 mL) light	25
Jell-O, diet, 1 cup (250 mL)	0
jelly beans, 10	100
Ketchup, 1½ tbsp (22 mL)	25
Lasagna, 4- x 3-inch (10 x 7.5 cm) piece	300
liquor, hard (rye, gin, rum, vodka), 1½ oz (45 mL)	75
Macaroni, plain, cooked, 1 cup (250 mL)	200
macaroni, Kraft Dinner, made per directions, 1 cup (250 mL)	400
macaroni and cheese, homemade, 1 cup (250 mL)	250
milk, skim, 1 cup (250 mL)	100
milk, whole (3.3%), 1 cup (250 mL)	150
milk, chocolate, 2%, 1 cup (250 mL)	200
muffin, commercial, 1 large	400
muffin, homemade, low-fat, 1 small	150
Oil, olive, canola or corn, 1 tbsp (15 mL)	125
olives, small green or black, 4	25
orange, 1 medium	50
orange juice, 1 cup (250 mL)	125
Pancake, 1 small, 4-inch (10 cm)	75
peanut butter, 1 tbsp (15 mL)	100
peanuts (shells removed), ½ cup (125 mL)	450
pie, apple, 2 crusts, ⅛ of a pie (1 piece)	300

pie, apple, 1 piece with 1 scoop ice cream	425
pineapple, 2 rings or ½ cup (125 mL), in juice	75
pizza, thin crust, 2 toppings, 1 piece	300
pizza, thick crust, 2 toppings, 1 piece	400
popcorn, air-popped, 3 cups (750 mL)	100
popcorn, movie-type with butter, large (20 cups/5 L)	1,500
pork chop, cooked, 5 oz (150 g)	300
potato chips, 1 small bag (45 g)	250
potato chips, 1 large bag (300 g)	1,625
potato salad, commercial, ½ cup (125 mL)	200
potato, 1 medium or 1 cup (250 mL) mashed (no butter)	150
potatoes, scalloped, from mix, 1 cup (250 mL)	250
prunes, 2 or ¼ cup (60 mL) prune juice	50
pudding, 2%, regular, ½ cup (125 mL)	150
pudding, skim, no-sugar added, ½ cup (125 mL)	50
Raisins, 2 tbsp (30 mL)	50
ribs, 4 ribs, roasted with sauce	500
rice cake, 1 flavored	50
rice, brown, long-grain, cooked, 1 cup (250 mL)	225
rice, fried, 1 cup (250 mL)	325
rice, white, long-grain, cooked, 1 cup (250 mL)	225
rice, long-grain, instant, cooked, 1 cup (250 mL)	175
Salad dressing, light, 1 tbsp (15 mL)	25
salad dressing, regular, 1 tbsp (15 mL)	75
salad, chef, large, homemade, 2 cups (500 mL)	250
salad, Caesar, restaurant-type, 2 cups (500 mL)	400
salad greens, tossed, 2 cups (500 mL)	25
sandwich, 1 slice of cheese/meat and 2 tsp (10 mL) margarine or butter	350
sausages, breakfast, cooked, 2 links	100
Slushee/Slurpee, small, 12 oz (341 mL)	175

Slushee/Slurpee, jumbo, 40 oz (1.1 L)	550
smoothie, specialty, large, 20 oz (568 mL)	500
smoothie, homemade, low-sugar, low-fat, 1 cup (250 mL)	100
soft drink/soda, 12-oz (355 mL) can	150
soft drink, diet, 12-oz (355 mL) can	0
soup, chicken noodle, ½ 10-oz (284 mL) can with water	100
soup, mushroom, ½ 10-oz (284 mL) can made with milk	150
soup, tomato, ½ 10-oz (284 mL) can made with milk	125
spaghetti sauce, jarred, ½ cup (125 mL)	100
spaghetti, cooked, 1 cup (250 mL)	100
steak, cooked, 5 oz (150 g)	275
strawberries, fresh, 1 cup (250 mL)	50
submarine sandwich, w/sauce & toppings, 12-inch (30 cm) sub	1000+
sugar, white or brown, 1½ tsp (7 mL)	25
sweetener, low-calorie, 1 tsp (5 mL)	0
Taco shell or 1 small corn tortilla	50
toast, 1 slice dry (28 g)	75
toast, restaurant, 1 slice buttered	175
tomato juice or vegetable juice, 1 cup (250 mL)	50
tomatoes, canned, 1 cup (250 mL)	75
tortilla, large, 8-inch (20 cm)	175
turkey, light and dark, cooked, 5 oz (150 g)	225
Vegetables such as broccoli, cauliflower, zucchini, cabbage, celery, turnip, onions & tomato, 1 cup (250 mL)	25
vegetables (peas, carrots, beets, or parsnips), ½ cup (125 mL)	50
Waffle, frozen, 1 small (4-inch/10 cm)	100
wine, dry, 4 oz (125 mL)	75
Yogurt, 2%, sweetened, ¾ cup (175 g)	175
yogurt, low-fat, no-sugar added, ¾ cup (175 g)	100

Regular Meals & Portion Control

Using a small plate serves up big results!

Enjoy smaller portions

Use smaller plates, smaller glasses and smaller bowls and even smaller spoons. Rather than eating potato chips right out of the bag, portion out your serving into a small bowl and put the rest away. This helps you eat less. The only exception is your water glass and salad bowl – they can be large! Portion out food servings in the kitchen on a plate rather than taking platters of food to the table. If buffets at home or in restaurants lead you to overeat, try to avoid them.

Eat at regular times to control hunger

Develop a routine of eating three meals a day, at regular times, to reduce hunger. If you get a little hungry, this is your body telling you that you are short of calories and that it will start using up some of your stored fat. Good for you! You want to burn fat.

Eat slowly

This gives your brain time to know that you are full. If you sit down to eat, this helps slow you down. Chew your food well, especially your first few bites. This sets the pace. Put down your fork between bites, and drink water during your meal.

Turn off the TV when eating

Research shows that we eat more while watching TV. Television distracts you – you don't realize how much you have eaten or that you are full. Also the TV ads for foods make you crave food whether or not you are hungry.

Meal plans show you the way

See pages 149–200 and the seventy additional meal plans in my book *Diabetes Meals for Good Health*. Choose from the wide variety of favorite meals and snacks. Depending on your calorie needs, choose either the large or small meals. With these meal plans you get lots of healthy food to fill you up, and the calories are controlled. These meals include lots of fiber and a small amount of protein at each meal, which keeps you going until the next meal or snack. When you start to eat more fruit and vegetables, and drink more water, you will feel more satisfied. Water replaces sweet beverages that quickly add on the calories and weight. You'll start to lose weight, and feel proud of your efforts. Now you'll be able to focus on healthy living, not dieting.

Small amounts of extra beverages or foods can cause weight gain when eaten regularly over many years. For example, you could gain 10 pounds (4.5 kg) a year by consuming each week an extra:

- *5 cans of soft drink, or*
- *5 bottles of beer, or*
- *2 Big Macs, or*
- *2 large servings of fries, or*
- *5 scoops of ice cream*

Cut out these extra foods and you are on your way to losing weight.

Pamela's story:

Pamela cooks for her husband and has helped him stick to the small meal plans in *Diabetes Meals for Good Health*:

"I had to do it. I put what portions were recommended right on our plates. I dished everything out and went by the measuring spoons and measuring cups. I made up my mind to do it. That's how we cook now. I cooked all the little desserts and stuff. I found that offset not having the seconds. Then there were times when the meals filled us up so nicely that we didn't even need the dessert."

Out of Sight – Out of Mind

The more you buy, the more you will eat!

Consider giving yourself a "treat budget"

First, keep track of how many treats you eat each week. This might include chips, chocolates, candy, donuts, ice cream, French fries, pie and so on.

Second, allow yourself one or two a week. It doesn't mean you have to eat them – but sometimes just knowing it's allowed in your budget makes it easier to make it through the week.

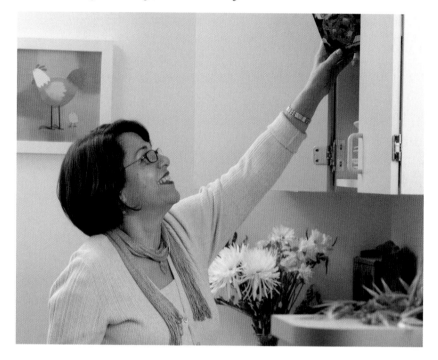

Put away tempting foods – or better yet, don't buy them. Instead, put low-calorie foods (such as fruit and vegetables) in easy to find places.

What is your weakness? White bread, sweet beverages, beer, potato chips, peanuts, cookies, ice cream or chocolates? Even apparently healthy choices, such as "100 calorie snack packs" become danger foods if you eat all the snack packages in the box. Avoid buying your "danger" foods.

Grocery shop with a list

- Don't shop when you're hungry.
- Only buy what you need.
- Stay away from the most tempting aisles.
- Don't linger near the bakery.
- Say no to buying chocolate bars at the check-out line.

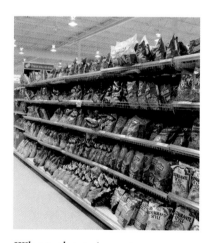

When shopping, stay away from the tempting aisles of chips and soft drinks.

Conquer your Cravings

Reach for improved blood sugar and weight loss.

Most people have experienced cravings and compulsive eating at one time or another. "I intended to eat one piece of chocolate, but before I knew it, I'd eaten the whole box." It's human and isn't just overweight people who overeat. Thin people eat compulsively too; they just usually do it less often.

What causes cravings?

Sometimes you're hungry. Sometimes things you see or smell will make your mouth water and make you feel hungry, even if you just ate. For example, TV ads of luscious looking food, seeing food in the store or on the counter can trigger cravings. How we feel can also set off cravings (happy, sad, angry, tired, lonely or bored).

"Three D's" of dealing with cravings

1. **D**eep breath – take a few!

2. **D**rink water – have a large glass.

3. **D**istract yourself – go do something else; eating is not the only thing in the world to do.

Establish a stop-eating routine

- Eat meals and snacks at about the same time.

- Consider "no eating" in the evening after you're finished eating dinner.

- Try to eat at the same place for each meal, whether you are home or in the workplace. The kitchen table or dining room is the old fashioned place to eat, and it works! Slowly you will stop associating the couch, the computer, the bedroom, or the car as places to eat.

- After a meal or snack, rinse out your mouth well. Brushing your teeth or dentures, and in the evening flossing your teeth, are also good ways to end the eating.

- Take a shower or bath to relax yourself for a good night's sleep. Adequate sleep is important for weight loss.

Of course, sometimes you'll overeat. That's okay, but start the next day with a healthy breakfast, and get right back to your healthy pattern, including practicing the "Three D's."

Pages 275–276 shows you many other practical ways to deal with cravings.

Do you feel that the more you eat, the less you enjoy it? Practice the "Three D's" to avoid second helpings or excess snacking.

Dine Out Sensibly

Dine out less often.

The most important thing about eating in restaurants is – not eating in restaurants, or at least, not very often. If you now eat in a restaurant daily, consider cutting back to one or two times a week. If you eat out once a week, try to cut it back to once or twice a month. Remember the old saying, "out of sight, out of mind"? Don't tempt yourself more than necessary. Studies show that taste influences us more than health. In other words, when sitting in a restaurant with many good things to choose, we quickly lose our willpower. If you only eat out rarely, then it's okay to splurge. If you are like most North Americans, you consume almost a third of your food budget outside of your home. In this case, what you eat in restaurants is critical to your health.

Studies show that families that eat together at home are both physically and emotionally healthier. Fast food restaurants and meals-on-the-run are very rushed. This kind of meal doesn't give families enough opportunities to learn to cook or talk together. Restaurant servings are larger, have fewer vegetables, and have more salt, sugar and fat than homemade meals.

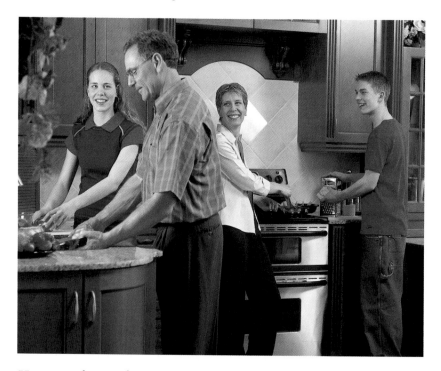

Homemade meals are easy, save you money, and can be made with healthy ingredients. You can cook a homemade meal in less time than it takes to go to a restaurant.

Adult baby food

Restaurants serve addictive soft processed hamburgers, soft buns with soft fries and large glasses of soft drinks. These are low-fiber foods that require little chewing, so they can be gulped down in large amounts.

Layers of food

Restaurants layer fatty or sugary foods on top of each other. This means that the height of the food, whether it is a burger, sub, dessert or cappuccino, grows and gets more mouth-watering.

Giving you more

Some restaurants constantly refill your basket of buns or bread, or refill your sweet beverages. Even before your meal comes, you will have overeaten on carbohydrates and calories.

This new way of eating excessive calories in a short time is causing weight gain and poor health in people around the world.

When you do dine out, eat sensibly.

1. **Plan ahead where and when you are going to eat.**
   Go to a restaurant that has some healthier food choices that you like. Restaurants with salad options or meal choices that aren't fried are good. Try to eat within an hour or two of your regular meal time. Late lunch or late dinner meals can result in overeating as you are too hungry.

2. **Plan ahead what you are going to eat.** If the restaurant has the nutrient information of their meals and food items available online, look it up before you go. You may be shocked at the amount of calories, fat, sugar and salt in many restaurant food items. Carefully go through the choices and choose a meal that fits into your approximate calorie range. For example, if you normally choose large dinner meals as shown in this book, then look for 700–750 calorie meals. Knowing what you want to order when you arrive at the restaurant means you won't have to browse through the menu – browsing can tempt you to change your mind and order something more.

   If you don't have nutrition information for the menu, look for healthy or smaller options. Sometimes it helps if you order first, so you are not tempted by what others order.

Have you ever ordered a "healthy" meal, for instance, a low-fat sub, then "rewarded" yourself with an unhealthy extra like cookies?

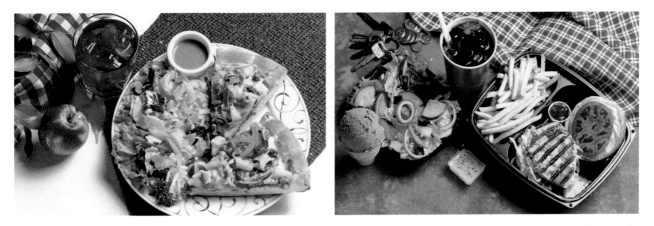

In my book *Diabetes Meals for Good Health,* there are examples of restaurant meals for each of the breakfast, lunch and dinner meals.

3. **Don't go to the restaurant hungry.** If you have a chance, before you go to a restaurant have a small snack (a fruit, some carrot sticks, 5–10 pecans or almonds, or a few crackers with cheese). Then you won't be so hungry and tempted to over-order and overeat.

4. **Order less and you will eat less!** Order smaller meals and avoid super-sizing and extras. Instead of calorie-packed "meal deals," order single items, senior meals, junior portions or half-size meals. Or share a meal, or part of a meal, with a friend or family member. For example, share an order of fries or a dessert, and save calories as well as cash. If the meal entrée choices look quite large, consider ordering a salad or soup with a small appetizer instead. Order a smaller steak than you would have in the past. We'd all love to eat more, but we just don't need it.

5. **Extra care at buffets.** Very few people can resist the temptation to overload their plate at buffets. Even salad buffets include "unhealthy choices" that might mysteriously end up on your plate and in your stomach. Try to stick to this buffet rule: go only once through the line, and choose smaller amounts all along the way.

6. **Ask the restaurant to bag it.** One large restaurant meal may be enough for two dinners. Solve your problem of what to have for dinner the next day!

Savara's story:

Savara talks about the challenges for her husband and herself when they eat out at buffets:

"For my husband, it was harder because he loves sweets and he was eating a lot of them. For the first six months he was not a very happy camper, but now if we go out he actually goes by the desserts and it doesn't even bother him. I think once he cut the sugars, he didn't crave them as much. He's a chocolate cake man, but now he can go by a piece of chocolate cake, and he says nay. When we go to a buffet, we try and eat healthy salads and stuff. He'll look for the reduced sugar desserts, and he'll have one once in awhile. He eats a lot of fruit. There are ways to get around. At salad bars, we just hold the dressings, hold everything… I find we're not overeating the way we used to, and we can feel it. If we overeat we don't feel so good, and the next day you go back to your regular habits and you feel a lot better."

7. Ask how foods are prepared and, if needed, request special items or substitutions.

- Choose fruit salad or a small glass of tomato or fruit juice instead of hash browns at breakfast. Ask for a poached or boiled egg instead of fried egg; ham instead of bacon or sausages; and toast (unbuttered if you don't mind) instead of a Danish or large bagel.

- With sandwiches, request bread or toast unbuttered. There often is mayonnaise added to the fillings so you don't need to double up on the spreads. My mother taught me "one spread per bread."

- Eat a submarine sandwich with no mayonnaise, but have just a little mustard instead.

- Drink diet soft drinks instead of regular.

- Try a small serving of low-fat milk instead of a regular soft drink, milkshake or smoothie.

- Order a single hamburger instead of the "meal deal" larger burger (see page 208).

- Consider getting small fries instead of large fries or choose a baked potato with no butter (or butter and sour cream on the side). Often mashed potatoes or rice are a lighter choice than fries, even though they usually have some fat added (see page 211).

Bagels and muffins

A 6-inch (15 cm) restaurant bagel is equal to four slices of bread. Low-fat muffins are often so large that they have significant calories, fat and sugar. See pages 204 and 214 (page 203 shows examples of egg breakfasts).

High-fat salads

A Caesar salad with the dressing can have as many calories as a hamburger and fries (see page 212). Mayonnaise-laden salads like potato salads and coleslaw are also high in fat and calories.

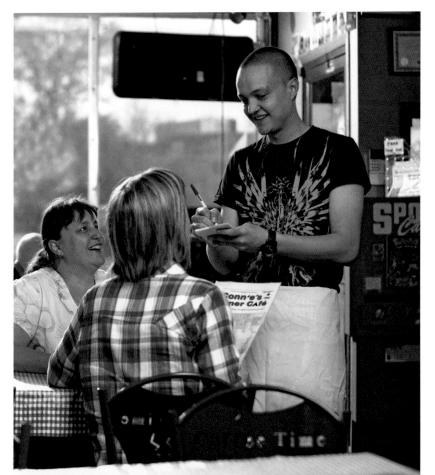

The "Eat This - Not That" section on pages 201–216 has tips on choosing restaurant foods.

- Get a double order of steamed vegetables (unbuttered) or a garden salad, or a broth-based vegetable soup or plain bun, instead of fries or garlic bread.

- Consider ordering a green or tossed salad. Ask for some grilled chicken on top and a bun on the side. For all salads, request a light salad dressing instead of regular dressing or ask for lemon on the side instead of dressing.

- Ask for no sauces, gravies and butter, or "on the side."

- Try plain rice instead of fried rice; burrito instead of a deep fried taco shell, vegetable stir fry instead of deep fried foods.

- Choose baked or grilled meat, chicken or fish instead of fried, deep fried or ribs.

- A thin crust pizza is healthier than a thick crust pizza. Try it topped with more vegetables and skip the fatty meats and extra cheese.

- Instead of a donut or Danish with a fancy coffee drink, have 2 or 3 donut bites ("holes") and a frothy cappuccino made with low-fat milk.

8. **Order water with your meal, and drink it.** It's free! Limit yourself when it comes to alcoholic beverages. Not only do these have calories, but when you drink, you are less likely to care about how much you overeat. Just a few cocktails can add 300–600 calories before you even start your meal. If you would like to order a drink, consider a glass of dry wine, a light beer or a hard liquor drink with a diet beverage. Alternatively, if you choose to have a non-alcoholic drink, order a diet soft drink, carbonated water or mineral water with lemon. If you make reservations or wait in the sitting area instead of the lounge, this removes the temptation to drink too much before your meal.

9. **Consider skipping dessert, except on your own birthday!** One lighter option if you are craving dessert is one scoop of ice cream, sorbet or ice milk, or share a dessert.

10. **After your restaurant meal, go for a walk.** This is especially important if you did overeat.

A Plan for Special Occasions

Celebrate holidays while limiting overeating.

The number of holidays celebrated across North America is as great as our ethnic origins. Regardless of the holidays you and your family celebrate, here are some tips for containing the holiday madness. These are ways to avoid weight gain and spiraling blood sugar!

Holiday feasting – longer holidays may cause us to overeat. My grandmother, who lived in Denmark as a child, spoke of how Christmas was very special. The family shared a carefully prepared five course meal on Christmas Eve, and on Christmas morning each child in the family received one imported orange plus a present. She celebrated Christmas over just two days, whereas today, holiday celebrations can last over a 2–3-month period. This means we have a lot more time and opportunity to overeat.

Holiday food – too much of a good thing? Another difference is the amount of food eaten over holidays. Most holidays now include homemade "traditional" foods supplemented with store-bought "celebration" foods, often candies and chocolates. Have you noticed how Christmas goodies line the shelves in October and early November, followed in February with chocolates for Easter, still two months away? An Easter bunny in the 1970s was the size of your hand, and now stands a foot tall. If you buy Halloween candy in September, it's all gone by the time October 31st rolls around – so you go buy more! The boxes of treats are getting bigger and bigger, so you may have candies and snacks left over after Halloween, Thanksgiving, Ramadan, Christmas, Super Bowl Sunday, Diwali, Passover, Chinese New Year, Mardi Gras, Easter or other celebrations. These "extras" then continue to tempt us for many days or weeks until we have eaten them all.

Holiday weight gain. An occasional indulgence or large meal causes a temporary blood sugar peak, but is manageable in the big picture. However, weeks of overindulgence and inactivity can lead to serious blood sugar and weight problems. On average, North American men gain 3–5 pounds (1.5–2.5 kg) over December, and women gain 2–3 pounds (1–1.5 kg). That's a lot more than one turkey dinner. Gaining 3 pounds (1.5 kg) equals an extra 10,500 calories. That means the overeating probably extended from November to early January. Trying to lose the extra pounds you've gained over a holiday is no fun, and definitely no holiday. Sometimes these pounds build year after year.

Birthday Parties

Do you have a large family with many birthday celebrations? This can be a challenge when you have diabetes as the calories and sugar add up. Could you decide on the special birthdays over the year that you want to celebrate with birthday cake, and have lighter choices at the others?

Are you taking rapid insulin?

If you are on a flexible insulin regime, you can take extra insulin for extra food. This works for a special day, but if you overeat over many days or weeks, the extra insulin and food will result in a weight gain.

Fight the holiday food frenzy.

1. **Try to contain your "holiday" feasting.** Some holidays do require a lot of cooking ahead of time. Decorations are good, but don't bring out the holiday foods until one or two days before the holiday begins if possible or for that day alone. Try to limit food shopping and baking of holiday goodies.

2. **Make a new tradition of healthy choices.** Consider adapting your traditional holiday recipes to make them lower in fat (see pages 100–108). Healthy choices can fit in your own home as well as when you bring food to other homes. See sidebar.

3. **Have regular meals.** You may be tempted to omit breakfast and lunch the day of a family gathering or party, so you can "save up your calories for later." Unfortunately this often backfires. You end up hungry, and then lose all good resolve. You dive into the snacks, followed by a meal which is too large. In addition to regular meals, have fruit before heading out, to take the edge off your appetite. Keep your stomach filled with water and low-calorie choices.

4. **Plan for your favorites.** Unless you have super-human willpower, don't plan on going without your favorites. Going without might make you feel deprived, and lead to overindulgence later. Go for the best, one or two of your favorites, in a moderate portion. You don't have to try everything.

5. **Limit the alcohol.** Drinking alcohol piles on calories and makes you less likely to say no to the extra foods. Choose lighter drinks from the list on page 137. Try soda with a touch of cranberry juice and lime.

6. **Smaller plates work.** Studies show that we eat more when people serve food on large dishes. For example, if the turkey is on a big platter we take more, and if the gravy is in a large gravy boat we pour more on our potatoes. If the host serves us from a small plate, we politely take less. If you are at a buffet, take a lunch plate rather than a larger dinner plate. This will automatically decrease your portion sizes. Try a variety of foods if you want, but less of everything.

7. **Festive fitness.** Holidays can be wonderful, but can also be stressful if there are family feuds. Exercise is a healthy way to help cope with this stress. Walk away from irritations. Getting out will also help you burn off some of the extra sugar and calories you may have eaten. After a heavy meal, ask, "Who'd like to go for a walk?" – getting out for even 15 minutes can help break the sitting and overeating. If you have a string of parties to attend throughout the holiday season, try to walk or exercise daily.

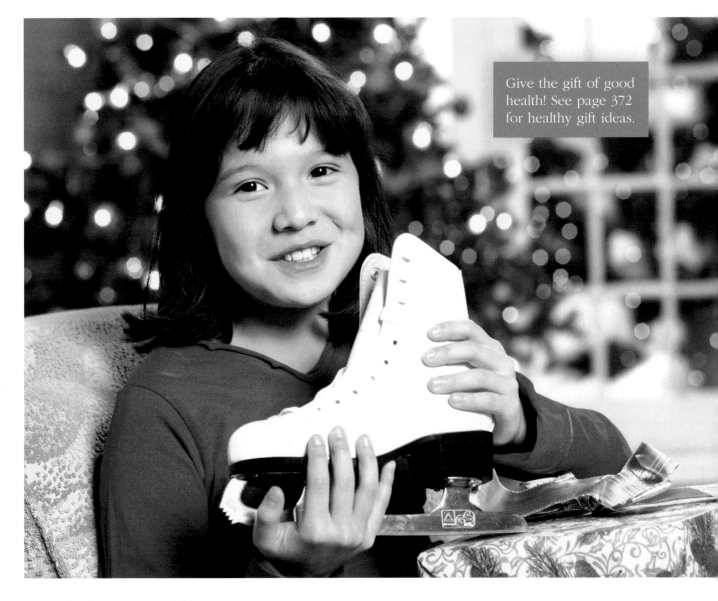

Give the gift of good health! See page 372 for healthy gift ideas.

Keep kids active and busy
If adults have been overeating, so have kids. They will need some fresh air and a chance to burn off some of their energy. Consider a swim or skate. Organize a game of football or another outdoor activity.

Manage Workplace Temptations

Create a healthy workplace for you and your colleagues.

At your workplace, do you have food tucked in your desk drawer? Are there food and goodies regularly sitting out in common areas, or at coffee breaks or during meetings?

This is a very common situation in many workplaces. It can mean by the time you get home you may have already eaten your daily limit of calories. Below are a couple of possible solutions. However, since you don't control all of your workplace, if you can get other work associates to come on board with you, your chance of success will be greater.

Decrease food in the office space

The office eating issue today is similar in some ways to the old office smoking issue. It wasn't really fair that the non-smoker had to breathe in second-hand smoke, so offices put policies in place to change this. Is it fair that a person who doesn't wish to eat during work confronts daily the smells and sights of others' irresistible foods?

Remove your own food from your office. Then talk to your co-workers. How many really want food constantly tempting them? If it's only a few people in the office, perhaps they might consider keeping their extra food out of sight.

Decrease food at coffee breaks

"Coffee breaks" were introduced more widely in the mid-1940s as a means for production line workers, who were standing on their feet all day, to sit down. If you work this type of job, then you do deserve a break. Yet today, many of us have an office type job where we are already sitting down most of the day! Although we may be craving a caffeine lift from coffee, our bodies and brains need exercise, not more rest. Exercise would help us return to our desks feeling fresh. Consider going for a 15 minute walk. If coffee is a must, bring it back to your desk with you. You may find you can even give up a coffee here and there and replace it with water.

Coffee breaks are a time to join your co-workers for light conversation. Convince one or several co-workers to join you for a walk and talk break.

Jody's story:

At work we have this thing called the Fit Wit: Fitness Wellness Initiative Team. We started at work using pedometers and having challenges. That's where I started using a pedometer. That was over a year ago. Now I know what it takes to walk at least 10,000 steps a day. It's excellent being on the Fit Wit committee at work. I'm learning more about nutrition, and exercise. I'm just walking, and doing portion control. Just those two things can change your life. That gets me excited. When you see positive changes happening it feels really good, and you want to keep doing it. You want other people to get involved too. If you've got information for them, it helps so much. Many people at work are doing things that they never did before – like taking the stairs instead of the elevator. We're in a four-story building. We have stair climb challenges regularly, where you mark off your flights. It's excellent, it's a team building thing. I haven't taken an elevator since we started. I'm just so happy about it…and I was someone who never really exercised before.

Decrease food at meetings

Many times food is the draw for employees to attend yet another meeting. When the meeting you are attending is less than exciting, eating seems a good way to pass the time! The problem is that once you and fellow workers have gorged on the sweet treats, your blood sugar goes up. Then you'll be feeling sleepy.

When someone serves food, most of us do not do very well with willpower alone. Ideally change needs to come from management. Do donuts and super-sized muffins, soft drinks, pizza and cookies need to be there? Meetings could be a great chance to serve fresh fruit and vegetable trays! Can meetings incorporate a 10 minute walk or exercise break? If you are a boss, you can make changes for the better, but as an employee you may feel you don't have much power to make changes. However, there is power in even one voice. You are likely not the only one in your group who wants to lose weight or who has high cholesterol or diabetes. Bring it up as a discussion point at a meeting. This is the starting point for others in your office to start making a change.

Healthier meeting snacks or meals:

- *fresh fruit trays with yogurt dip*
- *raw vegetable trays*
- *small muffins (2½-inch/6 cm or smaller)*
- *sandwiches on unbuttered whole-grain breads and made with less filling*
- *assortment of whole grain crackers, rice crackers and small chunks of low fat cheese*
- *soups and soda crackers*
- *sushi or spring rolls that aren't fried*
- *smaller serving sizes of desserts*
- *water jug and glasses with ice*
- *coffee and tea with low fat milk*

Travel and Still Stay on Track

See the world — and get healthier as you go.

If you drive a truck or RV, or have a job or lifestyle that you travel a lot, try these things to keep on track.

Make wise restaurant choices

Big meals mean big blood sugars! Try to choose smaller meals and space the meals out throughout your day. See pages 70–74.

Plan ahead when traveling – if driving, carry healthy foods in your vehicle

- Carry water or diet beverages. Forget the sweet drinks, desserts and junk foods. Just don't buy them. Chew gum!

- Carry a cooler or insulated bag, or perhaps you have a fridge in your vehicle. Keep your cooler stocked with fresh fruit, raw ready-to-eat vegetables (such as carrots, celery sticks or edible snap peas), hard boiled eggs, cheese slices, cheese strings or small containers of yogurt.

- Consider a stop at a grocery store instead of sitting down to a restaurant meal. Buy buns and meat or sliced cheese, and cucumbers to make a meal.

- For breakfast, bring along small plastic containers that you have prefilled with unsweetened cereals or plain oatmeal. These are then ready-to-eat with a spoon, and buy a 1 cup (250 mL) of milk from a vending machine or café. Mix the oatmeal with hot water from the tap or a coffee maker in a hotel room.

- Examples of easy travel meals or snacks to eat at a roadside picnic site or in the car include:
  - a peanut butter or cheese sandwich
  - a can of tuna or salmon for a fish sandwich or toss the fish in a bag of washed baby spinach with some chopped tomato and light dressing
  - hard boiled eggs with bread
  - cheese and crackers
  - small package of almonds
  - a small bag of sunflower seeds or peanuts with the shells on, not the big bag (see sidebar)
  - fresh fruit, packaged puddings or a few low-fat granola bars.

- If you have an RV or are a long-distance trucker, you may have a freezer and microwave in your vehicle. You can heat up a frozen dinner entrée or frozen leftovers brought from home. If you choose the large meals in this book, buy frozen entrees that have under 400 calories for lunch and under 700 calories for dinner.

Carry essential eating utensils:

A paring knife or pocket knife, some plastic cutlery, and a few reusable cups, bowls and plates.

Seeds and nuts:

A 1-cup (250 mL) serving of sunflower seeds with the shells on equals ⅓ cup (75 mL) of sunflower seeds without the shells. Either of these servings equals 240 calories.

Beware: *1 cup (250 mL) of ready-to-eat shelled nuts or sunflower seeds, or trail mix, has about 700–800 calories!*

Candies: *Instead of carrying a bag of candies that are a constant temptation in your vehicle, have a container of mini candies (e.g., Tic-Tacs).*

- When trucking and long-distance driving with a deadline, it can be hard to find time to stop regularly. Yet, if you go too long without eating you may get too hungry and then overeat when you get to that all-you-can-eat buffet or restaurant. Ideally, try to have a couple of shorter stops, rather than one longer stop. This will give you the chance to eat meals at consistent times. This is critical if you are on insulin or diabetes pills. See precautions in sidebar.

All-inclusive vacation and cruises:

The "free" food and drink is a temptation to overeat and over-drink because everyone else is doing it. While fun, these vacations can throw off your weight and blood sugar, and you'll be 5 pounds (2.5 kg) heavier when you return home. Remember the buffet rule: Go only once though the line, and choose smaller amounts all along the way. Vacations with an option for a kitchenette can be a good choice. Once at your destination, stock up on some staples for breakfast and lunch from the nearest grocery store.

Exercise when traveling:

When driving and you stop to get gas, a coffee or meal, take an extra 10 minutes to get out of your vehicle. Briskly walk up and down the parking area or rest stop area. Long periods of sitting cause blood sugar to rise, and blood and fluid to pool in your lower legs and feet. It's amazing how even 10 minutes of exercise can lower your blood sugar, and improve your circulation. These short exercise breaks also burn calories and help give your back a break.
Longer walks are even better.

When flying, get up and walk the aisles or do ankle rotations on long flights for better circulation to your feet.

Holiday exercising: Bring along a bathing suit or pair of shorts and T-shirt and stay at a hotel with a fitness room. Choose types of holidays that encourage walking and outdoor activity. Warm weather vacations provide an opportunity to do lots of walking, swimming and other exercise. Have fun!

Precautions

A low blood sugar when you are driving is extremely dangerous for you and other drivers and pedestrians. See pages 331–338 for more information.

High blood sugar can also be dangerous as it can make you feel tired and less alert.

If you are on diabetes or heart medication talk to your diabetes educator or doctor about adjusting your medications if flying through one or more time zones.

Keep Moving

Open the front door, not the fridge door.

Keep busy so you don't think about food. Instead of eating, get out of your home or office and go for a short walk. Make exercise a part of your daily life. If you have kids, get active outdoors with your kids. Indoors, walk up and down stairs and hallways, dance, or use your stationary bike or treadmill. Start with 5 minutes of continuous exercise and work up to 15–30 minutes, or more, a day. Watch less TV – those cooking shows and ads make you hungry. Screen time takes away from time spent moving around and being active. When you reach a weight "plateau" where you don't seem to lose any more weight, doing more exercise is crucial to boost your metabolism and help you burn extra calories.

Walking gives you energy

Studies show that people are more productive at work and home with exercise breaks. If you get into work early, try a short walk first thing in the morning, or go for a walk at lunch or in the evening. Your daily walk will be a great start to feeling fit and taking off some of those pounds.

Many of us live very busy lives. It's difficult to make health a priority. Yet exercising your body will give you more energy for everything else in your life.

Try not to use exercise as a reason to eat more: Have you ever said to yourself, "I went for a walk so I can eat a second helping." That kind of thinking defeats the purpose of the walk.

What's the secret to getting fit? Take time to do it. Every little bit counts. The goal is to do at least 150 minutes of aerobic exercise each week. That means at least 20 minutes of exercise such as walking each day.

Dorothy's story:

My life had taken a terrible loss and at that time, I turned to food for comfort. I gained over 30 pounds (13.5 kg). I was introduced to Karen's book *Diabetes Meals for Good Health*, and it became like a bible to me. As of today, I have lost this weight, and my blood levels are normal. I am keeping the weight off with the help of healthy eating, drinking my water and exercises. Doing exercises is a good part of keeping your weight in control. I have a dog and we walk all the time when weather permits. When I can't get outside I dance to music, and I have a tape called "Walk Off the Pounds."

Hang Out with Healthy Eaters

Healthy friends can help you be healthy.

Do you have friends and family who encourage you to overeat with them? This can be a big challenge, especially when it's your family. Surprisingly, sometimes when you start making positive lifestyle changes it can rub off on those around you. You may also need to look for some new hobbies, companions, and support groups or support persons that provide positive reinforcement for your good efforts. Even finding one new friend or support outside of your usual circle of friends or families can make a big difference.

Studies have shown that who you eat with makes a difference. If your family tends to eat a lot, that encourages you to also be a big eater. Men eat more when eating with their male friends than they do when eating with a spouse or girlfriend. Women often try and "outdo" each other at parties and get-togethers, which encourages overeating. Some people eat alone, and some look for companionship while eating. When you are trying to cut back on food, changing company may help.

There is strength in unity. *Having others in your house or in your community come on board with diet and exercise changes will give both of you positive benefits.*

Believe in yourself and your ability to make changes.

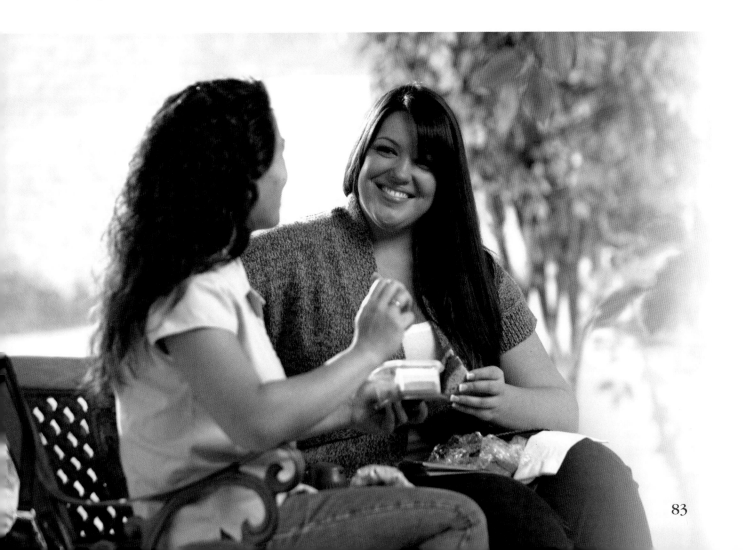

Paul's story:

My insurance has a counselor that calls every three months since the doctor diagnosed me. It's very helpful. The nurse answers any questions I have about my blood sugars and my food and diet, too. It helps because it's positive reinforcement.

Join the Team

Guidance and "cheerleaders" are essential for us all.

You may benefit from sharing your commitment for change with others. Your journey of weight loss and diabetes management is life-long. Developing a support team is important. This gives you motivation to keep on track and rewards you for your hard work and progress.

You choose your team. Visiting or talking on the phone or by email with a dietitian, an insurance nurse, a diabetes educator or a doctor on a regular basis acts as important incentive to keep on track. They can help you monitor your weight, blood pressure or lab test results. A friend, family member, co-worker, a walking buddy or a support group, such as a weight loss support group, can also help. If you are comfortable with using the internet, search out an online weight support or diabetes group. Key search words are "weight loss support."

Make one change at a time. With each change you'll move closer to your goals.

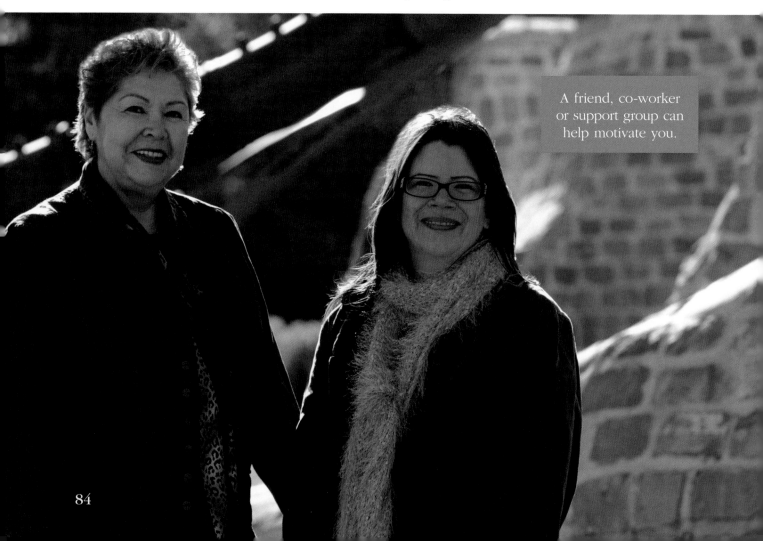

A friend, co-worker or support group can help motivate you.

84

2. Carbohydrates and your blood sugar

Most of the carbohydrates that we eat come from starches, sugars and desserts, fruits, milk and vegetables. This section explains how different carbohydrates affect your blood sugar.

On pages 85–89, you'll learn how eating less table sugar, sweet drinks and rich desserts will help reduce your blood sugar. These foods can raise your blood sugar quickly. If you eat a large portion, your pancreas will not be able to make enough insulin and your blood sugar will stay high for a long time.

Although it's wise to limit sugar and sweet drinks, eating carbohydrates such as starches, vegetables and fruits, and milk is an essential part of a healthy diet. On pages 90–93, you'll learn about carbohydrate foods that have a low glycemic index. These raise blood sugar slowly. In the right portions, these are healthy choices as they don't require your body to make as much insulin.

Limit sugar and sweet drinks

Added table sugar, sweet drinks, desserts and candies quickly turn into blood sugar. Fruit juice does have vitamins but is a liquid form of fruit sugar, and also needs to be limited.

Table sugar
- White or brown sugar, honey, corn syrup or maple syrup, and jam and jelly are all forms of sugar.
- Eating a *small* amount of added sugar at some meals or snacks is acceptable. Only eat 1–2 teaspoons (5–10 mL), or what would fit in the end of your thumb.

Rule of thumb:

At each meal, limit added table sugar, honey or jams to the amount that would fit in the end of your thumb.

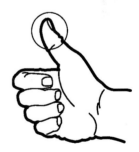

These are all words that mean sugar on food labels:			
• cane sugar • corn sugar • corn syrup	• dextrose • fruit juice concentrate • glucose	• high fructose corn syrup • honey • maltose	• molasses • sucrose • sugar • syrup
Sorbitol, mannitol and xylitol are a type of sweetener used in some diet products. These raise your blood sugar just half as much as regular sugar.			

Limit or avoid these sugar-sweetened foods

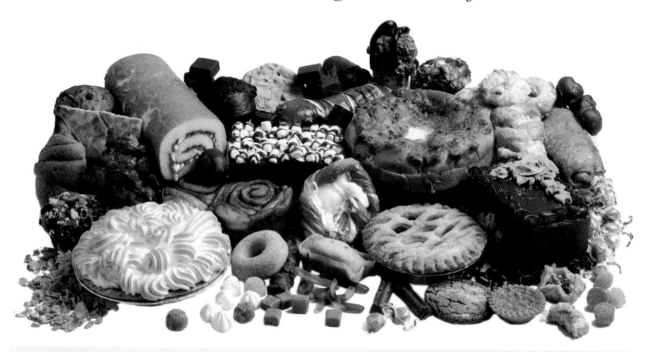

Remember, desserts and muffins are extra high in sugar (and fat) when they are mega-sized.

Choose the light desserts shown in the meal section of this book and in my first book, **Diabetes Meals for Good Health,** and other diabetes cookbooks.
Also see pages 100–108 for ideas on adapting recipes.

Limit or avoid these sugar-sweetened drinks and juices

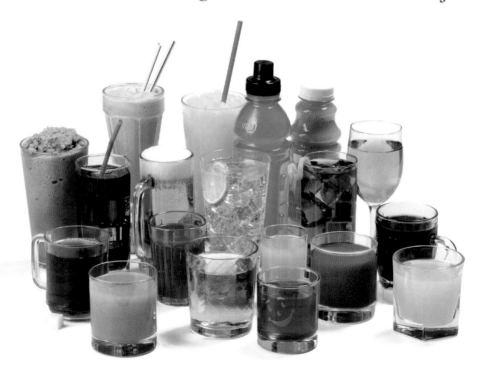

Skip the regular soft drinks

Each North American drinks about 26.5 gallons or 100 liters of soft drinks each year. That's equal to 42,800 calories. It takes about 3,500 extra calories to gain a pound (0.5 kg) of weight. This amount of soda can contribute to gaining more than 10 pounds (4.5 kg) in a year.

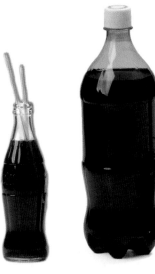

6-ounce
(170 mL) cola

4½ teaspoons
(22 mL)
of sugar

(80 calories)

32-ounce
(1 L) cola

25 teaspoons
(125 mL)
of sugar

(430 calories)

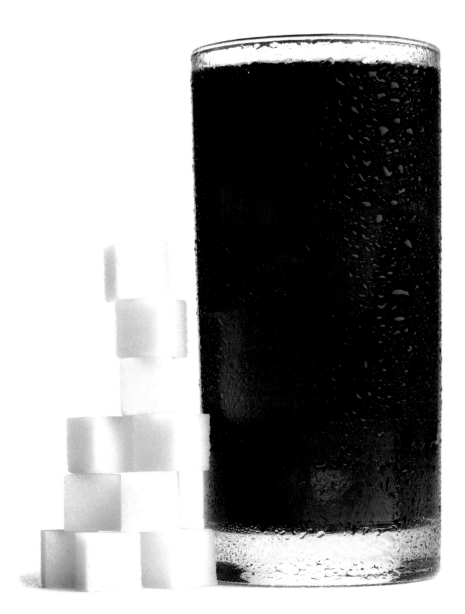

Portions are larger today.

In the 1960s, a 6-ounce (170 mL) cola was the most common portion of soft drink. This used to be an occasional special treat. The 32-ounce (1 L) portion is a common portion today. These are "empty calories" – sugar with no good nutrition.

Every time you drink a 12-ounce (355 mL) can of soda, you get 10 teaspoons (50 mL) of sugar that you don't need.

Unsweetened juices also have a lot of sugar

You may be surprised to learn that a 12-oz (375 mL) glass of unsweetened orange juice has the same sugar as a cola (10 tsp/50 mL of sugar). Apple juice has even a bit more. Juice does have vitamin C and other nutrients from fruit, but you should have only a small glass (4 oz/125 mL of apple, orange or cranberry juice, or 2 oz/60 mL of grape or prune juice). Large bottles of juice with several servings are too much to drink at once and make your blood sugar go up quickly. When thirsty, choose water or diet beverages or sugar-free drink mixes instead.

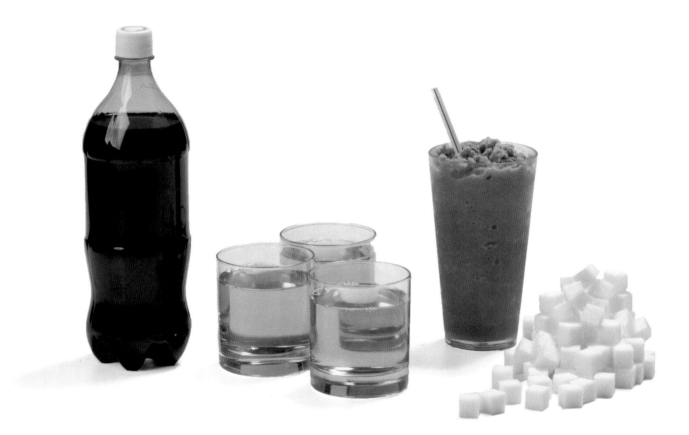

There are 60 teaspoons (300 mL) of sugar (or 1,200 calories) total in the beverages above:

One 32-ounce (1 L) bottle of cola, three 8-ounce (250 mL) glasses of unsweetened apple juice and a 16-ounce (450 mL) iced cappuccino.

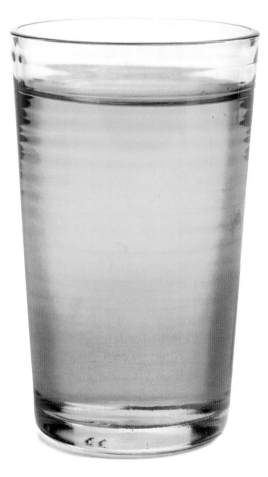

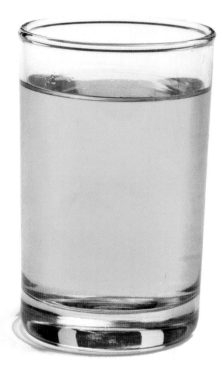

12 oz (375 mL)   4 oz (125 mL)

Every time you drink a 12-oz (375 mL) glass of unsweetened juice, you get 10 or more teaspoons (50 or more mL) of sugar that you don't need. Choose only the small glass on the right and count it as a fruit serving. Better yet, choose a fresh fruit instead and get all the benefit of fiber.

A 12-oz (375 mL) glass of apple juice has the equivalent of three or four apples' worth of sugar. You wouldn't eat this many apples at once, but it's easy to drink that much sugar in one glass of juice.

Don't be fooled into thinking that juices with herbs or other products added are healthier for you. They usually have all the sugar of regular juice.

Ways to slow down carbohydrate absorption

If you have eaten carbohydrate that is quickly absorbed, sugar will go into your blood quickly. Your pancreas will not be able to release enough insulin to bring down sudden increases in blood sugar. If the portion of carbohydrate you have eaten is large, your blood sugar will be high over several hours.

To reduce work for your pancreas and improve your blood sugar, here are things you can do.

Control your portions.
Use the meal plans on pages 149–200 as a guide. The "Eat This – Not That" section on pages 201–216 also has information on portions.

Divide your carbohydrates throughout the day.
Choose three meals a day, and snacks in moderation, if needed.

Eat less quickly-absorbed carbohydrates.
This means eating less table sugar, sweet drinks, juices, desserts and sweets. Also limit any food that you have found causes a spike or a sustained rise in your blood sugar when you test your blood at home.

To determine if a food causes a sustained blood sugar spike, you need to measure your blood sugar both before you eat and two hours after you eat.

At a meal or large snack, include some protein or fat with your carbohydrate.
For instance, if you have crackers with cheese, the protein in the cheese slows down the absorption of the carbohydrate in the crackers. The carbohydrates will be absorbed more slowly than if you ate the crackers on their own.

Choose low glycemic index carbohydrates daily.
Keep reading to learn more information about this.

Eat slowly.
This slows down the absorption of your carbohydrates.

Go for a walk half an hour to an hour after eating.
This uses up blood sugar from the food you just ate.

Certain diabetes medications help.
Insulin and some medicines can help reduce blood sugar rise that happens after you eat. See pages 315–330.

Choose low glycemic index carbohydrates daily

Glycemic index is a rating of how quickly a carbohydrate food raises your blood sugar. We call this GI as an abbreviation. Low GI foods raise your blood sugar slowly so are good choices. **See photo below and on page 93.**

Choose a variety of carbohydrates (starches, fruits and vegetables and milk) and try to include low GI choices daily. Keep portions reasonable – remember a *large amount* of even a low GI carbohydrate can make your blood sugar go too high because of the total amount of carbohydrate. For example, eating a low GI food such as whole grain bread in a *large amount* can cause a similar blood sugar rise as eating a high GI food such as white bread in a *smaller portion* or thinner slices. Portions are critical. Choose the meal and snack portions shown in this book as a guide.

A food that has a low GI ingredient does not mean the food itself will be low GI. For example, a granola bar made with oats and barley could have a lot of sugar added, which raises its glycemic index.

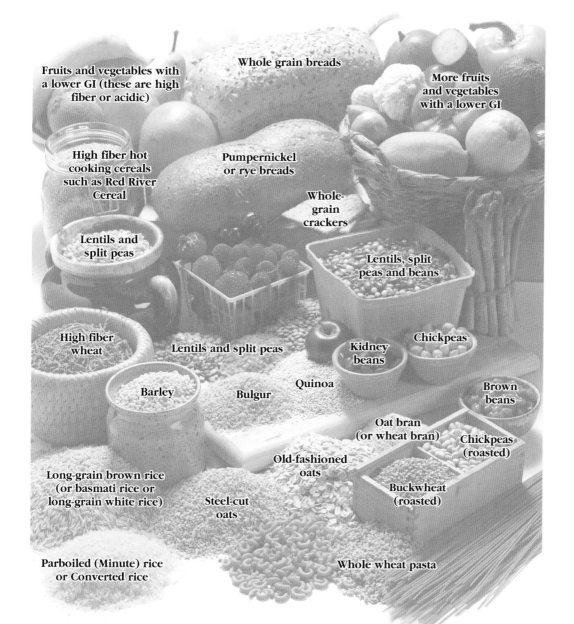

Fruits and vegetables with a lower GI (these are high fiber or acidic)

Whole grain breads

More fruits and vegetables with a lower GI

High fiber hot cooking cereals such as Red River Cereal

Pumpernickel or rye breads

Whole-grain crackers

Lentils and split peas

Lentils, split peas and beans

High fiber wheat

Lentils and split peas

Kidney beans

Chickpeas

Barley

Bulgur

Quinoa

Brown beans

Oat bran (or wheat bran)

Chickpeas (roasted)

Old-fashioned oats

Long-grain brown rice (or basmati rice or long-grain white rice)

Steel-cut oats

Buckwheat (roasted)

Parboiled (Minute) rice or Converted rice

Whole wheat pasta

What makes a carbohydrate low GI?

Lots of fiber! There are two main types of fiber.

- **Insoluble fiber** is in whole wheat, grains, fruits and vegetables. These foods have acids, such as phytic acid, that help slow down the absorption of carbohydrates. Phytic acid is also found in some foods high in soluble fiber such as beans and lentils.
- **Soluble fiber** is in oatmeal, barley and brown beans, and some fruits and vegetables. These fibers grab on to carbohydrates, slowing down their absorption. They also remove some cholesterol from the body.
- Look for food products with more fiber listed on the label.
- Have barley instead of potato or rice for a change.
- Choose thin slices of rye, whole wheat or whole grain bread (about 30 grams or 70 calories per slice).
- Try some of the low GI recipes such as Oatmeal (Breakfast 1), Taco Soup (Lunch 2) and salad with dandelion root (Dinner 3). In my book *Diabetes Meals for Good Health* try recipes such as Mexican Rice and Beans and Walnut Barley Medley.

Tartness or acidity: In addition to the acid in high fiber foods, other acids that slow down the absorption of carbohydrates include lemon or vinegar, or tannins such as in tea.

- Enjoy a cup of tea with your meal.
- Add lemon or vinegar on your vegetables (instead of added fat). Lemon is also nice on fish and in tea.
- Try vinegar and dill added to canned beets or sliced cucumbers for a low salt pickle.

Less processing: Blood sugar spikes less when the carbohydrate is raw (versus cooked), lightly cooked (as compared to overcooked), whole (rather than ground) and firm (firm fruit versus over-ripe fruit).

- Eat whole grain breads more often than white bread.
- Choose fresh potatoes instead of instant mashed potatoes.
- Make porridge out of slow-cooking oats instead of instant oatmeal.
- Enjoy mostly raw fruits and vegetables instead of juices or over-cooked fruit.
- Make homemade meals made from whole, fresh ingredients.

Fructose (fruit sugar) and lactose (milk sugar) convert more slowly to blood sugar than some other sugars or even some starches. Enjoy fresh fruit and milk or milk products as snacks or with meals.

Low GI carbohydrates – choose these!

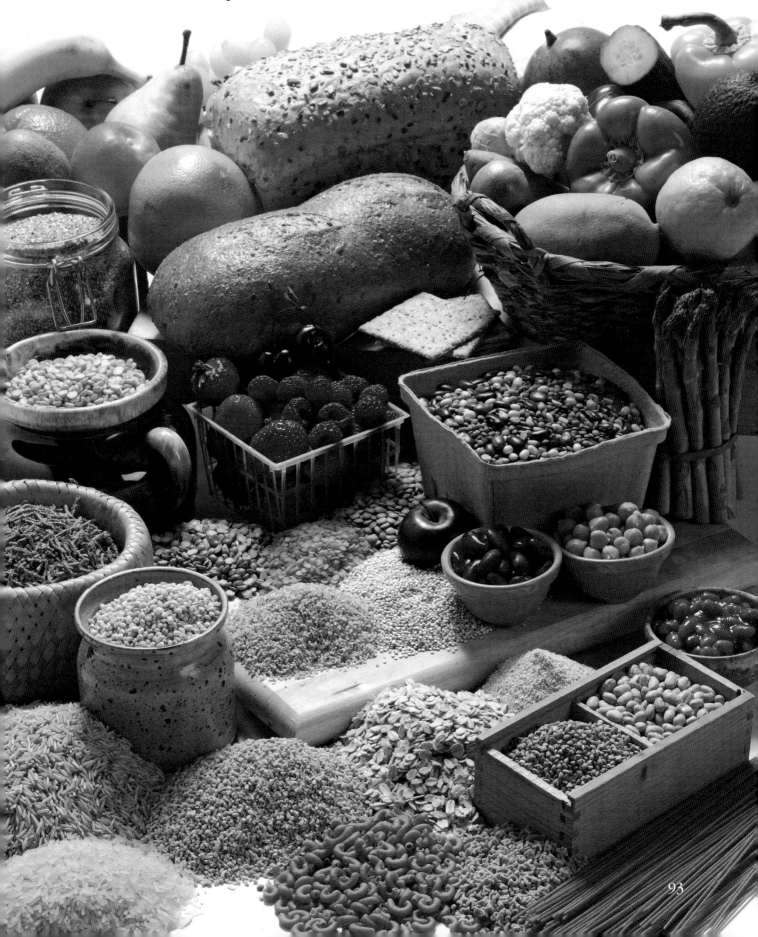

3. Food labels

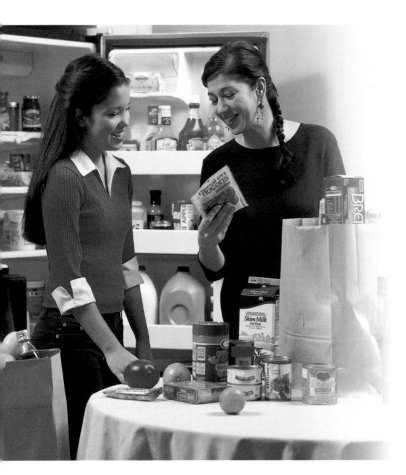

Healthy eating begins at the grocery store. The foods you buy are what you and your family will eat at home. Bring a list and stick to it. Healthier foods tend to be on the top and bottom of the shelves and around the outside walls of the supermarket. There is a large variety of food available – and this creates a lot of confusion as to what to buy. You don't need to try every new food. Read food labels and choose familiar foods that you know are good choices.

If you are trying to lose weight, it is important to look at the total calories and serving size of each product. Calories come from carbohydrates, protein and fat. Food products are a poor choice if they have too much added sugar, fat (especially saturated or trans fat) or salt. Things that are higher in vitamins and minerals are more nutritious choices.

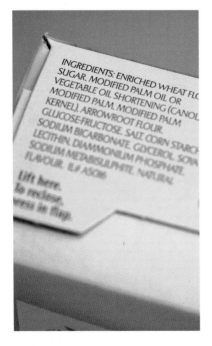

Ingredient List

Manufacturers list ingredients from the biggest to the smallest, based on how much the ingredient weighs. Heaviest food ingredients start the list and the lightest ingredients are last. If you see sugar, fat or salt listed first, this is usually a bad choice.

The ingredient list can be hard to understand. Sometimes the list includes similar ingredients with each one mentioned separately. For example, a label for canned fruit might list "peaches, water, sugar, syrup and cane sugar." At first glance it looks like sugar is the third ingredient. However, sugar, syrup and cane sugar are all different types of sugar. In fact, if you add up these three types of sugar, the total sugar might actually be the first or second ingredient. This is why it is a good idea to also look at the Nutrition Facts panel which will give you more information. Compare the amount of sugar per serving between different brands.

Nutrition Facts

Serving size

Look at the amount in a serving size. The company measures calories and other nutrition information based on this. The serving size listed isn't necessarily the same amount as you might eat...it's often smaller! For example, a chocolate bar may list the nutrition facts for only three squares, but most people eat the whole chocolate bar, so you get a lot more calories, fat and sugar than shown on the label. A cereal box might list 1 cup (250 mL), but you might have 2 cups (500 mL) for breakfast. If you eat double the serving size, then you will eat double the calories and nutrients.

The nutrients listed and their amounts

The amount of a nutrient in a processed food is listed as a percentage that an average person might need in a day. This amount is listed on food labels as "% Daily Value" which means percentage of your daily intake. For example, if a food serving has 30% vitamin C, that means eating that serving will give you 30% (about one third) of the vitamin C you need for the whole day. You could get the rest of your vitamin C (to make up about 100 percent) from fresh fruits and vegetables eaten during the day. The Daily Value percentage tells you if there is a little or a lot of a nutrient in one serving.

GET ENOUGH OF THESE:
- Fiber
- Vitamins and minerals
- Monounsaturated fat and omega-3 fat (not always listed)

GET LESS OF THESE:
- Calories (if you are trying to lose weight)
- Fat
- Saturated fat
- Trans fat
- Cholesterol
- Sodium
- Sugars (especially if they are added sugars)

If you are trying to lose weight, look for food with fewer calories and less fat. Your blood sugar will go up if the product is too high in carbohydrates (including starch, natural sugar in milk, vegetables and fruits, and added sugar such as table sugar or honey). Fiber is also a carbohydrate but doesn't increase your blood sugar.

As a general rule:
- 5% Daily Value or less is A LITTLE
- 15% Daily Value or more is A LOT (in the U.S., a 20% Daily Value is considered to be a LOT.)

Nutrition Facts Per 1 bar (14 g)		
Amount		% Daily Value
Calories 50		
Fat 0 g		0 %
Saturated 0 g + Trans 0 g		0 %
Cholesterol 0 mg		0 %
Sodium 5 mg		1 %
Carbohydrate 12 g		4 %
Fiber 1 g		3 %
Sugars 11 g		
Protein 0.2 g		
Vitamin A		0 %
Vitamin C		2 %
Calcium		0 %
Iron		0 %

Nutrition Health Claims (a few examples):

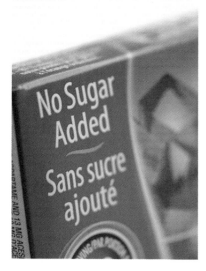

What it says on the label	What it means
Low in sugar	Has no more than 2 grams of sugar per serving (equal to just ½ teaspoon/2 mL of sugar), which is a good choice. **Caution**: If you eat more than one serving, the amount of sugar increases.
No sugar added or unsweetened	This doesn't have table sugar added to it. **Caution**: This food may have naturally sweet products added such as concentrated grape juice.
Sugar-free	This is very low in added table sugar (0.5 grams or less). **Caution**: It may contain sugar alcohols like sorbitol, fat, protein or salt.
Calorie-reduced	The food will have at least 50 percent less than the original product made by the same company. **Caution**: It may still have a lot of calories if the original product had a lot of fat or sugar.
Low calorie	It has 15 calories or less per serving. This is very low in calories. It will have little effect on your weight or blood sugar. **Caution**: It may be high in sodium (salt).
Low in fat	Less than 3 grams of fat. One serving would be a good choice. **Caution**: If you eat several servings, the fat adds up.
Fat-free	This is very low in fat with no more than 0.1 gram of fat per serving. **Caution**: It may be high in sugar or sodium.
Low in cholesterol	This product has little cholesterol. **Caution**: It may still have a lot of calories, and so can cause weight gain, which increases cholesterol.

Bottom line:

Read the Nutrition Facts table and compare products! The Nutrition Health Claim doesn't always tell you the whole story.

Tips for choosing healthy foods

Cereals

Fiber: A high fiber cereal will have at least 3 grams of fiber per serving.

Added sugar: Mostly choose cereals with 4 grams of sugar or less per serving. This means each serving contains no more than a teaspoon (5 mL) of added sugar.

Added fat: Choose cereals with 2 grams of fat or less per serving.

Compare labels: Read different cereal labels. If you're trying to lose weight, compare equal serving sizes. Try to choose the one with the lowest calories.

Bread and bagels

Bread: Choose bread that has about 70 calories per slice. This would equal 140 calories for 2 slices.

Bagels: Bagels are made from a dense dough so are higher in carbohydrates and calories than bread.

- A small bagel (about 3 inches/7.5 cm across) will have about 160 calories. That's equal to about 2 slices of bread.

- A large bagel (about 5 inches/12.5 cm across) will have about 320 calories and is equal to 4 slices of bread.

Bread and bagels:

- "Whole grain" means the entire grain kernel (the outside fiber and the inside wheat germ), with all its health benefits, is in the bread. This is a good choice.

- Whole wheat (60% or 100%), rye, or multigrain breads are usually good choices for fiber, although they may not include the wheat germ. If you buy a bag of wheat germ you can add it to your cereal, rice, yogurt or other foods.

- If you choose white bread or a bagel at a meal, complement the meal with high-fiber foods. For example, eat raw vegetables with your sandwich.

- Enriched means the manufacturer adds extra vitamins and minerals to the food.

Foods with lots of fiber are usually good choices.

Healthy cereal:

Nutrition Facts		
Per 1 cup (30 g)		
Amount	Cereal Only	Plus 125 mL Skim Milk
Calories	120	160
		% Daily Value
Fat 2 g	3 %	3 %
Saturated 0.2 g + Trans 0 g	2 %	2 %
Cholesterol 0 mg	0 %	0 %
Sodium 270 mg	11 %	13 %
Carbohydrate 22 g	7 %	9 %
Fiber 3 g	12 %	12 %
Sugars 1 g		
Protein 4 g		

Fiber on labels

Fiber goes through you without being absorbed. Therefore the calories and carbohydrates in fiber do not affect your blood sugar or weight. Yet manufacturers are required to list the carbohydrates and calories of fiber on the label. High fiber foods will actually have less carbohydrate and calories than what is shown.

Look at the cereal label above. The 3 grams of fiber means that there are actually only 19 grams of available carbohydrate (22 minus 3) that affect your blood sugar.

Canned fruit

Buy water-packed or juice-packed cans of fruit. If you buy fruit in syrup, rinse off the syrup to reduce your sugar intake.

Juices

A half cup (125 mL) of juice counts as a fruit serving (¼ cup/60 mL for grape or prune juice). Limit juice and choose fresh fruit most of the time. Light juices made with a low-calorie sweetener are a reduced sugar choice.

Milk

Choose skim or 1% milk. These are low in fat and a natural source of sugar (lactose). Avoid or limit milk with table sugar added such as chocolate and flavored (sweetened) milks. Look at the labels to compare the sugar content of sweetened milk to regular milk. If the label shows an *extra* 4 grams of sugar (carbohydrate) than regular milk, this means 1 teaspoon (5 mL) of sugar has been added to each cupful (250 mL). If the label shows 16 grams of *extra* sugar, this would mean 4 teaspoons (20 mL) has been added. Milk with vitamin D added to it is an excellent choice.

Cheese

Try to buy low-fat brick or sliced cheese most often. This is labeled as 20% or less MF (milk fat).

Sour cream

A great option is the fat-free kind (0% MF). The sour cream with 5% milk fat is the next best choice.

Soups, canned or packaged

The good news is that lower-salt soups are becoming more common. However, these still often have a quarter of the sodium that you need for the day (your "Daily Value"). The original product might have a third or more. Choosing the reduced salt variety is a better choice than the original, and is a good place to start. Keep in mind that some soups may also have a lot of added fat – check the label.

Chocolate Milk

1 cup (250 mL) of chocolate milk has 3 teaspoons (15 mL) of extra sugar added. If you want to choose chocolate milk, you can reduce the sugar by mixing it half and half with white skim milk.

Reduced-salt canned tomato soup:

Nutrition Facts
Per ½ cup (125 mL)

Amount	% Daily Value
Calories 80	
Fat 0 g	0 %
Saturated 0.2 g + Trans 0 g	0 %
Cholesterol 0 mg	0 %
Sodium 360 mg	15 %
Carbohydrate 19 g	6 %
Fiber 2 g	8 %
Sugars 11 g	
Protein 2 g	
Vitamin A	4 %
Vitamin C	15 %
Calcium	2 %
Iron	4 %

Pizzas, lasagnas and frozen entrées

These are often high in calories, fat and sodium. Some meals also have extra sugar added. Compare one brand to others before choosing the healthiest one. Consider eating ready-to-eat-meals less often.

Margarine, butter and oils

All three of these fats have similar calories, about 45 calories per teaspoon (5 mL). Fat is very concentrated in calories. Even a small amount gives you extra unwanted calories. If you are trying to lose weight, you need to cut back on all fat. It's also wise to look for products that are low in saturated and trans fats.

Light fats

Light butter and margarine have fewer calories, as the manufacturers make them with part water. They may be a bit watery if you put them on hot toast or popcorn, but taste good on cold sandwiches. Light oil may just be a "light color" rather than lower in calories. Check the food label to compare it to other oils.

Butter versus margarine

Butter and margarine are both mostly fat. If you eat too much of either, your total fat intake goes up. This can increase your weight and worsen your blood cholesterol and blood sugar. Go lightly with fats.

Olive oil and vegetable oils

These have healthy fat. Even so, use them sparingly because of their high calories.

Mayonnaise and salad dressings

Fat-free is the lowest fat choice. Choices with fewer than 30 calories per tablespoon (15 mL) are lighter choices than the regular varieties.

**Small changes in your food choices
can make a big difference over time.**

Make a fast homemade meal – where you control more of the ingredients.

Rule of thumb:

Measure the fat that you add to your meal. Eat no more than the amount that will fit in the end of your thumb (about 1–2 teaspoons 5–10 mL).

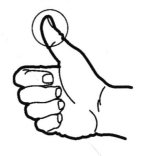

Healthy Fats

Olive oil especially, and canola oil, have a healthy type of fat called monounsaturated fat. Vegetable oils such as canola and soy bean oil include a small amount of healthy omega-3 fats.

4. Light desserts and sweeteners

Question and Answer about desserts with Karen Graham:

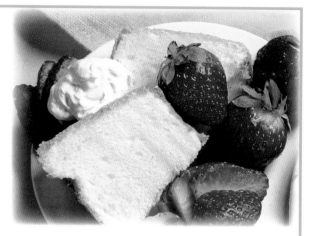

Amir: I found out I had diabetes last year. Since then I have lost 8 lbs (4 kg) and my blood sugar has improved. My problem is my wife. She has gone crazy about keeping me healthy and won't let me eat any sugar – no cake, no cookies, no pies, no jam, nothing. She's taken the fun out of eating. And, let's face it, I love eating, it's a big part of my life.

I know my wife is doing what she thinks is best, but this diabetes thing is frustrating both of us. Surely I can eat some sugar and desserts?

Karen's Answer: Congratulations on your weight loss and improved blood sugar! Cutting out obvious forms of sugar has certainly helped you improve your diabetes. Having diabetes doesn't mean you should never again eat dessert! It does mean switching to smaller portions and lighter desserts that are lower in sugar and fat.

Your wife's concerns about your health sound genuine. After all, she cares about you! It does also sound like she has taken control of your diet. She can lighten up a little, and here's why.

First, it's not just extra sugar and desserts that give you high blood sugar. You gain weight from eating and drinking too much food (meat, fat, starch and sugar) and then your blood sugar goes up. When you lose weight, your blood sugar goes down. And when you exercise, you use up the stored sugar in your body and your blood sugar goes down more.

So, I suggest you focus on eating the right portions of food. In my meal plans in this book and in my first book, *Diabetes Meals for Good Health*, the meals are in the right portions for healthy balanced daily eating. I include small portions of regular or light jam at breakfast, and regular sugar in some light desserts. Snacks and desserts include fruits, puddings and other lighter desserts, plain cookies, smaller portions of ice cream or sherbet, un-iced cake, and for snacks, occasional chocolates, hard candies and even marshmallows. Tips for reading dessert food labels are on pages 94–99. You or your wife may want to try some of my dessert recipes, or adapt your own favorite recipes (see pages 104–105).

When you eat smaller portions, then a reasonable amount of sugar can fit into your diet. Remember, a walk helps bring down blood sugar, especially an hour or so after a meal. A walk is a great thing you and your wife can do together. Good luck!

Using table sugar

Sugar is just one source of carbohydrate in our diet. You don't have to avoid it at the table and in baking but it should be limited. For example, if you want to use sugar in recipes, cut back on the amount you use. If you want to have some added sugar at a meal (such as honey, brown sugar or jam), use the tip of your thumb as a guide (1–2 teaspoons/5–10 mL). For some people, having a small amount of honey or jam can help satisfy a craving for sugar. This is certainly better than depriving yourself, and then binging. In terms of blood sugar management, your body can handle small amounts of extra sugar now and again. It's binging and overeating that is a problem.

Some people with diabetes choose to avoid as much added sugar as possible. Instead they use low-calorie sweeteners at the table and in baking. This is a personal preference, and either way works in a healthy eating pattern.

Cookies

All cookies have sugar and fat! Look for ones that aren't too thick or large. It's a better choice if each cookie has 40 calories or less. This is the same as three cookies having 120 calories. Limit yourself to 2 or 3 cookies.

Granola bars may seem healthier than cookies, but often they have lots of sugar and fat – compare labels.

Cookies with lower sugar and fat:

Nutrition Facts	
Per 3 cookies (22 g)	
Amount	% Daily Value
Calories 98	
Fat 3 g	5 %
Saturated 1 g + Trans 0 g	5 %
Cholesterol 0 mg	0 %
Sodium 94 mg	4 %
Carbohydrate 17 g	5 %
Fiber 1 g	4 %
Sugars 5 g	
Protein 2 g	

Yogurt

Choose yogurt with 100–120 calories per ¾ cup (175 g). These will be low in fat, and the sugar is replaced with a low-calorie sweetener.

Natural versus table sugar

Unfortunately, the Nutrition Facts table doesn't list natural sugar separately from added table sugar. (Natural sugar comes from milk, fruits and vegetables.) One way to know if there is any added table sugar in a product is to look at the ingredient list.

Puddings

Here's how you can tell if a boxed instant pudding is low in sugar. Pick up the box. If the weight of the box feels very light – it's the low-sugar kind. The box of regular pudding made with sugar is a lot heavier. When you look at the label, you will see the low-sugar kind has zero grams and the regular kind has 15–20 grams of sugar.

When buying ready-to-eat puddings, look for "no sugar added" on the label.

Ice cream:

Nutrition Facts	
Per ½ cup (125 mL)	
Amount	% Daily Value
Calories 120	
Fat 5 g	8 %
Saturated 3.5 g + Trans 0.2 g	19 %
Cholesterol 15 mg	2 %
Sodium 80 mg	3 %
Carbohydrate 17g Fiber 0 g Sugars 15 g	6 % 4 %
Protein 1 g	
Vitamin A	6 %
Vitamin C	0 %
Calcium	4 %
Iron	0 %

Most ice cream provides less than 5 percent of your daily calcium needs, so is not a replacement for milk.

Some of these "sugar-free" products actually have more fat and more calories than regular candies or chocolates.

Ice cream, frozen yogurt or sherbets

Choose brands that have 120 calories or less per ½ cup (125 mL). You will be shocked to know that some reduced-fat frozen desserts have more sugar, and some low-sugar ice creams have more fat than regular ice cream. The bottom-line is that these are all desserts. Only choose them occasionally and in a half-cup (125 mL) serving.

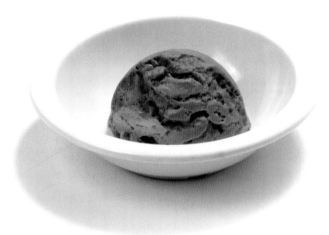

Sugar-free candy or sugar-free chocolates

These usually have little table sugar added, but may have other types of sugar added. For example, sorbitol, mannitol or isomalt. These sugars are called "sugar alcohols" but are not actually alcohol. Sugar alcohols are only half absorbed by your body, so only half the sugar and calories affect your blood sugar and weight. However, since sugar alcohols don't taste as sweet as table sugar, the manufacturer may add more or may add more fat to improve the flavor. It's important to check the food labels. Compare these sugar-free sweets to the regular products. Just because the label says "sugar-free" does not mean it is calorie-free and fat-free. Limit yourself to one or two pieces of candy or chocolate as an occasional treat.

Note: Having a couple of these sugar-free candies is fine. If you eat a lot of sorbitol candies, you might get diarrhea and bloating. This can happen if you eat 10 grams or more of sugar alcohols in a day. This is because the body isn't good at absorbing sugar alcohols. Some of it goes right through you.

Light syrups

These usually have less sugar and total carbohydrates than the regular syrup, so are a good choice. Light syrups are made with more water, and then are thickened with starch. They may also contain a sugar alcohol or a low-calorie sweetener.

Sugar-free jam

Some "sugar-free" jam can have as much sugar as regular jam. Concentrated grape juice sometimes sweetens sugar-free jam as a substitute for table sugar. When you concentrate grape juice, it's almost as sweet as regular sugar.

Other sugar-free jams contain extra fruit and less added sugar than a regular jam. You can also make homemade jams using reduced sugar pectin or no sugar recipes. These will have less sugar, and fewer calories per teaspoon, often as low as 5–10 calories per teaspoon (5 mL). However, as these jams don't taste as sweet as a regular jam, some people put more on their toast! Whether you eat one tablespoon (15 mL) of this diet jam or one teaspoon (5 mL) of regular jam, the calories will be about the same.

If you choose a light jam or syrup, and you limit your portion to the same amount as above, you will reduce your carbohydrates and calories.

Sugar-free gelatin, diet soft drinks or diet gum

Foods with a very low calorie level of 20 calories or less per serving, will not affect your weight or blood sugar. Choose these as a low-calorie snack or addition to a meal (also see page 197). Examples are diet gelatin, diet (or "zero") soft drinks or diet gum. Water is always a good option, as it has no calories!

As with puddings, a box of sugar-free gelatin weighs very little compared to the gelatin that is made with sugar.

Example of a good choice of no sugar added light syrup:

Nutrition Facts Per 3 tbsp (45 mL)	
Amount	% Daily Value
Calories 30	
Fat 0 g	0 %
Cholesterol 0 mg	0 %
Sodium 75 mg	2 %
Carbohydrate 7 g Sugars 6 g	2 %
Protein 0 g	

Rule of thumb:

At a meal, limit regular jam, syrup (or honey) to what fits into the tip of your thumb; this will generally equal 1–2 teaspoons (5–10 mL), or if you have a larger hand, 1 tablespoon (15 mL).

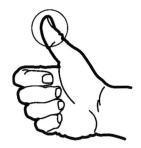

Making your dessert recipes lower in fat and sugar

Note: *Some cookbooks feature "light" recipes which have already had the fat, sugar or salt cut back. These may not require any more changes.*

- **Adapt your family or own recipes**
  The substitutions listed in the chart on page 105 will help you change your own recipes so they are lower in fat, sugar or salt.

- **Make one change at a time**
  Make recipe changes gradually – one ingredient at a time. If you change several ingredients at once, your recipe may not work out.

- **Small changes count**
  For proper rising and browning of cakes and muffins, you often need fat, sugar and/or salt. Some recipes depend on a certain ingredient such as butter, whipping cream, honey or molasses for good flavor. The goal isn't to cut out all fat and sugar and end up with a product you don't like! Rather, make small changes in your recipes to make them healthier. Over time, you will feel satisfied with desserts that are not as sweet or rich. Also, reducing the portion can make a variety of desserts fit in your plan.

- **Boost flavor with spices and flavorings**
  Once you've cut back on fat, sugar and/or salt, it's time to boost the flavor in other ways. Now try adding:

  - spices, such as nutmeg, allspice, cinnamon, cloves, cardamom or ginger

  - herbs like lemon balm or mint

  - lemon or lime juice

  - zest of lemon, lime or orange

  - flavoring extracts such as vanilla, coconut or peppermint

  - a sprinkle of drink mix powder (such as Kool-Aid)

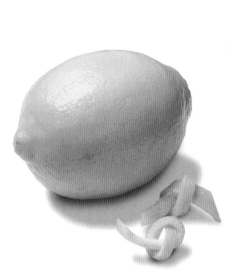

Recipe substitutions

If a recipe calls for:	Use this substitute or technique instead:
Sugar, honey, syrup or molasses	Sugar provides sweetness but is also important in tenderness, moistness and browning. If you remove all sugar the product is often flat and has a poor texture. To reduce the sugar and still get a tasty product: Cut the sugar or sweetener in half. If you find the recipe is not sweet enough this way, replace all, or part of the sugar that you removed with some low-calorie sweetener. Some low-calorie sweeteners lose their sweetness if baked at high temperature (for example, aspartame). Other sweeteners such as sucralose (Splenda) work well in baking.
Gelatin or pudding mixes made with sugar	Sugar-free gelatin or sugar-free pudding mixes
Whole or 2% milk (fresh or canned evaporated)	1% or skim milk Try one of these two ways to get a thickened milkshake or smoothie without the high fat milk or ice cream: 1) put skim milk or canned evaporated skim milk in a bowl and freeze it for half an hour or until crystals form on the top. Then beat with electric beaters or in a blender until thickened. 2) add ice cubes to your milk and blend. You can add yogurt or fruit to your drink for flavor and nutrition.
Half and half cream	Undiluted canned evaporated milk, or 1% or 2% milk
Fat – oil, margarine, butter, lard or shortening	Most cake-type recipes require some fat for a light texture, moistness and flavor. Start with decreasing the fat by half. Add an equal amount of applesauce, milk or yogurt in cakes and muffins, or pureed prunes in brownies. This will increase the carbohydrates slightly but decrease the fat and calories. NOTE: By reducing just one tablespoon of fat in your recipe, you cut out 100 calories. Starch-thickened products such as soup, sauces and desserts do not usually need any fat added.
Regular mayonnaise or regular sour cream (14%)	Fat-free or light mayonnaise, fat-free (0%) sour cream or light sour cream (7%), or plain low-fat yogurt (no gelatin-added is less watery), or 1% or 2% cottage cheese that you've blended until smooth.
Regular fat cheese (over 28% MF)	Low-fat (20% or less MF) cheese
Regular cream cheese	Light cream cheese (14% MF or less)
Salt, baking powder or baking soda	In your recipes, cut back on salt, baking powder and/or baking soda. All three of these products have a lot of sodium. For cakes, muffins or cookies to rise properly, you usually only need per cup (250 mL) of flour: ⅛ teaspoon (0.5 mL) of salt and 1 teaspoon (5 mL) of baking powder. For soda breads or biscuits, use only ¼–½ tsp (1–2 mL) of baking soda per cup (250 mL) of flour. Replace seasoning salt (such as garlic salt) with garlic powder, fresh garlic or herbs.
All purpose (white) flour	Replace half of the white flour with whole wheat flour, or add 2 tablespoons (30 mL) wheat bran to ⅞ cup (220 mL) white flour to make a cup (250 mL). Also, use whole wheat pasta and brown rice over white pasta and white rice.

Low-calorie sweeteners

Stevia

This is a low-calorie sweetener that comes from a plant source. In 2008, stevia extract was given partial approval as a food additive and table top sweetener in the USA. In late 2012, stevia was also approved in Canada. With these approvals in place you will start seeing stevia in more diet products, including soft drinks.

Less common sweeteners:

- *acesulfame-K (acesulfame potassium)*
- *saccharin*
- *cyclamates (not approved in the United States, approved in Canada but not for pregnancy)*
- *neotame (approved in the United States but not Canada)*

These sweeteners are sold as a variety of brand names. I suggest you do not have more than two packages a day, or choose alternatives. In some cases they are added to processed foods.

What are low-calorie sweeteners?

Both sucralose (Splenda) and aspartame (Equal, NutraSweet and Sweet 'N Low) are man-made chemicals that taste extremely sweet. You need only very small amounts to sweeten foods, making them low in calories. Grocery stores first sold aspartame in the 1980s. Sucralose came next. The government approved its sale in Canada in 1991 and the USA in 1998. These low-calorie sweeteners have been an amazing food product breakthrough because of their low calories and sweet taste. They allow us to drink zero-calorie drinks and desserts that are much lower in sugar and calories.

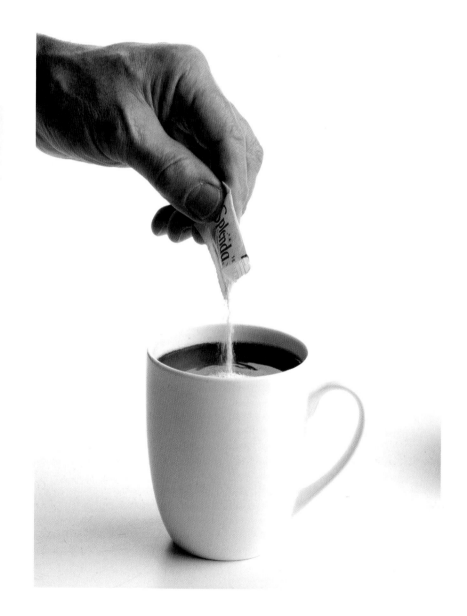

Sugar or low-calorie sweetener – which would be the best choice for a person with diabetes?

Drinking too many sweet drinks and overeating on sweet foods will raise your blood sugar. If you are trying to choose between a can of regular cola that has 10 teaspoons (50 mL) of sugar versus a diet coke with zero sugar, without question, I would recommend the diet cola. The diet cola won't raise your blood sugar. When your blood sugar is high, cutting out excess sugar helps bring it down as soon as possible.

If you drink 2 liters of cola daily, you would consume 50 teaspoons (250 mL) of sugar. The switch to 2 liters of diet cola will mean virtually no sugar. This will have a huge benefit on reducing your blood sugar.

The bigger question is *how much* diet products do we really *need* in the long-term? Do we need to be drinking diet soft drinks daily? Should we be learning to drink more water? While diet soft drinks have no sugar, they do have other ingredients that aren't good for us. In many cases, these include caffeine and phosphates (which draws important calcium out of our bones), and acids that are bad for our teeth.

Learning to eat our cereal without added sugar rather than adding low-calorie sweetener may make a big difference. Choosing a smaller amount of a sugar-sweetened product instead of a larger amount of diet product can also be worthwhile. For example, try eating ½ cup (125 mL) of regular yogurt rather than ¾ cup (175 mL) of yogurt made with aspartame or sucralose.

As you get used to a healthy diet, you may not feel such a need for low-calorie sweetened products. Replace some of your diet beverages with water, so that you can cut back on the total amount of low-calorie sweeteners you eat over the long-term.

In some of my dessert recipes, I use low-calorie sweeteners. I also give an option to use sugar if you want, but to use less. I believe in moderation and balance in everything in life. This same common sense applies to low-calorie sweeteners.

Do you actually lose weight using low-calorie sweeteners?

I have seen people manage their diabetes and lose weight by making changes that include low-calorie sweetened products. These products provide variety to their diet and help them maintain their lower calorie pattern. However, it is interesting that some studies show that people who consume a lot of diet products don't lose more weight. These people may compensate by eating more of something else. One scenario might be: "I'm having a diet pop, so I can splurge and have the large fries." Other studies suggest that eating diet products regularly may make you crave more sweets. This is another possible disadvantage of low-calorie sweetened products.

Water is the best beverage to quench thirst.

Are low-calorie sweeteners safe?

The US Food and Drug Administration and Health Canada think aspartame and sucralose are safe. The American Diabetes Association and the Canadian Diabetes Association also say these are safe foods.

This does sound reassuring. However, as a dietitian who has studied food additives, I think we may not yet have all the answers. The safety of a large number of people eating low-calorie sweeteners in larger amounts over many years is still unknown. When new evidence is gathered, recommendations change as a result.

The case of trans fat is a good example. Trans fat is a man-made product that was considered a "miracle" food by the food industry. Trans fats were first used commercially in the 1920s in England and more widely in North America after World War II. They quickly became part of nearly all processed foods. They were cheap, tasted good and could be fried and added to baked goods. Best of all, unlike vegetable oils and other natural fats, products made with trans fats could sit on the shelf for a long time and not go rancid.

We still may not know the long-term effects of low-calorie sweeteners.

It was not until the late 1980s, nearly thirty years after the common usage of trans fat in our foods that red flags went up. Those studies linked excess consumption of trans fats to heart disease. It took another ten years until comprehensive reviews of studies confirmed these bad effects. Then another ten years passed before countries began banning or putting restrictions on the use of trans fat by manufacturers. While trans fats are listed on foods, the American and Canadian governments haven't yet banned them. This may not be what happens with artificial sweeteners. However history has taught us that some caution and moderation is always valuable.

5. Reducing sodium

A small amount of sodium daily is essential to life

Salt, made up of sodium and chloride, is a mineral. Our body cells and tissues need salt. We use it for muscle and heart contractions, proper conduction of nerves and the transport of nutrients into body cells. Healthy kidneys efficiently get rid of excess sodium from the body. Athletes and manual laborers, especially those who work in hot and humid climates, need more sodium to replace what is lost in sweat. Table salt also has iodine added (it is not added to sea salt or kosher salt). Iodine is essential for brain development and helps keep your thyroid healthy. Your thyroid has a role in a healthy body weight.

Too much sodium is not healthy

As with all good things in life, you can have too much of a good thing. This is certainly the case with salt. Most of us get too much sodium in our diet, mostly from processed and restaurant foods. The total upper limit of sodium recommended for the average person is 2,300 mg. This is just less than 1 level teaspoon (5 mL) of salt a day. A teaspoon of salt may seem like a lot. However, some cans of soup have this much added to one can! Salt adds up quickly.

How sodium affects a person with diabetes

Eating lots of sodium and salty foods doesn't cause your blood sugar to go up, but it may increase your blood pressure. Eating lots of salt also contributes to osteoporosis, stomach cancer and kidney stones. And did you know? – a high salt intake might make it more likely for you to get dementia. Evidence shows that people with diabetes may not get rid of extra sodium as efficiently as someone without diabetes. Your insulin level may be part of this problem. Also, it relates to how your kidneys respond to hormones responsible for sodium excretion. Then, your body holds more sodium – and sodium holds water. Extra water in your body adds extra pressure inside your blood vessels. This damages your blood vessel walls, and puts you at risk for a heart attack or stroke. High blood pressure also damages your kidneys and eyes.

Sodium hides inside foods that are also high in fat (French fries and hamburgers, potato chips, bologna, etc.), so sometimes it's hard to tell whether sodium or fat is the greater villain. When you cut back on salty foods, you eat less fat too. Overall you'll feel healthier.

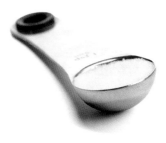

1 level teaspoon (5 mL) of salt is equal to about 2,300 mg of sodium. This is approximately your daily need for sodium (your Daily Value).

Other very important steps to improve blood pressure:

- *losing excess weight*
- *daily exercise*
- *eating potassium and calcium-rich foods (including fruits, vegetables, and milk)*
- *limiting alcohol*
- *being a non-smoker*
- *taking medications as prescribed*
- *managing stress*
- *anything that improves the health of your blood vessels such as eating foods low in saturated and trans fat and high in antioxidants (see pages 118–121).*

109

How do I cut back on sodium?

How much should we cut back?

The Canadian Hypertension Education Program and the American Diabetes Association recommendations for hypertension are that sodium be reduced even lower than 2,300 mg. However, this will be difficult to do until food manufacturers and restaurants start adding less salt to their foods. Also, further study is needed to ensure that this lower amount of sodium is healthy and safe. For example, will this lower intake give us enough iodine? Not all food manufacturers use iodized salt.

About three quarters of the salt in our diet is hidden in restaurant and processed foods. Sadly, there are no laws that require food processors or restaurant chefs to reduce sodium. They know that salty foods sell more, because sodium enhances flavor. Most don't want to decrease the sodium they add until all manufacturers and restaurants are required to do this.

Some food companies are beginning to reduce the sodium they put in their products. This is because of recent consumer demand for lower-salt products, but the change is frustratingly slow. We need to become savvy at comparing food labels and restaurant nutritional lists, and looking for the lowest sodium level.

Five tips to reduce sodium

1. Cut your overall portions – as you eat less, you reduce your total intake of sodium.

2. Choose less of the High and Very High Sodium Foods listed on pages 116–117. These include pre-packaged convenience foods and restaurant foods. Some of the saltiest foods are hot dogs, subs, hamburgers, pizzas, processed meats, soups, pasta dishes and potato chips. Also, consider whether the food item listed is part of a meal that includes other foods with sodium, or is it the entire meal? If the salty ingredient is part of a recipe, consider the sodium per serving. If you have a saltier food at one meal or snack, then choose lower-sodium foods at your next meal or snack.

3. Use less salt and salty seasonings at the table and in cooking. (On certain foods, you may really miss adding salt – if using salt occasionally, limit to no more than three shakes. That will equal about 50 mg of sodium.)

4. Replace salt with pepper, unsalted seasonings, herbs and spices, and lemon and lime.

5. Rinse and drain canned salted foods such as canned kidney beans or canned fish or corn. This reduces up to one third to one half of the added sodium.

The photograph on page 112–113 and the lists on pages 114–117 show the amount of sodium in different foods. There are five groups from lowest sodium to highest sodium. Very low sodium foods have very little salt. Very high sodium foods are loaded with sodium, ⅓ teaspoon (1.5 mL) or more per serving.

The portions shown in the charts are based on the Canadian Diabetes Association *Beyond the Basics* food choices. The only exceptions are:

- Portions of some salty low-calorie "extras" are shown in smaller amounts.

- Some portions of meat or starch are shown in more usual (larger) meal sizes than shown on labels or in the *Beyond the Basics.*

- Some portions in the high and very high sodium groups are based on standard restaurant or packaged portions.

When you look at a food label you will see sodium listed as a percentage. For example, under the column "% Daily Value" it might list sodium as 20%. This means that if you eat this food serving you will get 20% of the sodium that you need for the day. Other foods can contribute the other 80% of your sodium for the day.

Sodium amounts vary between manufacturers and restaurants, imported versus North American food products, and regular and new "reduced sodium" products. In some cases, sodium ranges are listed to reflect this variability. I developed the sodium lists on pages 112–117 from government nutrient lists, restaurant nutrient tables, as well as a survey of products lining the grocery shelves.

Pages 112–117	Amount of sodium in a food	
	milligrams (mg)	% Daily Value
Very Low Sodium Foods	0–24	less than 1%
Low Sodium Foods	25–140	1% to 6%
Medium Sodium Foods	141–480	over 6% to 20%
High Sodium Foods	481–720	over 20% to 30%
Very High Sodium Foods	more than 720	more than 30%

Example of a food that provides 20% of your daily sodium:

Nutrition Facts Per ½ cup (125 mL)	
Amount	% Daily Value
Calories 100	
Fat 0 g	0 %
Saturated 0 g + Trans 0 g	0 %
Cholesterol 0 mg	0 %
Sodium 482 mg	20 %
Carbohydrate 24 g Fiber 0 g Sugars 6 g	8 %
Protein 2 g	

Yes, it is possible to eat healthy delicious everyday meals and still not get too much sodium. Use the seven day meal plan on pages 149–200 as a guideline.

Very Low Sodium Foods

These portions each provide 0–24 mg sodium. This is less than one percent of your daily needs (less than 1% Daily Value). On labels, "sodium free" or "salt free" foods will have less than 5 mg of sodium per serving size shown.

100%
75%
50%
25%

These portions provide less than one percent of your % Daily Value.

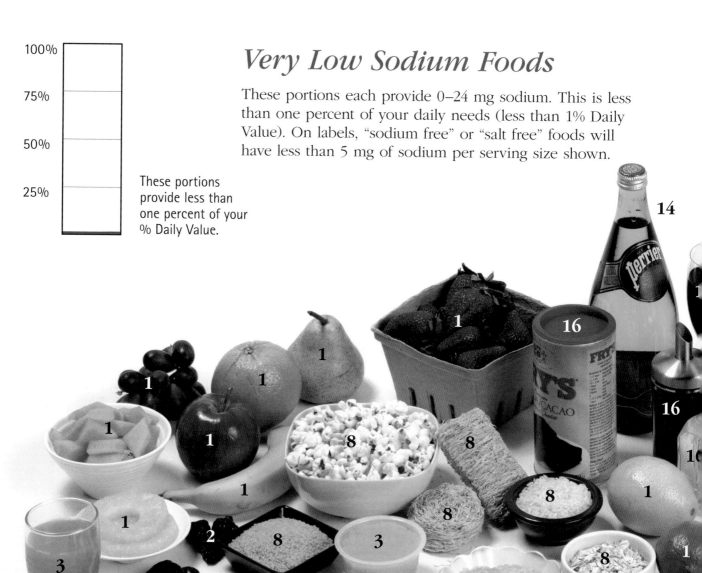

1. Fresh or canned fruit
2. Dried fruit
3. Fruit juice or applesauce
4. Fresh vegetables, raw or cooked
5. Canned or frozen unsalted vegetables

6. Garlic, onions, herbs, spices, pepper and no salt-spice blends
7. "No Salt" is high in potassium – ask your doctor if it is safe for you to use (it can interact with some medications)

Choose unprocessed food

The vast majority of unprocessed (natural) food is very low in sodium. This includes fresh and dried grains and starches, vegetables and fruits, dried beans and lentils, unsalted nuts and seeds, and unsalted fats. It also includes most frozen or canned vegetables and fruits with no salt added. Meats have some natural sodium, but in 1 ounce (30 g) portions are very low sodium foods.

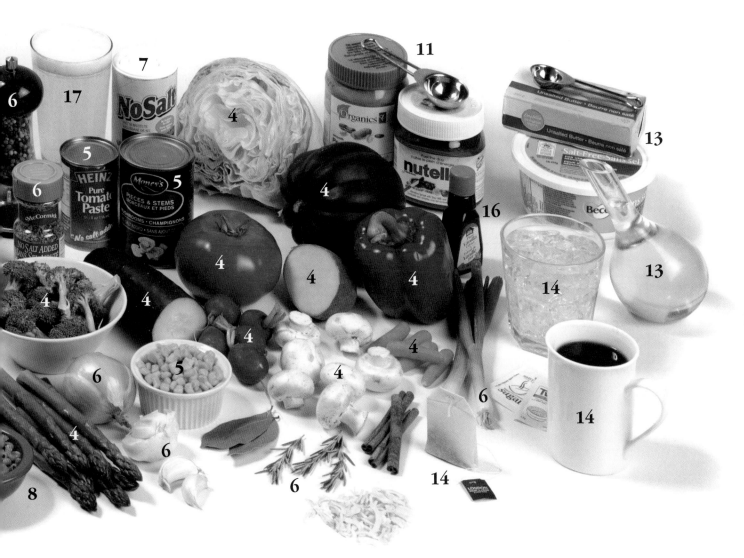

8. Grains and starches with no salt added (including wheat, pasta, couscous, rice, oats, flour, popcorn, etc.)

9. Dried beans and lentils

10. Nuts and seeds

11. Unsalted peanut butter and nut butters

12. Unsalted meat, 1 ounce

13. Oils and unsalted butter or margarine

14. Water, tea and coffee

15. Jams, sweeteners and plain candies

16. Condiments such as cocoa, flavorings or vinegar

17. Beer, wine and alcohol (not mixed drinks)

113

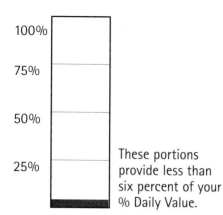

100%

75%

50%

25%

These portions provide less than six percent of your % Daily Value.

Low Sodium Foods

These portions each provide 25–140 mg sodium. This is one to six percent of your daily needs (1–6 % Daily Value).

On labels "low sodium" or "low salt" will have less than 140 mg sodium per serving size shown.

Starches
pancake, one 4-inch (10 cm): 110 mg

Vegetables
carrots, 1 cup (250 mL): 85 mg
celery, 2 medium stalks: 70 mg
mixed vegetables, frozen, 1 cup (250 mL): 75 mg
sweet potato, baked, ½ cup (125 mL): 45 mg
vegetable juice, low-salt, 1 cup (250 mL): 140 mg

Milk and milk products
hot chocolate mix, light, 1 package: 90 mg
soy beverage, 1 cup (250 mL): 30 mg
yogurt, low-fat, fruit with low-calorie sweetener,
    ¾ cup (175 mL): 110 mg
yogurt, plain, low-fat, ¾ cup (175 mL): 115 mg

Meats and proteins
chicken breast, baked, no skin, 4 oz (125 g): 85 mg
egg: 60 mg
fish, white, broiled, 4 oz (125 g): 65 mg
hamburger, 4 oz (125 g) cooked: 75 mg
peanut butter, regular (salted), 1 tbsp (15 mL): 65 mg
peanuts, roasted and salted, 2 tbsp (30 mL): 35–55 mg
tuna, canned in water, drained, ⅓ tin: 135 mg

Fats
butter, salted, 1 tsp (5 mL): 40 mg
margarine, non-hydrogenated, 1 tsp (5 mL): 35 mg
mayonnaise, light, 1 tbsp (15 mL): 110 mg

Soups
chicken noodle, low sodium, canned, 1 cup
(250 mL): 140 mg
cream of mushroom, low sodium, canned, 1 cup
(250 mL): 60 mg

Desserts and snacks
arrowroot biscuits, 4: 115 mg
chocolate bar, plain, milk chocolate, ½ bar: 35 mg
ice cream, ½ cup (125 mL): 65 mg
LifeStyle cookies, 2: 70 mg

Beverages
club soda, 12-oz (355 mL) can: 80 mg
diet 7-up, 12-oz (355 mL) can: 45 mg
diet ginger ale, 12-oz (355 mL) can: 120 mg

Condiments
barbecue sauce, 1 tsp (5 mL): 50 mg
ketchup, 1 tsp (5 mL): 50 mg
mustard, ready-to-serve, 1 tsp (5 mL): 65 mg
olives, green, stuffed, 4: 60 mg
sour cream, 1% MF, 2 tbsp (30 mL): 35 mg
Worcestershire sauce, 1 tsp (5 mL): 55 mg
Yum Yum pickles, 7 slices: 100 mg

Salts
Salts used just occasionally in tiny amounts (1⁄16 of
a teaspoon or about 4 quick shakes of a salt shaker):
    table salt: 145 mg
    sea salt: 135 mg
    Hys without MSG: 105 mg
    garlic salt or celery salt: 75 mg
    Half Salt: 65 mg
    Accent (MSG): 40 mg
Limit added salts and get most of your sodium from
nutritious food choices.

Medium Sodium Foods

These portions each provide 141–480 mg sodium. This is six to twenty percent of your daily needs (6–20% Daily Value).

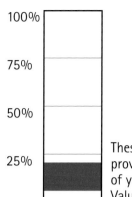

These portions provide 6–20% of your % Daily Value.

Low-fat varieties

Low-fat varieties, such as cheese and salad dressings, tend to be higher in sodium. This makes it a challenge when choosing products. If your main goal is weight loss choosing the lower calorie product may be your best bet. If your blood pressure is high or you have kidney problems, it's best to choose the lower salt variety but keep the portion small.

Starches
bagel, half 3-inch (7.5 cm): 155 mg
bannock, half of a 3-inch (7.5 cm) piece: 85–170 mg
bread, whole wheat, 1 slice: 170
cereal, dry, bran flakes, ½ cup (125 mL): 130 mg
cereal, dry, Special K or Cheerios, ⅔ cup (150 mL): 145–165 mg
French fries, fast food, no ketchup, small: 160–280 mg
oatmeal, instant, plain or sweetened, 1 pouch: 225–300 mg
pasta sauce mixes ("Side Kicks"), ¼ package: 350–370 mg
rice, converted, microwave (Bistro), flavored, ⅓ cup (75 mL): 140–200 mg
soda crackers, unsalted tops, 7: 160 mg (salted: 275 mg)
stuffing mixes, ¼ pouch (30 g): 410–460 mg
waffle, plain, frozen, 4-inch (10 cm): 260 mg

Vegetables
beans, wax, canned, 1 cup (250 mL): 225–340 mg
beets, canned, pickled, ½ cup (125 mL): 320 mg
corn, kernel, canned, salted, ½ cup (125 mL): 150 mg
mushrooms, canned, salted, ½ cup (125 mL): 350 mg
peas, frozen, 1 cup (250 mL): 150 mg (canned with salt: 450 mg)
salsa, ¼ cup (60 mL): 300–480 mg
spaghetti sauce, jarred or canned, ½ cup (125 mL): 360–480 mg
tomato juice, ½ cup (125 mL): 325 mg
tomato sauce, canned, 2 tbsp (30 mL): 195 mg

Milk and milk products
milk, chocolate, 1 cup (250 mL): 200 mg
milk, low-fat, white, 1 cup (250 mL): 125 mg
pudding cup, no sugar, ready-to-eat: 180 mg
pudding, light, made from a box, ½ cup (125 mL): 320 mg

Meats and proteins
bacon, 1 slice: 185 mg
baked beans, brown, canned, ½ cup (125 mL): 420–550 mg
cheese, cheddar, regular fat, 1 oz (30 g): 175 mg (low-fat: 205 mg)
cheese, feta, 2 tbsp (30 mL): 230 mg
cheese, processed, 1 slice (21 g): 310 mg
corned beef, Klik or Spam canned, 1/12 can (28 g): 225–400 mg
cottage cheese, 1% or 2%, ¼ cup (60 mL): 205–215 mg
pastrami or ham, deli, 1 oz (30 g): 330–375 mg
salmon, pink, drained, ⅓ can: 310 mg
sardines, canned in oil, drained, two 3-inch (7.5 cm): 240 mg
sausage, Italian, ½: 455 mg
sausages, pork and beef, 1 link (39 g): 315 mg
veggie burger, 1 (75 g): 480 mg
wieners, 1: 375 mg

Fats
salad dressing, creamy, light, 1 tbsp (15 mL): 190 mg
salad dressing, Italian, fat-free, 1 tbsp (15 mL): 210 mg

Desserts and snacks
chocolate bar, such as Oh Henry (67 g): 160 mg
corn chips or tacos, small bag (50 g): 335–430 mg
donut, cake type, 3-inch (7.5 cm): 260 mg
popcorn, microwave, 5 cups: 250–350 mg
potato chips, lower salt brands, 15 chips (25 g): 40–120 mg
apple pie, ⅛ piece: 210 mg
cake, from mix, 1/12 of a cake: 255–350 mg

Beverages
hot chocolate, restaurant, 10 oz (300 mL): 360 mg

Condiments or salts
baking powder, 1 tsp (5 mL): 300 mg
barbecue sauce, 1 tbsp (15 mL): 150 mg
HP sauce, 1 tbsp (15 mL): 160 mg
ketchup, 1 tbsp (15 mL): 140 mg
mustard, ready-to-serve, 1 tbsp (15 mL): 200 mg

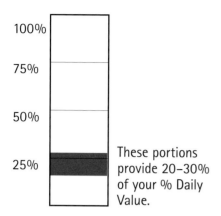

100%

75%

50%

25%

These portions provide 20–30% of your % Daily Value.

High Sodium Foods

These portions each provide 481–720 mg sodium. This is over twenty to thirty percent of your daily needs (20–30% Daily Value). Note: two servings from this group will add up to about half of your daily sodium needs.

Products differ between brands

The amount of sodium differs between brand names, and between Canadian and American producers. Check and compare the amount of sodium in your usual food brands and other available brands in your supermarket.

Starches
bagel: 6-inch (15 cm): 350–600 mg
French fries (fast food), large: 350 mg
      (570 mg with 2 ketchups)
Kraft Dinner, made without added fat, 1 cup (250 mL):
      615 mg
rice, Spanish or other flavors in a box, ⅓ cup (75 mL)
      cooked: 485 mg

Meats and proteins
beef jerky, one 9-inch (23 cm) strip: 570 mg
bologna, 2 slices: 550 mg

Soups
chicken noodle, canned, made with water, 1 cup
      (250 mL): 650–890 mg
chicken noodle, canned, 25% less salt, 1 cup (250 mL):
      485–660 mg (some brands 410 mg)
cream of mushroom, canned, made with water,
      1 cup (250 mL): 850–930 mg
cream of mushroom, canned, 25% less salt, 1 cup
      (250 mL): 630–650 mg
tomato soup, canned, made with water, 1 cup
      (250 mL): 695–800 mg (some brands 480 mg)
tomato soup, canned, 25% less salt, 1 cup (250 mL):
      720 mg

Meal items
cheeseburger (fast food): 640–750 mg
chili, canned, 1 cup (250 mL): 650 mg
Hamburger Helper, ⅕ package made with meat
      and milk, 1 cup (250 mL) prepared: 695 mg
pizza, ⅙ of 12-inch (30 cm) pizza: 350–650 mg
pizza, frozen, rising crust, ⅙ (128 g): 540 mg
TV dinners, light: 480–540 mg (also see Very High
      Sodium group)

Desserts and snacks
cheezies/cheese puffs, ¾ cup (175 mL): 440–520 mg
popcorn, theatre, large: 530 mg or more
potato chips, regular salt brands, 30 chips (50 g):
      600 mg

Condiments
dill pickle (Bick's), 1 (60 g): 570 mg
reduced salt bouillon, beef or chicken,
      1 sachet: 530 mg
reduced salt soy sauce, 1 tbsp (15 mL): 550 mg

Salts
Accent (MSG), 1 tsp (5 mL): 640 mg
table salt, ¼ tsp (1 mL): 580 mg

Sea salt, kosher salt and table salt are all salt!
Sea salt or kosher salt are typically not as refined and finely ground as table salt. Sea salt has about 2% other minerals by weight. The sodium content is very similar between all salts based on weight. However, by volume, sea salt or kosher salt are a bit less compact so the sodium level goes down just slightly.

Medications and sodium
Some medications contain sodium. Examples are some laxatives or antacids. Look for the word sodium in the drug name or ingredient list. Drugs that are effervescent (fizzy) also usually have sodium. Ask your pharmacist if any of your medications have sodium, and if so how much.

Very High Sodium Foods

These portions each provide over 720 mg sodium. This is thirty percent or more of your daily needs (30% Daily Value).

Foods with over 1,000 mg are marked with an asterisk (*).
Foods with over 1,500 mg are marked with two asterisks (**).
Foods with over 2,000 mg are marked with three asterisks (***).

Restaurant food is very salty! *Before you decide to eat out: request a copy of the restaurant's nutritional information (available for most chain restaurants) or search online.*

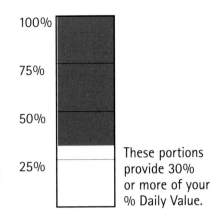

These portions provide 30% or more of your % Daily Value.

Soups
chunky beef, canned, ready-to-eat, 1 cup (250 mL): 770 mg
cream of mushroom made with water, 1 cup (250 mL): 800–850 mg
Cup-a-Soup, 1 pouch (11 g): 730–750 mg
Mr. Noodle in a bowl (110 g): 1,320–1,430 mg*
Mr. Noodle in a cup (64 g): 900–1,470 mg*
Mr. Noodles dry noodles (85 g): 1,340–2,640 mg***
soup, Subway or Tim Hortons, 10-oz (300 g): 820–1,390*

Other foods
corned beef or Klik, 4 oz (125 g): 900–1,140 mg*
ham or Spam, 4 oz (125 g): 1,500–1,600 mg**
pizza pop: 770 mg
ravioli, mini, ½ can: 830 mg
TV dinner, light: up to 900 mg

Restaurant meals
cheeseburger, double, with large fries and 2 ketchup: 1,720 mg**
cheeseburger with small fries and 1 ketchup: 1,020 mg*
chili, Tim Hortons, 10 oz (300 mL): 1,320 mg*
Chinese food (Panda Express), 10 oz (300 g) fried rice, 5 oz (150 g) BBQ pork and 1 Veggie Spring roll: 2,750 mg***
grilled chicken salad (fast food) with dressing: 990–1,350 mg*
hamburger (Whopper or Big Mac type): 930–1,020 mg*
KFC chicken breast: 1,050–1,310 mg* (grilled = 440 mg)
KFC Variety Big Box Meal (drumstick, 2 crispy strips, popcorn chicken, 2 home style sides and 32 oz/896 mL diet drink): 2,970 mg***
Macaroni and cheese, KFC, or store bought ready-to-eat, 1 cup (250 mL): 880–945 mg
Penne, baked, 3 cheese (Boston Pizza), small: 1,030 mg*
Pita, flat baked, Extreme Pita: 1,115–1,660 mg**
pizza, Hawaiian (Pizza Hut), 6-inch (15 cm): 1,180 mg*

popcorn chicken (KFC), large: 1,600 mg**
poutine, 1 serving fast food: 2,720 mg***
sandwich, Boston Pizza, with fries: 1,370–4,200 mg***
sandwiches, deli (McDonalds or Tim Hortons): 780–1,730 mg**
sub (Subway), 6-inch (15 cm): 1,160–2,850 mg***
taco salad: 1,400 mg*
wings, Boston Pizza, breaded barbecue, single order: 3,770 mg***
wraps, breakfast (Subway): 1,260–1,750 mg**

Snacks
muffin, large (Tim Hortons): 510–790 mg
potato chips, 350 g bag: 2,640 mg***
potato chips, lower salt brands, regular, 235 g bag (117 chips): 300–960 mg
potato chips, ripple, 235 g bag (117 chips): 1,270 mg*
potato chips, salt and vinegar, 235 g bag (145 chips): 2,915 mg***
pretzel twists, 12 (50 g): 720–1,000 mg*

Condiments
oyster sauce, 1 tbsp (15 mL): 750 mg
sauerkraut, ½ cup (125 mL): 825–1,650 mg**
soy sauce, 1 tbsp (15 mL): 1,030 mg*

Salts and salt substitutes:
baking soda, 1 tsp (5 mL): 1,285 mg*
garlic salt or celery salt, 1 tsp (5 mL): 1,170 mg*
Half Salt, 1 tsp (5 mL): 1,040 mg*
Salt substitutes: Most salt substitutes are made with potassium chloride instead of sodium chloride. Using these can interfere with certain high blood pressure pills: talk to your doctor or pharmacist.
Hys seasoning salt without MSG, 1 tsp (5 mL): 1,700 mg**
sea salt or kosher salt (coarse ground), 1 tsp (5 mL): 2,130 mg***
table salt, 1 tsp (5 mL): 2,325 mg***

6. Lowering cholesterol levels

Question and Answer about cholesterol with Karen Graham:

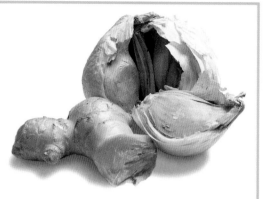

Rosita: I have had pre-diabetes and high blood pressure for several years. My doctor recently did some tests and told me that now I also have high cholesterol and high triglycerides. I was shocked when he told me this. Even though I have put on weight over the years (I am 5'2" and I weigh about 160 lbs/73 kg), I didn't think it was so bad. He is considering starting me on a cholesterol pill. I hate to have to take more pills though, so he suggested I try and lose some weight and improve my diet to see if I can bring my levels down. He said I may still need some new medications at some point. He wants to reassess my levels in three months. I would like to do this without medications, what would you suggest? How do I cut cholesterol out of my diet?

Karen's Answer: Your doctor is absolutely right. While medications are very important, being healthy in the long-term means a lot more than just popping pills. It means changing the problem that caused your blood sugar, cholesterol, triglycerides (blood fat) and blood pressure to go up in the first place. All these things are related.

You need a certain amount of cholesterol in your blood. It's an essential part of your body's cells and nerves. It also has a role in making bile for digestion, certain hormones and vitamin D. When you have too much though, it can block your blood vessels. There are many factors that can cause cholesterol to go up, not just the cholesterol in foods. Your liver makes the majority of cholesterol in your body. When you lose weight, this can reduce how much cholesterol your liver makes. Weight loss also improves your body's ability to remove excess cholesterol from your blood.

Complete the Checklist on pages 119–121. Learn about other factors that also help improve cholesterol, such as reducing stress, exercise and reducing saturated and trans fats. Eating less added sugar and drinking less alcohol can improve triglycerides. Cutting back on salt is an important part of reducing high blood pressure. After you complete the Checklist, focus on improving the things you "never" do or only do "sometimes." One or two changes is a great start. Good for you if you are already doing the things in the Checklist "most of the time."

Do you need additional help with food planning?

Ask your doctor to refer you to a Registered Dietitian.

Checklist for Cholesterol, Triglycerides and Blood Pressure

Do You...

1. Eat smaller portions of food?
This will help you lose weight. When you weigh less, your heart doesn't have to work so hard, and your cholesterol, triglyceride and blood pressure usually come down. Your liver will make less cholesterol.

❑ most of the time
❑ sometimes
❑ never

2. Eat more soluble fiber?
This reduces your blood cholesterol. Find soluble fiber in foods such as oatmeal and oat bran; psyllium; barley; peas, beans and lentils (such as kidney beans, brown beans and chick peas); apples, pears, artichoke hearts, chicory and dandelion roots, onions, leeks and garlic.

❑ most of the time
❑ sometimes
❑ never

3. Eat less meat and unhealthy fats?
Choose smaller portions of meat and eat more vegetables. Add less fat to your meals. Eat less French fries, donuts, potato chips, cookies and fried chicken.

❑ most of the time
❑ sometimes
❑ never

4. Eat more healthy fats?
Choose foods that have polyunsaturated omega-3 fats and monounsaturated fat. Have fish or seafood twice a week or choose ground flaxseed (or flaxseed oil), wheat germ, omega-3 eggs or omega-3 milk. In small amounts, choose foods such as olives and olive oil, canola or soybean oil, avocados, walnuts, almonds, hazelnuts, pecans, peanuts, pistachios, cashews, macadamia nuts, soy nuts, pumpkin seeds, sunflower seeds or sesame seeds. **Note:** An added benefit of these foods (along with legumes, grains, vegetables and fruits) is that they naturally include something called plant sterols. These help remove some of the "bad" cholesterol from your blood. Some new products on the market also have plant sterols added (such as some yogurts or margarine).

❑ most of the time
❑ sometimes
❑ never

5. Eat foods rich in B vitamins?
Some B vitamins such as folic acid lessen blood vessel damage and stroke by reducing the buildup of a chemical called homocysteine. Choose dark leafy green vegetables, whole grains, beans and legumes. Other sources of folate are flour, many dry cereals (check the label), orange juice, green peas, corn, beets, green beans, nuts and seeds.

❑ most of the time
❑ sometimes
❑ never

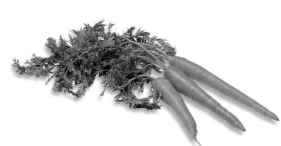

6. Eat lots of antioxidants?

Antioxidants are plant compounds and vitamins that help reduce inflammation of your blood vessel walls. Eat a rainbow of colors of fruits and vegetables:

- apples with the peel, cherries, plums, prunes and raisins
- all berries
- orange and red vegetables and fruits such as carrots, squash, pumpkin, sweet potatoes, bell peppers, oranges, red grapefruit, mangos, watermelon and guavas
- grapes and pomegranate and their juices – limit to ⅓ cup (75 mL) a day; and red wine in moderation
- dark green vegetables such as spinach, broccoli and kale
- garlic and onions, broccoli, cabbage, Brussels sprouts, bok choy, cauliflower, turnip and rutabagas
- herbs and spices such as rosemary, thyme, marjoram, sage, peppermint, tarragon, oregano, sweet basil and cinnamon
- peas, beans and lentils
- avocado, nuts and seeds, especially walnuts
- fortified soy milk, soy protein, soy nuts and tofu
- tea – especially green and black tea
- hot cocoa, or an occasional small piece of dark cocoa-rich chocolate

7. Eat less sodium & more potassium?

Less sodium: Limit salty foods, like snack foods, processed meat, canned and packaged soups, and all pre-packaged convenience and restaurant foods. Put away the salt shaker. Take out the pepper grinder, herbs and spices.

More potassium: Choose fruits and vegetables such as banana, melons, dried fruit, orange, kiwi, mango, pear, artichoke, avocado, beet greens, beets, Brussels sprouts, celery, mushrooms, parsnips, potato, pumpkin, spinach, carrots, yams, tomatoes and squash. Also find potassium in bran cereals, beans and lentils, meat and milk.

8. Include calcium?

Studies show low-fat calcium foods in your diet can help improve your blood pressure and reduce "bad" cholesterol. They also may play a role in helping you lose weight and reduce blood pressure. Choose low-fat milk, low-fat yogurt or pudding, and 20% or less milk fat (MF) cheese.

9. Limit sugars and sweet drinks?
Juice, soft drinks, other sweetened beverages, desserts
and candies increase your blood sugar and triglycerides.

❏ most of the time
❏ sometimes
❏ never

10. Limit alcohol?
Two or more drinks a day increases your blood pressure.
Any amount can worsen triglycerides.

❏ most of the time
❏ sometimes
❏ never

11. Limit coffee?
Limit specialty coffees loaded with fat and sugar. Avoid
perked coffee as it has been shown to increase cholesterol
because of a chemical called terpenes; filtered coffee is a
better choice. There is some evidence that excess caffeine
may increase heart arrhythmias and homocysteine. Limit to
3–4 cups (750 mL–1 L) per day. Choose more water instead.

❏ most of the time
❏ sometimes
❏ never

12. Keep active?
Being active improves blood flow and increases your
metabolism to help burn calories. Doctors recommend
at least 20–25 minutes of exercise a day. Try walking or
using an exercise bike. Start slowly and gradually do more.

❏ most of the time
❏ sometimes
❏ never

13. Avoid smoking?
Try to cut back or quit. You may have tried to quit before –
please think about trying again.

❏ most of the time
❏ sometimes
❏ never

14. Manage your diabetes?
Improving your blood sugar can improve your blood
cholesterol and triglycerides, and your blood pressure.

❏ most of the time
❏ sometimes
❏ never

15. Manage your stress?
Stress harms the inside lining of your blood vessel walls.
Stay busy to take your mind off your problems. When you
exercise or laugh, "happy hormones" go through your body
to help you relax. A walk in the evening will help tire you
out and help you sleep better. Seek help from a friend
or professional if your stress bothers you too much.

❏ most of the time
❏ sometimes
❏ never

How did you do?

If you checked "most of the time" often – you are doing well.

If you checked "never" often – then consider trying to make some changes in these areas.

7. Herbs and vitamins

Herbs and Spices

Herbs (fresh or dried) and spices are nutritious additions to your diet. Buy them at a grocery store or grow them in your garden or in a pot on your windowsill. Perhaps the greatest benefit of herbs is their flavor. When you add them to other foods, you can cut back on your use of salt, sugar or fat as flavorings.

Beneficial herbs and spices

Antioxidants (*protect against heart disease and cancer*): *Garlic, onions and chives, rosemary, thyme, marjoram, sage, peppermint, tarragon, oregano, sweet basil, cinnamon, curry powder and paprika.*

Mild blood thinners: *Garlic, onions and chives.*

These may be of benefit to blood sugar (*however, concentrated extracts made from these are not yet recommended, see pages 125–128*): *cinnamon, allspice, black pepper and fenugreek.*

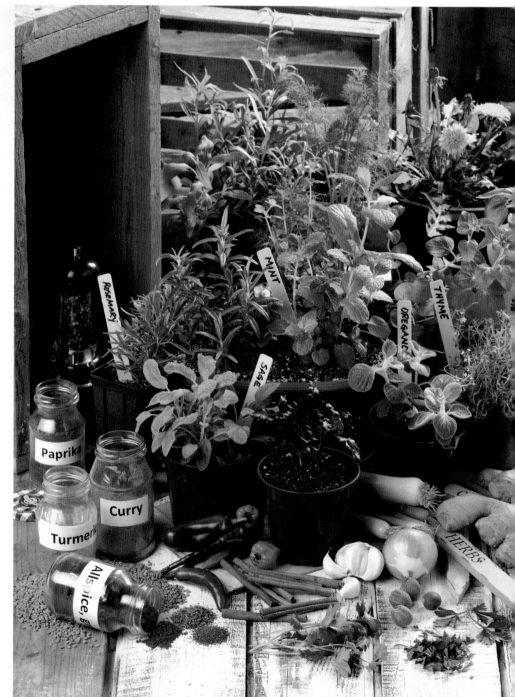

Tea

People around the world have consumed black, green and oolong brewed teas for thousands of years. After water, tea is the second most common beverage in the world. Its antioxidants may help clear out the blood vessels of unwanted chemicals. Early research indicates that tea may even help insulin work better. Tea has tannins (the dark color of tea) that help reduce the glycemic index of food at a meal. Perhaps the greatest benefit of tea is that it has a soothing taste and helps family and friends relax.

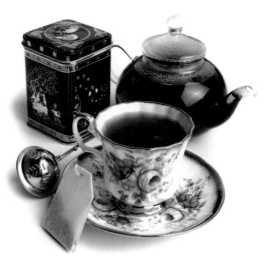

Go for hot, not iced

Powdered ice tea and bottled ice tea have lots of sugar (except for sugar free varieties). Brewed tea, whether it's hot or cold, has more health benefits.

Herbal Teas

Herbal teas are beverages made from any part of a plant except tea bush leaves. Herbal teas sold in grocery stores are safe, calorie-free and usually caffeine-free. Homemade herbal teas made directly from herbs, roots or leaves may be more potent and therefore have benefits and risks as do herbal supplements. Herbal teas gain strength through prolonged steeping. If you want a refreshing beverage, steep briefly. If you're seeking a medicinal dosage, most teas require at least 10–15 minutes of steeping. Herbal teas (other than those sold in supermarkets), like herbal supplements, should be used on the advice of your doctor.

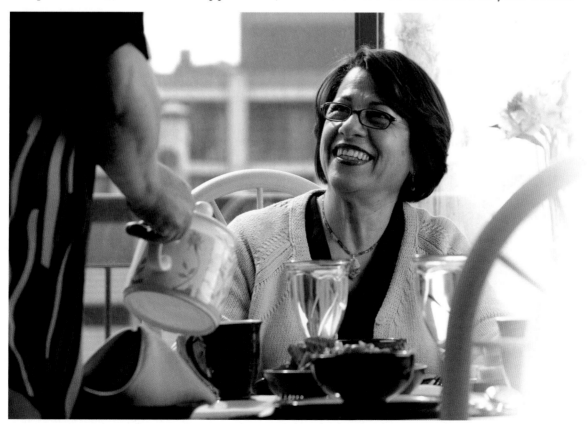

Herbal supplements

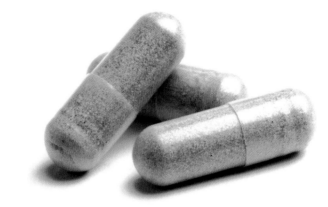

Benefits of herbal supplements

About a quarter of prescription medications have active ingredients that come from plants. Herbal supplements are generally not as strong as most prescription medications. For this reason, they may be your "drug" of choice. Some people may react strongly to prescription and/or over-the-counter drugs and may find the less potent herbal supplements of some benefit. For example, for a mild muscle ache, you may find a cup of peppermint tea can help you feel better with fewer side effects than a commercial pain killer.

While the medical community recognizes the potential of herbal supplements, they have a difficult time recommending them because they are poorly tested and regulated. Unlike prescription drugs that come from a laboratory, herbal supplements are not standardized. Therefore, their benefits and risks will vary. If you test your blood sugar at home, monitor to see if there is any difference in your blood sugar with the use of herbal supplements. You will want to know if herbal supplements make you feel better, otherwise there is no reason to spend money on them.

What is the diabetes placebo effect:

You are taking an herbal supplement (or vitamin pill) that you believe will help your blood sugar. This belief may help you feel happier, less stressed and more in control of your health. This in turn could help your blood sugar! The name for this is the placebo effect. It shows that our minds and beliefs have a role in keeping our bodies healthy.

Concerns about herbal supplements

Inadequate testing and regulation

Herbal supplements are not tested and regulated in the same rigorous way as prescription medications. In most cases, we can't confirm the safety or health benefits of herbal supplements. Herbs are plants and are affected by variable growing seasons, contaminants in the earth and water, and pesticides and fertilizers. For this reason, it is hard to create standardized dosages in supplements. Some concentrated supplements may contain uneven amounts of beneficial or toxic components.

Also, the following problems have been found in many containers of imported herbal supplements:

- The container didn't contain the stated product.
- It was in a stronger or lesser dosage than on the bottle.
- There were contaminants, such as lead or arsenic.

All these factors increase your potential health risks when you take an herbal supplement.

There are many herbal supplements that claim to help lower blood sugar. The truth is we simply don't know if this is true. There hasn't been enough research done on herbal supplements. The risks and benefits aren't clear. In North America, the government and drug companies don't yet regulate or market most herbal supplements in a scientific way. Therefore, their effects on your blood sugar can vary.

If in doubt—don't take it.

Interactions with medications

Be aware that herbs can cause side effects or interact with other medications. Your pharmacist has access to herbal dictionaries. The pharmacist can tell you of any known potential benefits and risks, and possible interactions with other herbs or drugs. This is more reliable than the claims you may hear about or read on a package.

Herbal supplements with known drug interactions:

- If you are on a blood thinner such as warfarin or aspirin, increased bleeding can occur if you also take willow bark, devil's claw, alfalfa, chamomile, evening primrose oil, feverfew, garlic, ginger, ginkgo biloba, ginseng or red clover. Devil's claw might also increase blood sugar.

- St John's Wort interferes with antidepressants such as fluoxetine, e.g., Prozac. It also interferes with some cholesterol medications.

- If you take a drug that makes you sun-sensitive (for example, glyburide), St. John's Wort can worsen the sun-sensitivity.

- If you take the heart drug digoxin or a thiazide diuretic (for blood pressure), dried aloe, cascara sagrada, senna or licorice can cause low potassium levels.

- Blood pressure can go up with ginseng, licorice, yerba mate and yohimbine. For information on yohimbine, see page 401.

Dangerous herbal supplements

You shouldn't take these because of adverse health risks (this is not a complete listing):

Chaparral, coltsfoot, comfrey, ephedrine (ephedra or ma huang), germander, jin bu huan, lobelia, phenylalanine, sassafras, *Timospora crispa,* and L-tryptophan.

> **Natural does not necessarily mean safe.**
>
> **If you are taking herbal supplements, please advise your doctor or pharmacist. Doctors do not recommend herbal supplements if you are pregnant due to insufficient information about whether they are safe for your growing baby.**

Herbs and kidney disease:

If you have kidney damage stop taking all herbs (unless your doctor tells you to take them). Your kidneys filter out excess drugs and herbs into your urine. If your kidneys are not working fully, herbs can build up in your body.

These herbs are known to be unsafe when you have kidney disease:

bucha leaves

juniper berries

uva ursi

parsley capsules

Artemisia absinthium (wormwood)

autumn crocus

chuifong tuokuwan

horse chestnut

periwinkle

sassafras

star fruit

tung sheuh

Vandellia cordifolia

126

Example of seven diabetes herbal supplements

Ginseng root or berry extract

- **Potential benefits:** Some studies show American ginseng root and Asian ginseng root or berry extract have benefits in decreasing blood sugar rise after a meal. However, other studies have not shown ginseng to improve A1C levels. It may also improve cholesterol and triglycerides.

- **Potential side effects:** Ginseng's side effects are not clear due to the large varieties of ginseng used in different studies. Some ginseng species (other than American ginseng) have significant side-effects at high doses, including high blood pressure. Ginseng can interact with your diabetes medications and can cause low blood sugar. Ginseng can also interact with pills you are taking for depression or to stabilize your mood, or water-losing pills.

Ginkgo biloba leaf extract

- **Potential benefits:** Some evidence suggests that ginkgo leaf extract may help protect blood vessels walls and improve circulation. It's used in Europe and sold as an approved drug, but not yet regulated in North America.

- **Potential side effects:** Ginkgo is known to interact with some antibiotics, cholesterol medication, and blood thinners – it can cause bleeding if you take it in large amounts.

Cinnamon

Chinese cinnamon or cassia (*Cinnamomum aromaticum*) is the variety of cinnamon most available in stores.

- **Potential benefits:** Some studies show mild benefits to reducing blood sugar from eating about ½–1 teaspoon (2–5 mL) of cinnamon daily. Other studies show no benefit to blood sugar from eating cinnamon. If more study confirms that cinnamon is beneficial, then the next step is to try and extract the beneficial compound and concentrate it for safe medicinal use.

- **Potential side effects:** Cinnamon contains something called coumarin, a moderately toxic compound. One or more teaspoons (5 or more mL) of cinnamon a day may result in excess coumarin. Coumarin isn't the same as the drug "coumadin" and isn't a blood thinner. Yet, in certain situations, coumarin converts to one. Therefore don't eat too much cinnamon if you are on a blood thinner such as aspirin or coumadin.

> **Caution**
> Most doctors don't yet recommend ginseng and ginkgo due to insufficient testing and regulation. Their potential for interacting with other drugs is mostly untested and therefore unknown.

> **Recommendation:**
> Doctors don't recommend you take more than 1 teaspoon (5 mL) of cinnamon a day (2.3 grams), or equivalent in capsules. Smaller amounts can be included as a healthful and tasty addition sprinkled on your hot cereal, cocoa or light desserts.

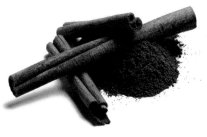

Caution

Always tell your pharmacist or doctor what herbs and medications you are taking and find out how much is safe for you. Herbs, like medications, can cause side effects if taken in large amounts.

This herb comes from the leaf of a woody plant that grows in India.

Bitter melon is a vegetable that grows in the tropics that is also called balsam pear or karela. This vegetable is cooked in stir-frys or made into a juice.

Prickly pear cactus and Aloe vera

The scientific name for prickly pear cactus is *Opuntia streptacantha*. You may know *Aloe vera* as a common house plant. These herbs are usually sold as capsules.

- **Potential benefits:** Both plants are known for their gel like sap found in their leaves, and this sap contains soluble fiber. Short-term studies have shown that their main benefit may be that they have soluble fiber. Soluble fiber can lower fasting blood sugar by slowing down the rate that you absorb carbohydrates. Please see Glycemic Index, on page 91–93, for effective and safe sources of soluble fiber, such as oatmeal, barley and brown beans.

- **Potential side effects:** Prickly pear cactus and *Aloe vera* can interact with diabetes medications. If you take water-losing pills such as lasix or hydrochlothiazide, or a heart pill called digoxin, you must talk with your pharmacist or doctor. Prickly pear cactus has been known to cause some unwanted skin changes, like eczema. *Aloe vera* can cause diarrhea in some people.

Gymnema sylvestre

- **Potential benefits:** It may help diabetes in three ways: 1) decrease the absorption of sugar from your gut, 2) improve how your body uses blood sugar, and 3) stimulate your pancreas to make more insulin.

- **Potential side effects:** As with some other herbs that may lower blood sugar, *Gymnema* may also interact with other diabetes medications. More studies are needed to know its benefits and side effects.

Bitter melon

Its scientific name is *Momordica charantia*.

- **Potential benefits:** Animal studies have suggested that it may help reduce an animal's blood sugar by three possible ways: 1) help the pancreas make more insulin, 2) help tissues pick up blood sugar more easily, or 3) reduce how much sugar the animal's liver makes. However, there is no clear evidence yet that it is helpful in people with diabetes.

- **Potential side effects:** If you are taking this you may need to adjust your diabetes medications. Bitter melon may cause your body to lose too much potassium. This is a concern if you experience diarrhea or take laxatives or certain blood pressure pills that also pull potassium out of your body. Bitter melon is not recommended if you are pregnant, as it might cause a miscarriage.

Vitamins and Minerals

Food is the best source for vitamins and minerals

If you eat a variety of foods as shown in my "Hands-On Food Guide" on pages 55–59, and in the meal plans in this book, you will get all your vitamins and minerals. The chart on pages 132–133 shows you good food sources of common vitamins and minerals, and their roles in your body. These foods help you prevent and manage diabetes complications. When you eat whole foods, vitamins and minerals are in safe amounts. Also, they are in a healthy combination with other nutrients including fiber, antioxidants, and factors that help the absorption of nutrients. This is why food is the best way to get your nutrients. If you take too much of one vitamin or mineral pill, it can affect another in an unhealthy way.

You do not need to take vitamin and mineral pills unless your doctor or dietitian has prescribed them. If a doctor prescribes a vitamin or mineral pill for you, be sure to ask why, and know how many you should take. Also remember the importance of eating healthy foods and regular exercise.

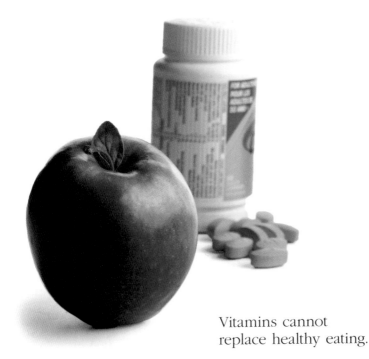

Vitamins cannot replace healthy eating.

Food supplies what you need

You only need tiny amounts of vitamins and minerals to keep you healthy. For example, you need 70–90 milligrams of Vitamin C every day. You'll consume that in one large orange. If you also take a pill of 1000 milligrams (or 1 gram) of Vitamin C every day, your kidneys have to work harder to flush out the extra Vitamin C.

Benefit of supplements is questioned

A very large 2009 research review study (Archives of Internal Medicine Journal) of women ages 50–79 showed that multivitamins didn't protect against heart attack, stroke, cancer or an early death. These results came as a shock. Nearly half the population of women (and nearly as many men) takes a multivitamin pill believing they are getting a benefit. In addition, large studies using vitamin C, E, beta carotene (which turns into vitamin A) and selenium, don't show conclusive benefits. For diabetes, chromium studies have failed to show any significant benefit for blood glucose levels except for those malnourished and deficient in chromium. Vitamins B_1, B_6, and B_{12} have failed to show conclusive benefits in treating diabetic neuropathy.

When supplements do benefit

For someone with a vitamin or mineral deficiency or who is malnourished, a supplement can definitely help. Here are some examples of when supplements may be given to people with diabetes:

- to help heal a foot or lower leg wound
- to counteract the side effects of certain medications
- to try to slow down macular degeneration
- prenatal supplements during pregnancy (see page 385)
- with kidney disease due to dietary restrictions

More is not better

Your healthy body looks after you, storing the vitamins and minerals that you need for later. For example, Vitamins A, D, E and K and iron are stored in your fat and liver. If you take vitamins or minerals in large amounts (mega doses), you may end up with more than you need. Vitamins A and D, folic acid and vitamin B_6, iron, zinc, calcium and selenium are toxic at high doses.

Hemochromatosis: Some people have a rare genetic condition called hemochromatosis. They get a build-up of iron in their body. This can lead to diabetes and heart disease and a variety of other problems. It is life-threatening if not treated.

Do you live in Canada or a northern location with low winter sunlight?

As you get older, your skin does not make vitamin D as well. The government of Canada recommends a daily supplement of 400 I.U. of vitamin D if you are over 50 years old. Some doctors may recommend up to 1,000 I.U.

What is a mega dose?

It is a larger dose – more than what your body needs.

For each vitamin and mineral, the Recommended Dietary Allowance (RDA) is the amount you need for good health. If you take a dose of supplement that is at, or above, the Upper Limit (UL) you are more likely to get adverse effects. This is a mega dose. To determine the RDA and UL of each vitamin and mineral search these words on the internet "DRI tables." Multivitamin pills do not generally contain mega doses. However, when you buy vitamins or minerals individually, each pill will usually have a higher amount. Then if you take too many pills each day, your total intake goes up, and you can get a mega dose.

Examples of the side effects from taking mega doses of supplements over an extended time:

- Beta carotene (vitamin A) increases the risk of lung cancer (especially in smokers and ex-smokers) and prostate cancer. Mega doses are not safe if your kidneys are not working well.

- Vitamin C can increase your risk for kidney stones, and cause excessive absorption of iron (especially in males).

- Vitamin D can cause a high blood calcium level, kidney damage and affect growth in children.

- Vitamin E can cause an increased risk of bleeding, lung cancer or heart failure.

- Folic acid increases the risk of prostate cancer and some breast cancers.

- Magnesium can worsen kidney problems, and cause stomach upset and diarrhea.

- Chromium can cause weight gain, headaches, sleeping problems and stomach upset.

- Selenium may increase the risk of diabetes and high cholesterol.

- Zinc can cause stomach upset and depress your immune system.

- Some recent studies suggest that healthy older women who take excess calcium pills may have an increased risk of a heart attack.

- Excess iron will be stored in your liver, and can increase your risk for a heart attack.

Vitamins	What food is it in?	What does it do in the body?
Vitamin A (beta carotene can convert to vitamin A)	It's in organ meats, eggs, fish, milk, dark green and yellow/orange vegetables such as carrots, squash and sweet potatoes. Also Vitamin A is in tomatoes, mangos, pink grapefruit and cantaloupes. Manufacturers add it to milk, margarine and butter.	It's important for good vision; for healthy teeth, nails, hair, bones and glands. Vitamin A helps protect your body cells against infection and is an antioxidant. This vitamin helps wounds heal.
Vitamin B1 (thiamin)	B1 is in whole bran (wheat and rice), enriched flour and cereals, wheat germ, meats, green peas, dried peas and legumes and nuts.	B1 helps your body use carbohydrates for energy and growth. It has a role in proper muscle coordination and the maintenance of nerves.
Vitamin B2 (riboflavin)	B2 is in milk, green vegetables, meats – especially organ meats, legumes, cheese, eggs, yogurt, cottage cheese, whole grains, enriched flour and cereal.	B2 helps your body turn protein, fat and carbohydrate into energy. B2 helps maintain healthy skin and eyes and builds and maintains body tissue.
Vitamin B3 (niacin)	B3 is in meats – especially organ meats, poultry, fish, peanuts, legumes, corn, whole grains, enriched flour and cereals.	B3 helps to break down protein and turn food into energy. It helps keep your gut and skin healthy.
Vitamin B6 (pyridoxine)	B6 is in meats – especially organ meats, eggs, fish, legumes, walnuts, green leafy vegetables, bananas, grapes, watermelon, carrots, peas, potatoes, whole grains and wheat germ.	B6 is necessary to make and to use certain proteins. It helps your nervous system work properly and protects you against infection. You need B6 for a healthy heart.
Vitamin B12	B12 is in meats – especially organ meats, shellfish, eggs, fish – especially salmon and herring, milk and milk products – especially blue cheese. Some soy products have B12 added to them.	B12 is necessary in the making of hemoglobin and healthy red blood cells and helps maintain a healthy nervous system.
Folic Acid (folate)	Folic acid is in organ meats, beans and legumes, spinach, kale, parsley and other green leafy vegetables, asparagus, corn, green peas, fruits such as oranges, orange juice and melons, nuts, whole grains and yeast. It is also in flour and pasta (and some rice) marked "enriched."	Folic acid is necessary to make certain proteins and genetic materials for your cells and keeps your blood cells healthy. Taken during pregnancy, it reduces the risk of some birth defects. Both folic acid and vitamin B12 may help reduce a chemical called homocysteine, and may play a role in reducing your risk for heart attack and stroke.
Vitamin C	Vitamin C is in fruit, especially citrus fruits and juices, strawberries, kiwi, cantaloupe and guava. Tomatoes, cabbage, sweet peppers, potatoes, onions, broccoli and green leafy vegetables including dandelion greens also have Vitamin C.	Vitamin C helps in the production of collagen and is necessary for healthy skin, gums, blood vessels, muscles, teeth and bones. It aids in the absorption of iron. It works as an antioxidant and helps wounds heal.
Vitamin D	This is the "sunshine vitamin" – our skin makes it when we go out in the sun. It's in fish – especially fatty fish such as salmon or sardines, liver and eggs. Milk, margarine and butter contain added Vitamin D.	Vitamin D works together with calcium and phosphorus to build and maintain strong bones and teeth. It also has a role in muscle strength. It may help your insulin work better and is important for diabetes. Low vitamin D may be a risk for diabetes, hypertension, multiple sclerosis, cancer and arthritis.

Vitamin E	Vitamin E is in vegetable oil, nuts and seeds, peanut butter, wheat germ, green leafy vegetables, avocado, legumes, eggs, margarine, butter, liver, milk, whole grains and fortified cereals.	Vitamin E is an antioxidant and helps protect your cell coverings. It is important in healthy blood cells and body tissues.
Vitamin K	Vitamin K is the "bacteria vitamin" – in a healthy person, it's produced in the gut by bacteria. Green leafy vegetables are the best food source. It's also in fruit, cereals, dairy products, meat and vegetable oils.	Vitamin K is necessary for clotting of blood and healthy bones.

Minerals	What food is it in?	What does it do in the body?
Calcium	Calcium is in milk and milk products, dates, blackstrap molasses, oysters, scallops, salmon and sardines with bones, fish heads, legumes, almonds, green leafy vegetables and broccoli. Manufacturers add it to some tofu, soy beverages and orange juice.	Calcium is important for bone and tooth formation. Also, helps in blood clotting. It's important for the functioning of your nerves, muscles and heart. It plays a role in keeping a healthy weight and blood pressure.
Iron	Iron is in liver and organ meats, meats, eggs, shellfish – especially oysters, nuts, sardines, legumes, broccoli, peas, spinach, prunes, raisins, bran, enriched cereals, blackstrap molasses and wheat germ.	Iron is important for healthy blood and muscle cells and in the prevention of iron-deficiency anemia. Also, it helps in the formation of enzymes which have different roles in your body.
Magnesium	Magnesium is in green leafy vegetables, whole grains, nuts and seeds (including peanut butter). Also, it's in legumes, peas, fish and seafood, yogurt, brown rice, oat bran and cocoa.	Magnesium is helpful in bone and tooth formation and the functioning of the nerves, muscles and blood vessels. Some studies, but not all, have suggested magnesium may have a role in improving fasting blood sugar and helping insulin work, especially in people who are low in magnesium.
Chromium	Chromium is in cereals and whole grain bread especially those with lots of bran. Some beer, red wine, and grape juice contain chromium. It's also in meats, especially processed meats, poultry, fish, egg yolks and green vegetables.	Chromium helps insulin work. It may improve blood sugar, blood cholesterol and blood fat levels.
Potassium	Potassium is in fruit, especially orange juice, bananas, pomegranates and dried fruits. Vegetables such as carrots, potatoes, spinach and tomatoes, meats and milk contain potassium.	Potassium is necessary for nerve and muscle function, and for maintaining acid-base and water balance in the body. It plays a role in a healthy blood pressure.
Selenium	Selenium is in brazil nuts, cashews, meat, seafood and poultry. There are smaller amounts in grains, dairy products and legumes.	Selenium is an antioxidant. It helps regulate thyroid hormones, which are important in weight maintenance.
Zinc	Zinc is in meats, liver, eggs, shellfish – especially oysters, sardines, cheese, green leafy vegetables, oranges, prunes, strawberries, whole grains and nuts and seeds.	Zinc is part of enzymes and insulin. It's also important for healthy skin and growth. It helps wounds heal. Zinc in combination with antioxidant vitamins *might* slow down advanced age-related macular degeneration (eye disease) for some people.

133

8. Alcohol

Question and Answer about alcohol with Karen Graham:

Matthew: Both my partner and I have put on weight over the years. We like to sit out on our deck in the evenings and talk, have a few drinks and eat peanuts or mixed nuts. My partner usually prepares the drinks and snacks. How should we change our routine now that I have diabetes?

Karen's Answer: All forms of alcohol including wine, liqueurs, coolers, beer, and hard liquor (spirits) have calories. Whether you have the alcohol with your meals or as a snack, it adds extra unneeded calories. Cutting back on alcohol helps you lose weight. It sounds like you and your partner need to consider different drinks and snacks.

You might both be surprised that three drinks and half a cup of peanuts or mixed nuts can add up to 920 calories (see below). In comparison, the large dinner meals in this book have 730 calories, and the large snacks have 200 calories.

Show your partner the purple snack sections on pages 196–200 (more snack ideas are in my book *Diabetes Meals for Good Health*). You'll find a wide selection of choices. Perhaps start by replacing one or two of your alcoholic drinks with a diet beverage or iced water with lemon. Then switch to a small or medium snack, and just occasionally eat a large snack. Try homemade popcorn where you control the amount of fat and salt. Popcorn makers with motorized stirring rods make great popcorn – ⅓ cup (75 mL) kernels plus ½ tsp (2 mL) oil makes 8 cups (2 L) popped. Your partner may even consider joining you on these changes.

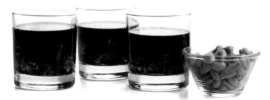

½ cup (125 mL) peanuts and
3 rum and coke (1.5 oz/45 mL rum
and 4 oz/125 mL cola each)

920 calorie meal!

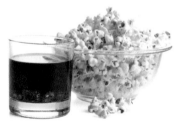

4 cups (1L) lightly oiled popcorn,
1.5 oz (45 mL) rum and diet cola,
and iced water with lemon

250 calorie snack

One other thought is to consider going for a walk in the evening. It's also a nice way to pass the time. Ask your partner to join you for your walks.

I hope some of these suggestions help you in your goals of cutting back. Keep up the good work. Next time you see your doctor, ask your partner to come with you, and hear recommendations directly from your doctor.

Risks of alcohol

Alcoholic drinks are fattening

Alcohol is more fattening than carbohydrates. Alcohol has 7 calories per gram compared to 4 calories per gram of carbohydrate (fat is the highest at 9 calories per gram). One and a half ounces of whiskey, rum or vodka has over 100 calories. Beer, liqueurs, coolers and sweet wines also contain sugar, boosting calories even more. See the table on page 137.

Alcohol can cause or contribute to many health problems

Alcohol is a highly addictive substance. Weigh any potential benefit of alcohol against the risk of addiction. Your liver recognizes alcohol as a toxin. It can handle small amounts, but large daily amounts of alcohol contributes to many health problems. These problems include:

- high blood pressure, high triglycerides and stroke

- liver disease and pancreatitis

- diabetes retinopathy, an eye disease

- diabetic neuropathy, a nerve disease

- alcohol during pregnancy increases the risk of fetal alcohol syndrome

- Your risk is greater for certain cancers, such as breast or liver cancer even with low to moderate drinking of one or two drinks a day, including wine.

- If you are elderly and unstable on your feet, drinking alcohol can increase your risk of falling and breaking a hip or other bone.

- significant interactions with medications, causing unwanted side effects

Do not drink alcohol if you:

- or close family members have a history of binge drinking or other alcohol problems.

- are on certain medications or have a condition where alcohol is not recommended – talk to your doctor.

- are planning to drive.

- are pregnant or trying to get pregnant, or breastfeeding.

- have pancreatitis, liver disease or very high triglycerides.

Bottom line:
Alcoholic drinks add extra calories to your waistline. Plus, you may eat more when you drink, so now there are extra calories from the drinks and the extra food. Just one drink (a bottle of beer or 1½ ounces/45 mL liquor with mix) a week can result in a 2 lb (1 kg) weight gain over the year. Five drinks a week can result in a 10 lb (4.5 kg) gain over the year.

Non-drinker –
zero drinks

Moderate drinker –
one drink a day for women; two drinks a day for men.

Heavy drinker –
more than three drinks a day.

Do not drink and drive.

If you don't drink — don't start. The risks outweigh the benefits.

Alcohol and energy drinks

Do not mix energy drinks with alcohol. Most energy drinks are high in caffeine. Both caffeine and alcohol are diuretics. They can cause dehydration and heart irregularities. You are particularly susceptible to dehydration when your blood sugar is high.

Low blood sugar if you are on insulin or medications

You can get a low blood sugar if you drink alcohol and you are taking insulin or certain types of diabetes medications. See below and low blood sugar information on pages 331–338. Over-drinking puts you at serious risk for low blood sugar that can occur up to 24 hours after drinking. If you have drunk too much, make sure you eat or drink some carbohydrate, and someone should stay with you and check your blood sugar every 2–4 hours, even during the night.

Avoiding low blood sugar when drinking alcohol:

- limit drinks to one or two
- do not drink on an empty stomach
- have extra sugar handy
- if also exercising, (e.g., dancing and drinking) have a snack to make up for the effect of the exercise

Does alcohol have benefits?

Research shows that drinking alcohol in moderation, especially red wine, has some benefits in reducing heart disease. In part this may be due to an antioxidant called resveratrol. This is in the skin and seeds of grapes, especially dark red and purple grapes. Some of these same benefits can come from having a ½ cup (125 mL) portion of red grapes or a small glass of red grape juice (limit to 2 ounces as a serving). Another possible benefit of moderate alcohol intake is that for some people, it may help insulin work better.

Moderate consumption may help some people manage occasional stress, by helping them relax and have fun. This is a good thing, but the key is moderation.

Alcoholic Drink	Portion (in most common drink size)	Alcohol (1 ounce = 9.6 g)	Sugar (Total carbohydrate is converted into tsps of sugar)	Calories
Spirits (hard liquor) For example, whiskey, rum, brandy, vodka or gin. 40% alcohol by volume = 80% proof				
On ice, or mixed with water or diet soft drink	1½ oz (45 mL)	1½ oz (45 mL)	0	100
Mixed with 4 oz (125 mL) soft drink or fruit juice (based on cola)	5½ oz (165 mL)	1½ oz (45 mL)	3¼ tsp (16 mL)	150
Mixed with 4 oz (125 mL) tomato or clamato juice	5½ oz (165 mL)	1½ oz (45 mL)	1¼ tsp (6 mL)	120
Beer				
Canadian beer (7% alcohol)	12 oz (341 mL)	2 oz (60 mL)	2½ tsp (12 mL)	185
American beer (5% alcohol)	12 oz (341 mL)	1½ oz (45 mL)	2½ tsp (12 mL)	140
Light beer (Canadian 4% alcohol)	12 oz (341 mL)	1 oz (30 mL)	1 tsp (5 mL)	100
Light beer (American 4% alcohol)	12 oz (341 mL)	1 oz (30 mL)	1 tsp (5 mL)	100–110
Low carb beer (4% alcohol)	12 oz (341 mL)	1 oz (30 mL)	½ tsp (2 mL)	90
Low-alcohol beer (0.5% alcohol)	12 oz (341 mL)	0.1 oz (3 mL)	2½–4 tsp (12–20 mL)	65
Wine Alcohol content of wine can vary a lot. A light white wine may have 9%, a full bodied red wine may have up to 12% and sherry and port have around 20% alcohol. Champagne might not have a high alcohol content but the bubbles in it cause it to be absorbed into your blood more quickly.				
Dessert wine, sweet (15–18% alcohol)	5 oz (150 mL)	1¾–2½ oz (52–75 mL)	4–5 tsp (20–25 mL)	210–275
Dessert wine, dry (18% alcohol)	5 oz (150 mL)	2½ oz (75 mL)	½ tsp (2 mL)	165
Table wine, red or white (12% alcohol)	5 oz (150 mL)	1½ oz (45 mL)	¼–½ tsp (1–2 mL)	100–110
Champagne (8–14% alcohol)	5 oz (150 mL)	1½ oz (45 mL)	1 tsp (5 mL)	105
Low alcohol wine (0.5% alcohol)	5 oz (150 mL)	0.1 oz (3 mL)	3½ tsp (17 mL)	65
Ciders				
Sweet cider (6% alcohol)	12 oz (341 mL)	1¾ oz (52 mL)	3½ tsp (17 mL)	170
Dry cider (6% alcohol)	12 oz (341 mL)	1¾ oz (52 mL)	3 tsp (15 mL)	130
Coolers				
Vodka cooler (5% alcohol)	12 oz (341 mL)	1½ oz (45 mL)	7 tsp (35 mL)	220
Citrus Cooler (5% alcohol)	12 oz (341 mL)	1½ oz (45 mL)	9 tsp (45 mL)	240
Light cooler (3% alcohol)	12 oz (341 mL)	¾ oz (22 mL)	6–11 tsp (30–55 mL)	170–250
Cocktails (made to standard size recipes and sizes)				
Daiquiri	4 oz (125 mL)	2 oz (60 mL)	2 tsp (10 mL)	140
Margarita	4 oz (125 mL)	2 oz (60 mL)	1½ tsp (7 mL)	150
Mojito	4 oz (125 mL)	2 oz (60 mL)	1½ tsp (7 mL)	160
Piña colada (also high in fat)	8 oz (250 mL)	2 oz (60 mL)	3 tsp (15 mL)	325
No-alcohol drink – Bloody Mary	4 oz (125 mL)	0	2 tsp (10 mL)	40
No-alcohol drink – Strawberry daiquiri	4 oz (125 mL)	0	12 tsp (60 mL)	200
Liqueurs				
Cream-based (34–53% proof)	1½ oz (45 mL)	1 oz (30 mL)	3–6 tsp (15–30 mL)	135–165
Non-cream based (80% proof)	1½ oz (45 mL)	1–1½ oz (30–45 mL)	1½–2½ tsp (30–55 mL)	115–135

- **High blood sugar.**
  Your blood sugar is
  consistently above
  15 mmol/L (270 mg/dL)
  and you feel very unwell.

- **Low blood sugar.**
  You are having continual
  lows, and you are unable
  to keep your blood
  sugar above 4 mmol/L
  (70 mg/dL).

- **Dehydration.** Symptoms
  include being very thirsty,
  your mouth and skin is
  dry and when you pinch
  your skin it doesn't
  bounce back. You have
  muscle cramps, reduced
  sweat and urine, and
  you may feel dizzy or
  confused. Dehydration
  can happen because of
  vomiting, diarrhea, fever
  and high blood sugar.

- **Fever.** You have a fever
  over 100° Fahrenheit
  (37.8°C).

- **Bleeding**. You have
  blood in your urine,
  stool or vomit.

- **Unusual symptoms
  such as numbness
  or stiff neck.**

- **Concerns that you feel
  sicker.** You worry about
  your illness and your
  symptoms get worse.

9. What to eat when ill

This section provides five guidelines for coping with a brief
illness. It also includes photographs to give you ideas of
what to drink or eat when you are sick. A brief illness might
include the flu, a cold, food poisoning, or a bout of severe
pain lasting one or several days. You may be vomiting,
have diarrhea, a cough, sore throat, fever, pain or infection.
For guidelines on when you should see a doctor, see sidebar.
For extended illnesses, consult your doctor or diabetes
educator for guidelines.

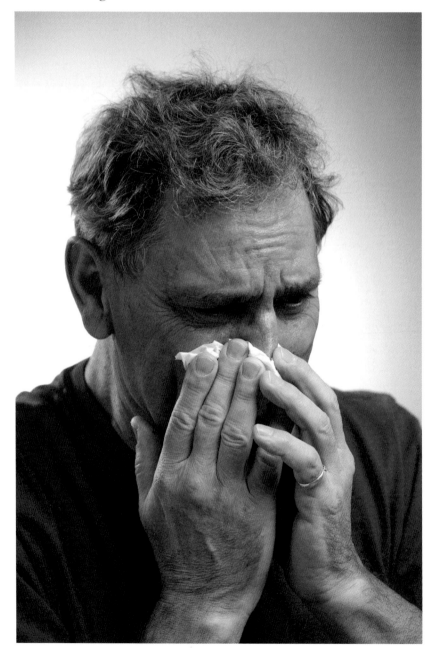

1) *Take your insulin and medication*

When you're sick, blood sugar most often goes up, even if you aren't eating much. The reason blood sugar usually goes up is that illness or pain increases stress hormones in your body. These hormones increase your blood sugar.

Occasionally, blood sugar can go low, especially if you aren't eating and have severe diarrhea and vomiting.

Adjusting insulin

- If you take insulin and adjust it yourself, then follow your adjustment guidelines.

- If you don't adjust your own insulin, contact your doctor or diabetes educator for recommendations.

Diabetes pills

- Don't change your dosage of diabetes pills during a short illness.

Other medications

- If a doctor prescribes any medication for short-term illness such as pain killers, antibiotics or decongestants, ask if it will affect your blood sugar. Also, over-the-counter medications can affect blood sugar or blood pressure. Ask your pharmacist or doctor about these.

Cough drops and syrups and cold medicines

- Check labels of cough or cold medicines for sugar (carbohydrate). One teaspoon of sugar will equal 4 grams of carbohydrate. If you can't tolerate most foods, then take regular sugar-containing cough drops or cough syrup as part of your daily carbohydrate intake, see page 142.

- If you are able to eat other foods, or your blood sugar is high, use sugar-free cough drops or cough syrup.

Sugar-free products can cause diarrhea

Be aware that sugar-free products usually have alcohol sugars in them (see page 102) such as sorbitol or isomalt. These can cause mild diarrhea if you eat 10 g in a day, and severe diarrhea if you eat 20 g or more in a day. A typical sugar-free cough drop can have 2–4 grams of sugar alcohol each, so just 3–4 sugar free cough drops could cause or worsen diarrhea.

Take your medication

Keep taking your insulin or diabetes pills, unless your doctor or nurse tells you otherwise.

Plan ahead

Talk to your doctor or diabetes educator before you get sick, and learn how to adjust your insulin if you are sick.

If you live on your own:

Tell a family member or friend that you are sick. They may need to come and stay with you or call or check on you periodically.

Gargle a salt and water solution to help relieve a sore throat.

If you don't test your blood sugar at home

Learn the signs and symptoms of high and low blood sugars, see page 18 and 333. Also see treatment of lows on pages 334–336.

One cup an hour

As a general rule, try to drink a cup of fluids every hour that you are awake.

Limit or avoid red liquids and foods

This includes red foods such as red Jell-O, cranberry juice, red Popsicles, cream soda, red cough candies or beets. These can be confused with blood if you are vomiting or have diarrhea.

2) Check your blood sugar

How often you need to check your blood sugar will depend on how sick you are. To be safe, check your blood sugar every 4 hours and more often if they are going too high or too low. Write down your blood sugar numbers. Call your doctor or diabetes educator for guidance about adjusting your insulin dosage.

3) Drink lots of water and sugar-free fluids

It's easy to become dehydrated when your blood sugars are high, or if you run a fever, vomit or have diarrhea. Therefore, extra sugar-free fluids are essential.

Examples of sugar-free fluids are on page 141.

- You may tolerate diet soft drinks better if they are flat (without bubbles). Stir with a spoon and let sit for an hour before drinking it.
- Avoid caffeine or limit coffee, strong tea and caffeinated colas to less than 4 cups (1 L) a day. Their caffeine can cause you to lose further water.

> **If you are not able to drink enough fluid, call your doctor.**
>
> Your doctor may tell you to stop certain pills to protect your kidneys.

4) Eat lightly

If you aren't up to eating your usual meals and snacks, substitute lighter foods or drinks. Examples of light foods or drinks when you are ill are on page 142. These will help provide you with some carbohydrate as well as electrolytes (sodium and potassium). Do not drink alcohol unless recommended by your doctor. Alcohol can contribute to a seriously low blood sugar.

5) Rest and sleep

If you can, move your limbs and walk around a little to help your circulation. If you feel nauseated, keep your head and shoulders raised when resting. Wear loose clothing or pajamas, and put a cool cloth on your face and neck.

Sugar-free fluids – Sip on these throughout the day and evening.

1. Mineral water or soda water
2. Water
3. Crystal Light or Sugar-Free Kool-Aid
4. Diet soft drinks (caffeine-free)
5. Sugar-free Jell-O
6. Weak tea
7. If you can't keep anything down, try sipping on ice chips
8. Herbal tea (such as ginger tea)
9. Sugar-free Popsicle or Freezee
10. Broth or consommé

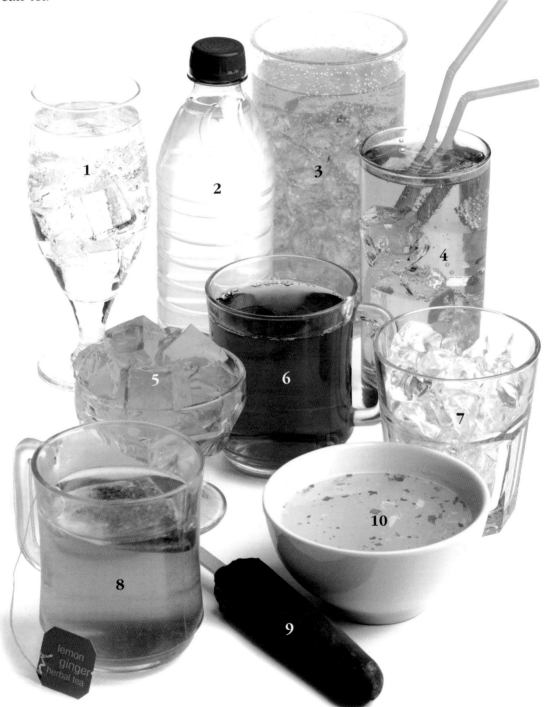

Examples of some lighter foods or drinks each having 15 grams of carbohydrate – try to choose one of these every hour.

1. Kool Aid – 1 pouch (¾ cup/175 mL)
2. Ginger ale or 7-up (regular) – ¾ cup (175 mL)
3. Pedialyte (pediatric) – 2½ cups (625 mL)
4. Gatorade (regular) – 1 cup (250 mL)
5. Orange juice – ½ cup (125 mL)
6. Nutritional supplement for diabetes – 1 cup (250 mL)
7. Yogurt (plain or diet) – ¾ cup (175 mL)
8. Hot tea or lemon with 3 tsp (15 mL) of honey or sugar
9. Apple juice – ½ cup (125 mL)
10. Ice cream, sherbert or frozen yogurt – ½ cup (125 mL)
11. Cola, caffeine-free – 1 cup (250 mL)
12. Rice cake – 1
13. Toast or bread, plain or lightly buttered – 1 slice
14. Applesauce – ½ cup (125 mL)
15. Soda crackers – 7
16. Melba toast – 4
17. Plain crackers (larger) – 3
18. Fruit roll-up – 1
19. Chicken noodle soup – 1 cup (250 mL) or ½ cup (125 mL) noodles
20. Cough syrup (regular) – 1–2 tsp (5–10 mL)
21. Banana – 1 small
22. Arrowroot biscuits – 3
23. Ginger cookies – 3
24. Jell-O (regular) – ½ cup (125 mL)
25. Rice Krispies, Special K or Corn Flakes with milk – ½ cup (125 mL)
26. Popsicle or frozen juice bar – 1 double stick
27. Lemon candies – 3

28. Cough candies (regular) – 4
29. Scotch mints (regular) – 4
30. Digestive cookies – 2
31. Jelly beans – 6

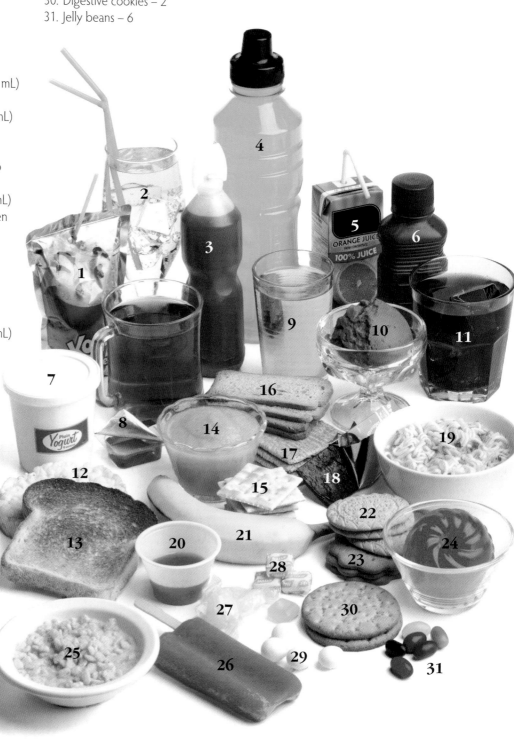

10. How to gain weight

Ten percent of people with type 2 diabetes are lean when diagnosed. Of this ten percent, some will be underweight at the time of diagnosis while others will become this way due to weight loss. If you are underweight, gaining weight will help you feel better. Weighing too little can make you more likely to get an infection or have poor strength or break a bone. High blood sugar, poor appetite, or inadequate food intake can all cause weight loss. There may also be an underlying health problem that may cause you to lose weight, so please talk to your doctor. This section provides guidelines as to how you can gain weight without raising your blood sugar a lot. Eating more as well as taking insulin or diabetes pills may help you gain needed weight. Moderate exercise helps build muscle.

First, determine if you are underweight

Are you truly underweight or just think you're too skinny? People on average weigh 25 lbs (11 kg) more now than 40 years ago, so it's important to not compare yourself to others. If you were a healthy weight as a young adult, use this weight as a guide. Also talk to your doctor or dietitian.

Diabetes medications may help with weight gain

High blood sugar can cause weight loss due to loss of large amounts of sugar in the urine. In order to stop losing weight and to regain lost weight, you need to bring down your blood sugar. It is likely you need diabetes pills or insulin. Talk to your doctor.

Small changes in how you eat makes a difference

When your appetite is poor, making small eating changes can make a difference. As with all people with diabetes, you will benefit from spreading your calories and carbohydrates across three small meals. You'll likely also need small snacks in between so that you get enough calories. It's helpful to add extra protein and fat to meals and snacks as this will give you calories with little increase to your blood sugar.

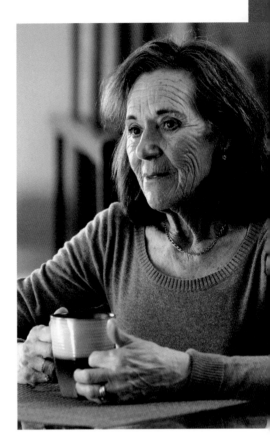

Body Mass Index (BMI)

You can also determine if you are underweight or at a healthy weight by comparing your weight to a chart called the Body Mass Index (search "BMI" on the internet). Also see page 340.

143

Tips to gain weight

Sample Meal Plan, below: shows you a healthy day's intake from the reduced calorie Seven Day Meal Plan, with ideas on how to boost the calories. This is just an example of a meal. Vary the portions and foods as necessary.

Ways to Boost Calories, pages 145–146: Choose from lots of ideas and foods. Foods high in saturated animal fat such as whole milk and cheese rather than the light varieties are marked here as "EXTRA FATS." If your cholesterol levels are good, choose these extra fats until you regain your lost weight.

Other things to help you gain weight, pages 147–148.

Sample High Calorie Meal Plan
Ways to increase calories at the meal or snack

Breakfast 1: Oatmeal (pages 152–153)	• Use whole milk or cream instead of skim milk • Add 2–3 teaspoons (10–15 mL) of oil, butter or margarine to your porridge • Put extra chopped nuts on top
Morning Snack: Small banana	• Spread some peanut butter on your banana
Lunch 1: Deluxe Sandwich (pages 160–161)	• Put margarine on both slices of bread • Add extra avocado or sliced olives to your sandwich • Have a piece of cheese with your apple
Afternoon Snack:	• Add a handful of peanuts to your small or medium snack
Dinner 1: Minute Steak and Potato (pages 168–171)	• Add extra margarine or butter, and/or shredded cheese to your potatoes • Use a high fat gravy instead of a fat-free variety • Choose a larger portion of meat • Fry onion in extra fat • Top your peas and carrots with some roasted sunflower seeds • Use a regular fat pudding when making the English Trifle • Add extra almonds to your serving of English Trifle
Evening Snack:	• Supplement a small to large snack with a diabetic nutrient bar or half a diabetes nutritional supplement beverage

Ways to boost calories

- Increase your portion of protein at all your meals and snacks. Protein includes lean meat, fish, skinless chicken, eggs, seafood, nuts and seeds.

- Add white beans or kidney beans to soup or casseroles. This will add some carbohydrate but will also boost protein.

- Try to always include a protein at breakfast. For example, an egg, a slice of low-fat cheese (less than 20% MF) or lean meat, or chopped nuts on cereal.

- Add a slice of cheese to make meat sandwiches higher in calories.

- Use sockeye salmon canned in oil, and tuna or sardines canned in oil.

- Boil and peel a few eggs and put them in the fridge. Several times a week, grab one for a snack or with a meal. Scramble eggs with added fat and cheese.

- Swirl a beaten egg into soup or into macaroni and cheese while it is cooking.

- Add sliced or shredded cheese to soups, salads, sandwiches and casseroles, stews, mashed potatoes, ravioli and tacos. Have cheese as a snack with crackers or a muffin.

- Add a cheese sauce to vegetables.

- Add almonds, pistachios, walnuts, pecans, peanuts, hazelnuts, cashews or soy nuts, or pumpkin seeds or sunflower seeds, to casseroles, salads, and desserts. Also choose these as snacks or on the side with your meals.

- Top pancakes or cereal with crushed nuts.

- Have a spoonful of peanut butter straight from the jar! Look for trans fat-free peanut butter. Add peanut butter to fruit smoothies or milkshakes, or to a stir fry, tomato soup or casseroles. Try a half peanut butter and cheese sandwich as a snack or a spoonful of peanut butter stirred into ½ cup (125 mL) of sugar-free vanilla yogurt or vanilla pudding.

- For a snack have a half sandwich or one piece of bread with any protein added: meat and cheese, salmon or peanut butter.

- Rather than eat fruit on its own, eat it with a piece of cheese, a spread of peanut butter or a few nuts. Try half a small banana spread with peanut butter, or apple slices with 1–2 ounces (30–60 g) of cheese or a spread of light cream cheese.

ADD EXTRA FATS
(if your cholesterol levels are normal)

MEATS: Choose medium to fatty cuts of meat, and chicken with the skin.

CHEESE: Use regular fat cheese.

EGGS: Eat eggs daily.

YOGURT: Some yogurts are made with cream (5% or more MF) rather than milk and so are higher in fat and calories.

PUDDING: Make your pudding with whole milk or even half and half cereal cream. Whole fat sour cream can be mixed in to the pudding.

BUTTER OR CREAM CHEESE: Choose butter or regular cream cheese instead of light cream cheese.

MILK: Drink whole (homogenized) milk (not low fat milk). Use whole evaporated milk.

MILK POWDER: Use a whole milk powder instead of skim milk powder.

CREAM INSTEAD OF MILK:

Put half and half cream or whipped cream on your cereal, in your coffee or tea, and on puddings and canned fruit.

CREAM DRINK:

Drink a small glass of whipping cream flavored with a bit of vanilla or your own favorite flavoring. Sip with a straw.

ADDITIONS TO RECIPES:

Add butter, full-fat cream cheese, gravy, full-fat sour cream and whipping cream to recipes and foods.

- Olives have healthy monounsaturated fat; enjoy a few.
- Avocado is low in carbohydrates and also rich in monounsaturated fat. Slice it up and add it to a sandwich, tortilla roll, tacos or in a salad. Try halving an avocado and eating it with a spoon. It is nice served with a dash of Worcestershire sauce, or lemon or lime juice.
- When making sandwiches or toast or having a slice of bread, crackers or a muffin, top it with some margarine or other fat such as cream cheese. Try a slice of raisin bread with 2–3 teaspoons (10–15 mL) of spread on top.
- Drink 1% or 2% milk instead of skim.
- Greek yogurt (unsweetened) is high in protein and some varieties are also very high in fat, further boosting calories.
- You can also use low-fat evaporated milk full strength. A half cup (125 mL) will equal 1 cup (250 mL) regular milk. You can add this to cereal, puddings or coffee or tea, or hot cocoa.
- Add skim milk powder to soups, stews, casseroles, mashed potatoes, cereals and scrambled eggs.
- Add ¼ cup (60 mL) of skim milk powder to each cup (250 mL) of milk to double the protein. Also, stir 1 tablespoon (15 mL) of skim milk powder into a cup of yogurt or pudding. If using a plain yogurt, you can sprinkle in some sugar-free drink crystals for flavoring.
- Add protein supplements, such as Beneprotein, to a variety of foods.
- Add dried unsweetened coconut to desserts, or coconut milk to curries or to beverages such as smoothies. New evidence indicates that coconut milk has a healthy type of fat, as long as it is not hydrogenated.
- Add extra oil such as olive, canola, corn or soya oil, margarine, mayonnaise, and salad dressings to recipes and foods such as mashed potatoes, rice or pasta, oatmeal, scrambled eggs, TV dinners or casseroles. Fry foods to get extra calories from the fats.
- Buy diabetes nutritional supplement beverages or snack bars at pharmacies or some large food stores, sometimes called "meal replacements." Look for brands that say they are especially for people with diabetes. These will usually be high in fiber.

Remember, these additions to your diet are just if you're trying to gain weight. Take care not to feed your family members extra fat if they do not need the additional calories.

Other things to help you gain weight

Eat three small meals **plus** snacks

- Have your meals and snacks at regular times. You may want to set an alarm to remind yourself to eat.

- Have a full meal at the time of the day when your appetite is best.

Take a multivitamin pill if you are not eating well

If you have lost a lot of weight or aren't eating well, a "one-a-day" vitamin and mineral pill may be helpful. Ask the pharmacist for a vitamin pill that does not interact with any other medications you take.

Slowly increase your food

Slowly increase your food intake to allow your body some time to get used to the extra food.

Don't fill up on low-calorie foods

Limit plain coffee, tea, clear soup, diet drinks or raw, bulky vegetables. These fill you up but don't give you the calories that you need. However, drinking water is still so important to help flush out your bladder and empty your bowels, and so you don't get dehydrated.

If you get tired easily, use quick and easy foods

- Keep easy-to-make and favorite foods on hand and in sight.

- Buy ready-to-eat meals and foods such as instant oatmeal, ready-to-eat puddings or fruits cups. Try occasional frozen entrees or pre-cooked foods, or salads from the deli.

- Cook meals in advance and freeze them in single portions.

- Order some extra meals to be delivered. Consider signing up for Meals on Wheels or ordering a pizza delivery.

- Share a meal with a friend, neighbor or family member. It's nice for a change to eat out at a restaurant, senior center, or a meal program at an apartment block or personal care home.

If you are a senior:

Getting out more often may improve your appetite overall. Talk to friends or call the senior center to find out if there is anything going on that interests you. If you need a ride, call your local seniors' centre and ask them if they offer rides.

Mouth rinse

Rinse with club soda or make this homemade rinse: mix ⅛ teaspoon (0.5 mL) of salt (or ¼ teaspoon/1 mL baking soda) in 1 cup (250 mL) of water.

Boost your appetite

Dress it up: Make your meal look good by using a colorful place mat, table cloth or napkin. Place a flower or candle on the table. Change these often. You deserve the best.

Flavor it up: Foods will taste better if you add herbs and spices. Ask your doctor or dietitian if it's okay for you to add a bit of salt to your food, as this also helps with flavor.

Sunlight helps: If possible, dine by a window to get some sunlight. Choose a comfortable chair to sit in when you eat. If you eat meals in your bed or in a big chair, prop yourself up with pillows so that you can see your food and eat easily.

Fresh air too: Try to get some fresh air every day. If you can't get outside, open a window briefly to allow stale smells to leave and to let in fresh air. When the weather is nice, try eating some meals outside on a deck, balcony or bench.

Drink wine or a tart drink. Ask your doctor if an occasional 3–5 ounce (90–150 mL) glass of wine before or with a meal would be okay. This could help lift your appetite. Instead of wine, you could start your meal with a tart drink such as tomato juice. Beware – regular alcohol consumption could make you disoriented and increase your risk of a fall.

Freshen up your mouth: Some medications can cause a bad taste in your mouth and take away your appetite. Try chewing on a sprig of mint or parsley. Cinnamon or mint flavored sugar-free gum might also help. Also, see the section on proper tooth and mouth care on pages 297–300.

Keep active

Do some physical activity – even a short walk can help improve your appetite. Lifting small weights also helps you gain muscle as weight. This also brings down blood sugar and is good for your overall health. Walking, swimming and biking build muscles and weight – increase exercise gradually. See pages 247–251 for ideas on a Level 1 or 2 strength training and exercise program.

Monitor your weight and request regular lab tests

- Have your weight taken at the doctor's office. Write down your weight. Also ask when your last weight was taken and how much you weighed.

- Tell your doctor or dietitian if you have lost more than 10 lbs (4.5 kg) in the last 6 months.

- Have your blood sugar A1C done (see pages 340 and 343–344).

Seven Day Meal Plan with Recipes

Breakfast Meals

1.	Oatmeal	152
2.	Fruit Crepes	154
3.	Cereal with Berries	156
4.	Poached Egg & Toast	158

**All small breakfast meals have 250 calories
and all large breakfasts have 370 calories.**

Lunch Meals

1.	Deluxe Sandwich	160
2.	Taco Soup	162
3.	Luncheon Wrap	164
4.	Pizza Bun	166

**All small lunches have 400 calories
and all large lunches have 520 calories.**

Dinner Meals

1.	Minute Steak with Potato	168
2.	Nuts and Bolts Stir Fry	172
3.	Hot Chicken Salad	176
4.	Vegetarian Sauce & Pasta	180
5.	Seafood Chowder	184
6.	Chicken Curry & Rice	188
7.	Vegetable Omelet & Beans	192

**All small dinners have 550 calories
and all large dinners have 730 calories.**

Snacks

Low Calorie (20 calories or less)	197
Small (50 calories)	198
Medium (100 calories)	199
Large (200 calories)	200

149

Nutrient Analysis

Nutrient analysis for the recipes and meals were calculated by Food Intelligence (Toronto, Ontario) with the assistance of Genesis R&D software using the Canadian Nutrient File 2007b and USDA Nutrient Database for Standard Reference.

The calculations based on imperial weights and measures (pounds, cups, tablespoons, etc), used:

- skim milk
- lean ground beef (hamburger) with less than 17% fat
- rice, pasta and hot cereals without the addition of salt
- 3 medium or 4 small boiling potatoes per pound (500 g), and approximately 3 large or 4 medium baking potatoes per 2 pounds (1 kg)
- granulated white sugar unless otherwise specified
- large eggs
- typical addition of unmeasured ingredients (e.g., tomato in sandwich).

If there was a choice of ingredients, the first listed was calculated. If there was a range of quantity, the smaller amount was calculated.

Carbohydrate Choices
Carbohydrate Choices for the meals were based on the Canadian Diabetes Association *Beyond the Basics Poster.* Each carbohydrate choice has 15 grams of available carbohydrate (total carbohydrate minus fiber).

Small breakfasts: 2–3
Large breakfasts: 3–4

Small lunches: 2.5–3.5
Large lunches: 3.5–4.5

Small dinners: 3–4.5
Large dinners: 4–5.5

Should I choose the large or small meals?

If you choose a small breakfast, lunch and dinner, you will get 1200 calories.

If you choose a large breakfast, lunch and dinner, you will get 1,620 calories.

Mix and match your meals. If you want, add in snacks to get a meal plan from 1200–2200 calories a day. See chart below.

A. Daily Meal Plan Chart

small meals with no snacks	1,200 calories
small meals with two small snacks	1,300 calories
small meals with one small and two medium snacks	1,450 calories
small meals with one small, one medium and one large snack	1,550 calories
large meals with no snacks	1,620 calories
large meals with two small snacks	1,720 calories
large meals with one small and two medium snacks	1,870 calories
large meals with one small, one medium and one large snack	1,970 calories
large meals with three large snacks	2,220 calories

Calories for the small meals:
- breakfast has 250 calories
- lunch has 400 calories
- dinner has 550 calories

Calories for the large meals:
- breakfast has 370 calories
- lunch has 520 calories
- dinner has 730 calories

Calories for the snacks:
- low-calorie snack has 20 calories or less
- small snack has 50 calories
- medium snack has 100 calories
- large snack has 200 calories

All the small and large meals in this book have the same calories as the seventy meals in my other book, Diabetes Meals for Good Health. These recipes and meals will give you more choices when planning your day's intake.

151

BREAKFAST 1

Oatmeal

For an added health bonus, this breakfast includes:

- *Cranberries. These may help reduce cholesterol. If you don't have cranberries, have chopped apple or another fruit instead.*

- *Cinnamon. Due to its flavor, when you use cinnamon you don't need as much sugar to sweeten food. A ½–1 tsp (2–5 mL) serving of cinnamon a day may help reduce blood sugar.*

- *Pecans. These provide protein to keep you feeling full through the morning. Pecans, almonds, peanuts, hazelnuts, walnuts, pistachios, and sunflower or pumpkin seeds are all a great source of healthy fats.*

- *A sprinkle of bran cereal for extra fiber.*

All forms of oatmeal have soluble fiber which slows down blood sugar and helps lower cholesterol. Slower cooking types of oatmeal are in a more whole, unprocessed form, and are the healthiest. This includes steel cut oats and large flaked oats. They take longer to digest, meaning a slower rise in blood sugar. For more information on absorption rates of different carbohydrates, see glycemic index on pages 90–93. Follow the package directions for cooking your oatmeal.

Steel cut oats – slowest cooking (10–20 minutes)
These are whole oats (including the hull) chopped in several pieces. They look like little pellets. Scottish Oatmeal cooks a bit faster as it has smaller chopped pieces of oats.

Large flaked oats (5 minutes to cook)
These oats have been flattened (rolled). They look like flakes.

Quick cooking oats (2–3 minutes to cook)
The processing of these rolled oats lasts longer than the large flaked oats. They are smaller flakes. They cook up in 2–3 minutes.

Instant oats – fastest cooking (ready to eat with hot water added)
The processing of these oats rolls them so much that it crushes them. They still have some of the benefits of oatmeal but have the highest glycemic index so will raise your blood sugar the fastest.

Your Breakfast Menu	Large Meal (370 calories)	Small Meal (250 calories)
Oatmeal or other hot cereal Topped with:	1½ cup (375 mL) cooked (9 tbsp/135 mL)	1 cup (250 mL) cooked (6 tbsp/90 mL)
• cranberries (dried and sweetened)	1½ tbsp (22 mL)	1 tbsp (15 mL)
• cinnamon and bran cereal	sprinkle	sprinkle
• brown sugar	1½ tsp (7 mL)	1 tsp (5 mL)
• pecans or other nuts, chopped	1 tbsp (15 mL)	1½ tsp (7 mL)
Skim or 1% milk	1 cup (250 mL)	1 cup (250 mL)

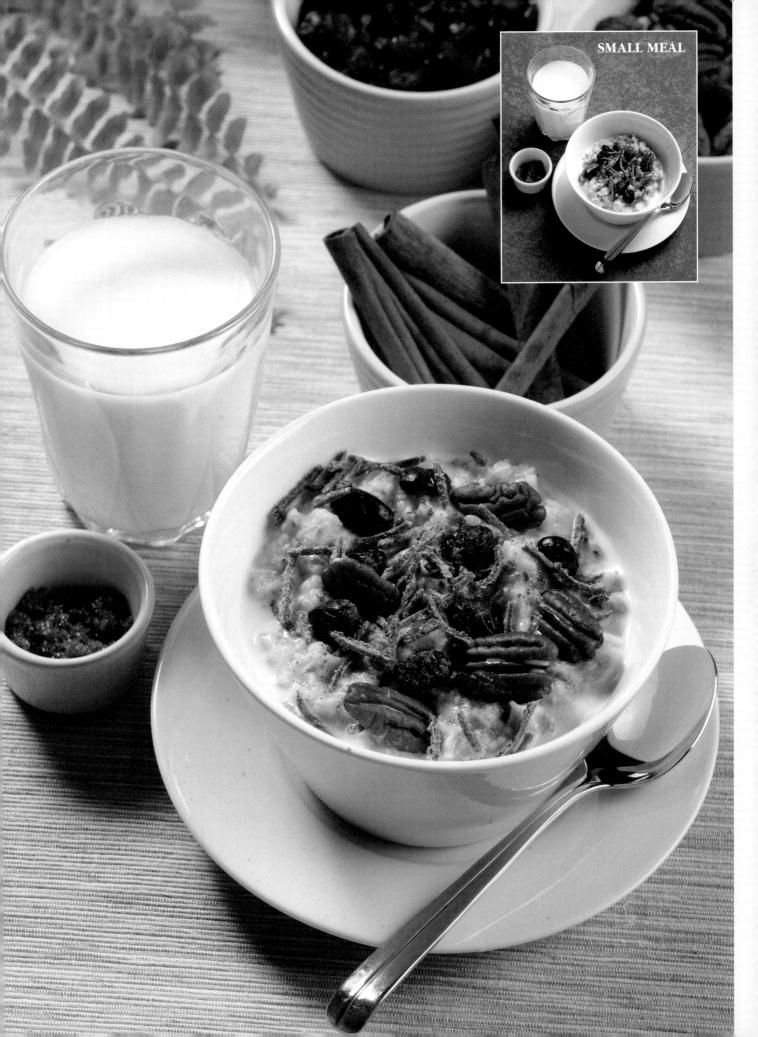

SMALL MEAL

BREAKFAST 2

Fruit Crepes

Crepes

Makes ten 8-inch (20 cm) crepes

1½ cups (375 mL) flour
½ tsp (2 mL) salt
1 tsp (5 mL) baking powder
1 tbsp (15 mL) sugar
2 eggs
1 cup (250 mL) skim milk
1 cup (250 mL) water
2 tbsp (30 mL) margarine or butter (for coating the pan)

Per crepe	
Calories	117
Carbohydrate	17 g
Fiber	1 g
Protein	4 g
Fat, total	4 g
Fat, saturated	1 g
Cholesterol	38 mg
Sodium	193 mg

Crepes are like thin pancakes. Fill them with a variety of fillings.

Crepe fillings:

- *cottage cheese, shredded cheese, yogurt, low sugar pudding*

- *fruit such as sliced peaches or pears, chopped apple, blueberries or strawberries, orange pieces or chopped banana, or dried dates or figs*

- *chopped peppers, mushrooms or salsa*

- *smoked salmon or shrimp*

1. In a large bowl mix together the flour, salt, baking powder and sugar.

2. In a medium bowl, beat the eggs with a fork or whisk. Add the milk and water to the eggs, and mix well.

3. Add the egg mixture to the flour mixture. Whisk until smooth.

4. Heat a stick free pan or crepe pan on medium to high heat. Using a pastry brush, lightly coat the pan with butter or margarine

5. Ladle a thin layer of crepe mixture into the pan. For a 12-inch (30 cm) frying pan you will need just under ¼ cup (60 mL) per crepe. Immediately tip the pan to even out the layer of batter. Cook until the edges are a little brown. Flip over and quickly cook the other side.

6. When making your next crepe, spread some more fat on the pan using your pastry brush.

7. Put some filling in your cooked crepes (see sidebar for a few examples), then roll up or fold, and cut in half. Sprinkle with low calorie sweetener if desired.

Your Breakfast Menu	Large Meal (370 calories)	Small Meal (250 calories)
Crepes	2	1
1% or 2% cottage cheese (or shredded cheddar cheese)	½ cup (125 mL) (or 3 tbsp/45 mL)	½ cup (125 mL) (or 3 tbsp/45 mL)
Peach	1	1
Tea	1 cup (250 mL)	1 cup (250 mL)

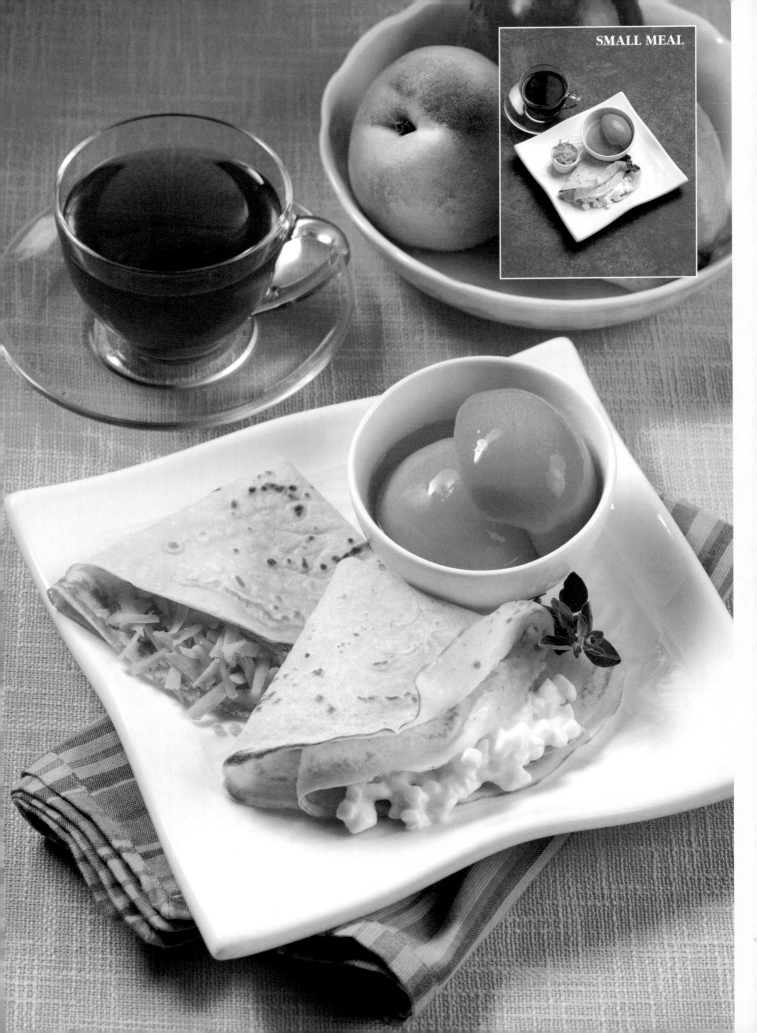

SMALL MEAL

BREAKFAST 3

Cereal with Berries

Shredded Wheat is an excellent cereal choice. It is a good source of fiber and has no added fat or sugar.

Other examples of healthy dry cereals include:

- Wheetabix or Muffets
- Fiber 1
- Bran Flakes
- Kashi Heart to Heart

Rice Krispies, Puffed Wheat or Special K are also low-fat cereals so are good. However, these ones are low-fiber so if you want, you could add a teaspoon of wheat germ, bran or ground flax seed to your bowl.

Tips when you are shopping:

- Buy food products with a shorter ingredient list. These are often more healthy and have fewer additives.

- Fill your cart up with lots of foods that don't have labels – especially fruits and vegetables, and grains. These are Mother Nature's foods. Foods without labels will usually have more nutrients and fiber and less fat, sugar and salt.

- When buying cereals remember that
  1 tsp (5 mL) of sugar = 4 g
  1 tsp (5 mL) of fat = 5 g

- For more label reading tips about cereals go to page 97 and 202.

Are you looking for a caffeine-free hot drink to have with breakfast? Try a cup of herbal tea or grain beverage with chicory (such as Caf-Lib). You probably won't need to add any sweetener as the flavoring from the herbs or chicory root gives a natural sweetening. Add a small amount of milk if desired.

½ cup (125 mL) spoon size shredded wheat equals 1 biscuit.

Include a fruit with your cereal to start your day off right:

Blueberries and other berries have lots of antioxidants. These help keep your blood vessels healthy by reducing inflammation. Fresh and frozen (thawed) berries are equally nutritious.

Nuts add protein to make you feel full through the morning.

Your Breakfast Menu	Large Meal (370 calories)	Small Meal (250 calories)
Shredded Wheat or other cold cereal	1½ biscuit	1 biscuit
Skim or 1% milk	1 cup (250 mL)	½ cup (125 mL)
Blueberries or other berries	1 cup (250 mL)	½ cup (125 mL)
Chopped nuts (walnuts and almonds)	2 tbsp (30 mL)	2 tbsp (30 mL)
Cup of grain beverage with chicory (or coffee or tea)	1 cup (250 mL) (1 tbsp/15 mL of beverage blend)	1 cup (250 mL) (1 tbsp/15 mL of beverage blend)

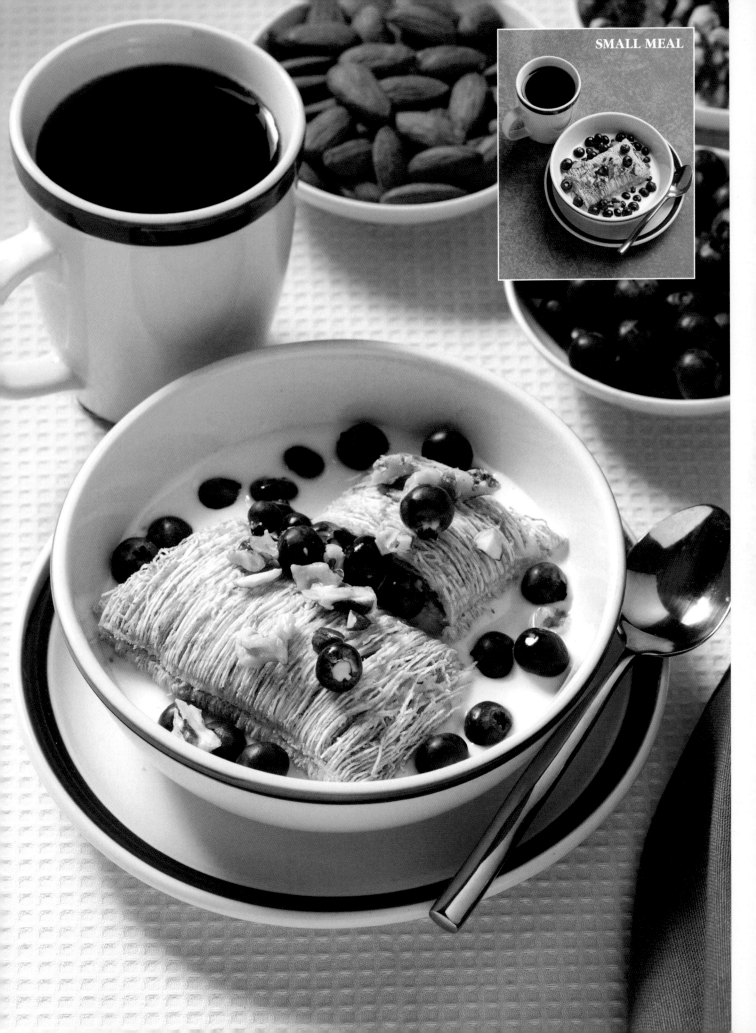

SMALL MEAL

BREAKFAST 4

Poached Egg & Toast

Choose whole grain and skinny bread!

Thinner sliced bread is best! If you want to decrease your carbohydrates and calories from bread, check the label for ones that have no more than 28 grams and about 70 calories per slice. Thinner sliced bread (whether white or whole wheat) will have less effect on your blood sugar. Some breads that are marketed as "healthier" with lots of grains in them are actually cut very thick, and in some cases can have double the calories and carbohydrates of a regular sliced bread. Over the past ten years, bakers decided to slice bread slices thicker, without us even knowing it.

Want a bagel instead of toast?

Look for whole grain, small bagels. A 3-inch (7.5 cm) will equal 2 slices of bread. A typical 5-inch (12.5 cm) coffee shop bagel will equal almost 4 slices of bread. See page 203 and 204 for more information about an egg or bagel breakfast.

Now that you have your toast, top it with a protein:

- 1 egg
- 1 ounce (30 g) of cheese or 28 g cheese slice
- 1 tablespoon (15 mL) of peanut butter
- 1 tablespoon (15 mL) Nutella (hazelnut spread) can be chosen occasionally – it has more sugar, but less fat than peanut butter

Alternatives to 1 tomato:

- ½ cup (125 mL) tomato or vegetable juice
- 1 small mandarin orange
- ½ peach, pear or apple

Mom was right all along!

Studies have shown that eating breakfast can help you learn better. Eating in the morning starts your engine (your metabolism) so you begin to burn calories. This can help you lose weight – and keep it off. Also, when you eat breakfast and other regular meals you don't get as hungry and are less likely to eat more later. When you cut back on evening snacking, you wake up feeling ready for breakfast.

Oregano

Fresh or dried oregano adds nice flavor to eggs!

Your Breakfast Menu	Large Meal (370 calories)	Small Meal (250 calories)
Toast	2	1
Margarine or butter	2 tsp (10 mL)	1 tsp (5 mL)
Jam or jelly, or honey	1–2 tsp (5–10 mL) (or 1 tbsp/ 15 mL if low sugar jam)	1–2 tsp (5–10 mL) (or 1 tbsp/ 15 mL if low sugar jam)
Egg	1	1
Sliced tomato	1 medium	1 medium
Kiwi	1	1
Coffee	1 cup (250 mL)	1 cup (250 mL)

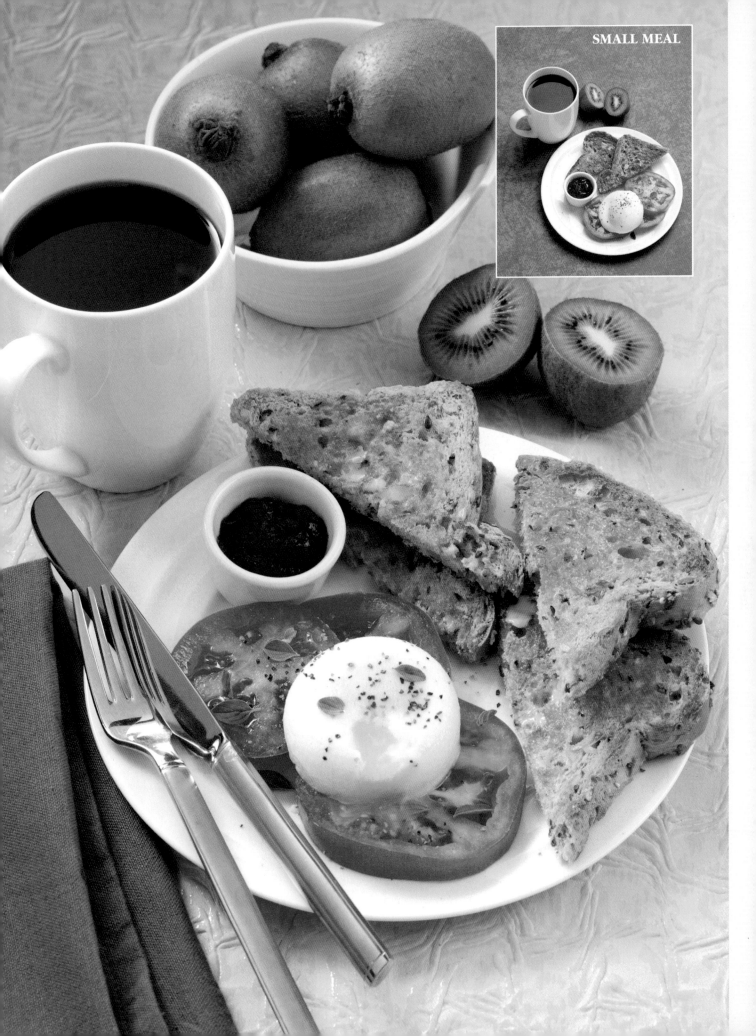

SMALL MEAL

LUNCH 1

Deluxe Sandwich

Try one of my three favorite sandwich fillings for 2 slices of bread. The large meal photo shows a half of each.

Grilled cheese:
1 ounce (30 g) of cheese
2 tsp (10 mL) of margarine spread on the outside of the sandwich

Fry sandwich in a frying pan or sandwich grill, on both sides, until golden brown.

Avocado and turkey bacon:
1 tbsp (15 mL) of light ranch or blue cheese dressing
½ small avocado
thinly sliced red onion
1 strip of cooked turkey bacon or 1 tbsp (15 mL) bacon bits

Ham and cheese:
1 ounce (30 g) ham or turkey
1 ounce (30 g) your favorite cheese
1 tbsp (15 mL) light mayonnaise
lettuce and tomato

Other sandwich options:

For protein: leftover chicken, turkey, beef or pork, or tuna, salmon, shrimp, crab or sardines, peanut butter or sliced egg.

For toppings: slices of red onion, fresh mushrooms, thinly sliced peppers (or roasted peppers), lightly cooked asparagus spears, salsa, sliced olives or pickles, hot peppers or alfalfa sprouts.

Instead of salt on your sandwich: black pepper, fresh basil, dill, parsley or coriander, or basil pesto (available in a jar or squeeze tube), green onion or red pepper jelly.

In a rush?

Pick up a hot, cooked rotisserie chicken, bring it home and remove all the skin. Slice it up for a fast filling for sandwiches or wraps. Also use it for your main course protein. No salt added rotisserie chickens are sold in some locations.

See page 205 for information about deli sandwiches.

Your Lunch Menu	Large Meal (520 calories)	Small Meal (400 calories)
Sandwich of your choice	1½ sandwiches	1 sandwich
Celery	2 stalks	2 stalks
Apple	½	1

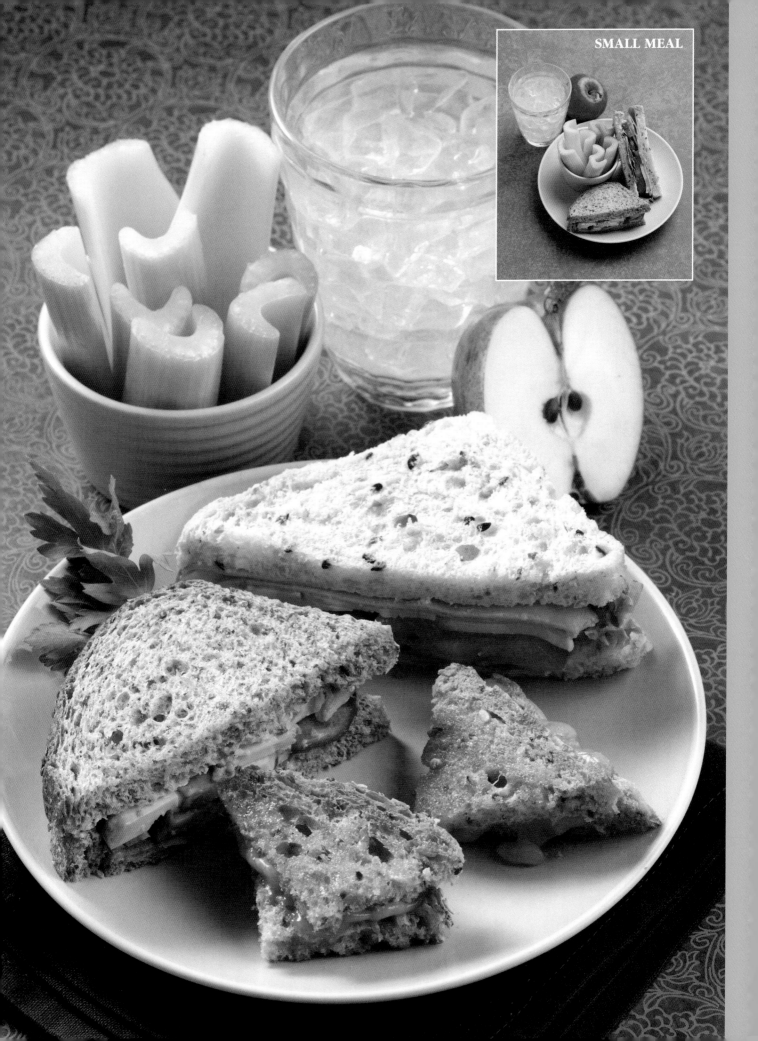

LUNCH 2

Taco Soup

Your favorite hearty bowl of soup with crackers makes a great lunch on a cold or hot day! Make this taco soup ahead, and freeze any leftovers. It is great for another lunch or for dinner.

Taco Soup

Makes 13 cups (3.25 L)

1 lb (500 g) of lean ground beef
1 medium onion, chopped
2 large stalks of celery, chopped
1 green pepper, chopped
28 ounce (796 mL) can tomatoes, diced or whole
19 ounce (540 mL) can kidney beans, rinsed
19 ounce (540 mL) can black beans, rinsed
2 cups (500 mL) of frozen kernel corn
2 tsp (10 mL) chili powder
1 tsp (5 mL) each of cumin, oregano, paprika and garlic powder
½ tsp (2 mL) of black pepper
2 cups (500 mL) water
Garnish: dollop of fat-free sour cream

1. Brown the hamburger meat at low-medium heat. Drain off any fat.

2. Add the onions, celery and green pepper. Cook until soft.

3. Add the rest of the ingredients. Add water if soup seems too thick.

4. Bring to a boil, then cover and simmer for 30 minutes. Add extra water if getting too thick.

Per cup (250 mL)
Calories 160
Carbohydrate ....21 g
Fiber .... 5 g
Protein ....12 g
Fat, total .... 4 g
Fat, saturated .... 1 g
Cholesterol........ 18 mg
Sodium..........283 mg

Tips to reduce salt

- *Reduce one third to one half of the salt from canned beans when you rinse them in cold water.*

- *Frozen corn has no salt added, whereas canned corn is quite salty. If using a can of corn, rinse the corn, and if available use a low sodium variety.*

- *Commercial taco mix is salty, so the mixture of spices in this recipe is a great replacement.*

- *Compare the salt in this soup to canned soup, see page 206.*

In this soup, you can use a combination of beans, such as navy, white and pinto.

Your Lunch Menu	Large Meal (520 calories)	Small Meal (400 calories)
Taco Soup (or other hearty soup)	2 cups (500 mL)	1 cup (250 mL)
Soda crackers	4	4
Carrot sticks	½ cup (125 mL)	½ cup (125 mL)
Skim or 1% milk	1 cup (250 mL)	1 cup (250 mL)
Grapes	15 (½ cup/125 mL)	15 (½ cup/125 mL)

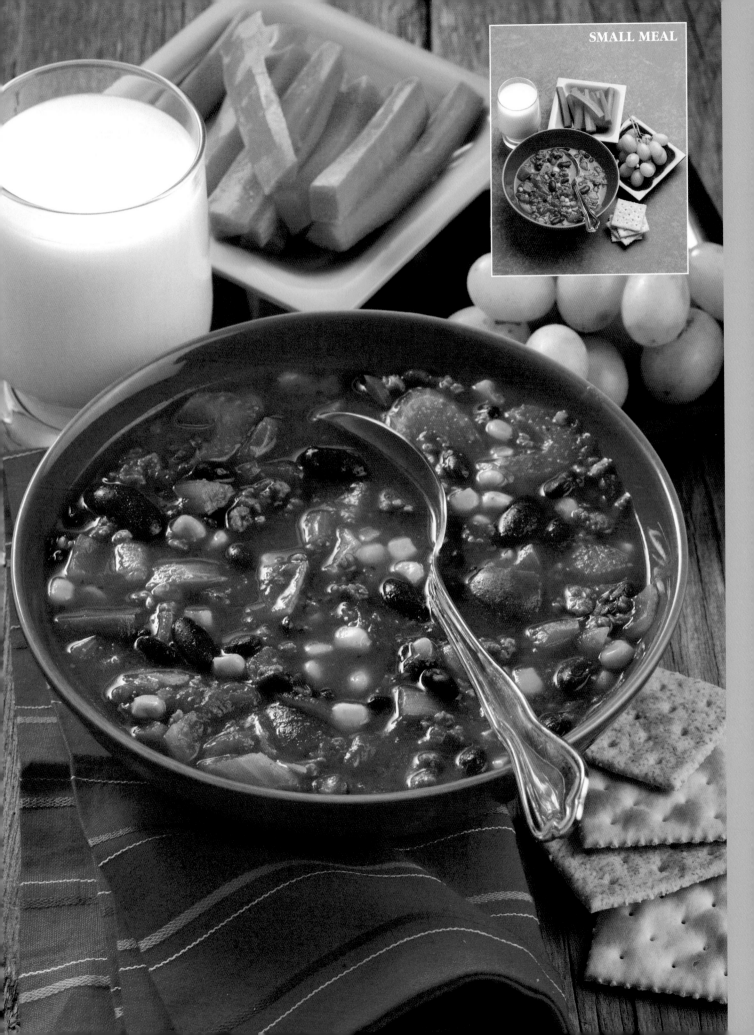

LUNCH 3

Luncheon Wrap

Serve these wraps cold. Enjoy them fresh or make them a day ahead and store in your fridge. Different kinds of tortilla shells include plain, or spinach, dried tomato or cheese flavored. Fill your wrap with some protein such as fish or shrimp, egg, meat, chicken or cheese, and some vegetables.

Cream cheese spread

Look for a lower fat variety with about 15% milk fat (M.F.) and 30 calories per tablespoon (15 mL). They come in a large variety of flavors. Types with herbs and garlic go well with a sandwich tortilla, but you can choose your own favorite flavor.

Restaurant wraps

A variety of fast food restaurants now carry wraps. If you are on the run for lunch, try to find a wrap that has 400 calories for the large meal or 300 calories for the small meal.

Luncheon Wrap

Here are the recipes for the three wraps shown in the photograph. The portions given below are for one 10-inch (25 cm) wrap (3 pieces).

Fish or seafood filling:

½ cup (125 mL) tuna, salmon, crab or shrimp, drained
2 tbsp (30 mL) light mayonnaise or fat-free mayonnaise
1 green onion (or chives) sliced or chopped

Egg salad filling:

2 hard boiled eggs, cooled and sliced or mashed
1 tbsp (15 mL) light mayonnaise or 2 tbsp (30 mL) fat-free mayonnaise
½ dill pickle, chopped

Meat and cheese filling:

1 tbsp (15 mL) of light cream cheese herb and garlic spread
2 ounces (60 g) of precooked chicken, turkey or meat
2 tbsp (30 mL) shredded light cheese
red pepper strips (roasted or raw) or shredded carrots
cooked asparagus spears

1. If using cream cheese, spread evenly on one side of the tortilla shell. If using mayonnaise, blend with your protein ingredient.

2. At one end of the tortilla shell, place the protein and vegetables. Add black pepper to taste.

3. Starting at the end with the filling, roll up the wrap into a tight roll.

4. Cut on an angle, in thirds, for a nice effect.

Your Lunch Menu	Large Meal (520 calories)	Small Meal (400 calories)
Wraps	1 wrap (3 pieces)	⅔ wrap (2 pieces)
Radishes	5	5
Skim or 1% milk	½ cup (125 mL)	½ cup (125 mL)
Pear	1	1

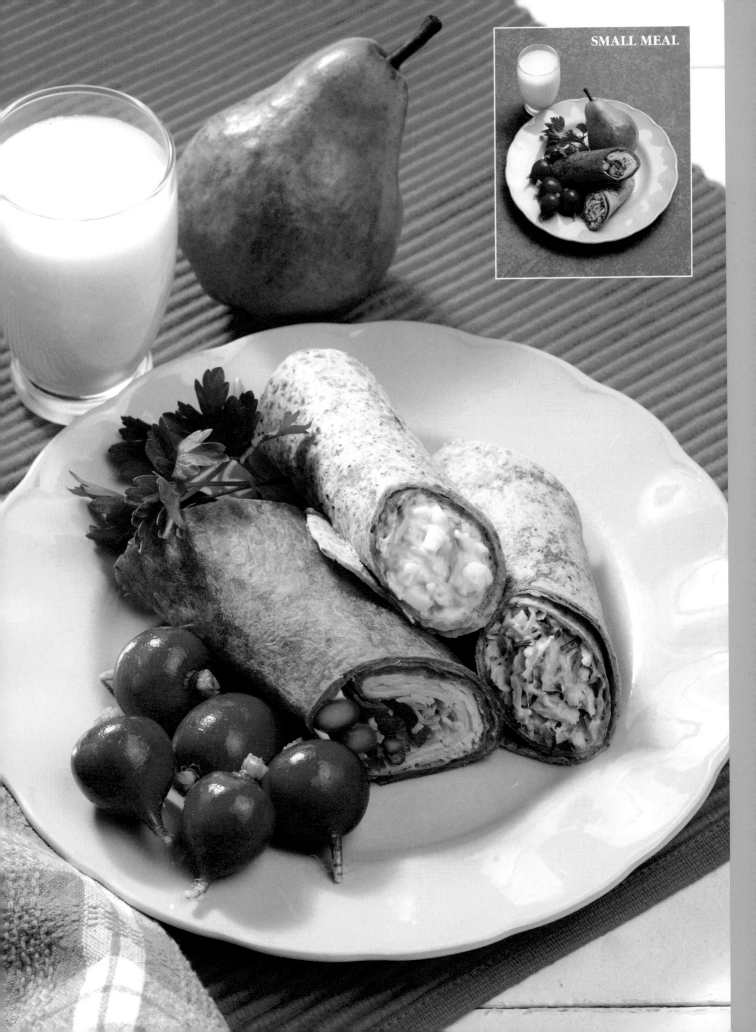

SMALL MEAL

LUNCH 4

Pizza Bun

Pizza bun

On one side of each half bun add 1 tablespoon (15 mL) of pizza or pasta sauce, tomato sauce or salsa. Then add your own favorite toppings – try one of these varieties.

Additions for each half bun:

Vegetarian Ranch:
- 2 tbsp (30 mL) brown beans, black beans or kidney beans (drained)
- a sprinkle of kernel corn (frozen or canned)
- red pepper strips
- 1 tbsp (15 mL) shredded mozzarella or other cheese
- for extra flavoring (optional): chopped cilantro or basil

Hawaiian:
- 1 ounce (30 g) of chopped ham
- chopped peppers and pineapple tidbits
- 1 tbsp (15 mL) of shredded mozzarella or other cheese

Classic:
- ½ ounce (15 g) cooked lean hamburger; chicken or pepperoni
- chopped peppers, mushrooms or other fresh or frozen vegetables
- 2 tbsp (30 mL) shredded mozzarella or other cheese

  1. Toast your bun (or bread) either in the toaster or in the oven.

  2. Place cut bun or English muffin (or slice of bread) on a baking sheet. Spread with tomato sauce.

  3. Top with the beans, chicken or meat, and cheese, vegetables and flavorings.

  4. Broil for a few minutes until the cheese bubbles.

You can make your pizza bun on an open-face hamburger or hot dog bun. Even using a slice of bread is good!

For a lower salt option than tomato sauce, chop up a tomato and mix with a dash of oregano and basil.

Your Lunch Menu	**Large Meal** (520 calories)	**Small Meal** (400 calories)
Pizza buns	3 halves	2 halves
Cucumber	½ medium	½ medium
Diet beverage	12 ounce (355 mL)	12 ounce (355 mL)
Pudding, no sugar added	½ cup (125 mL)	½ cup (125 mL)

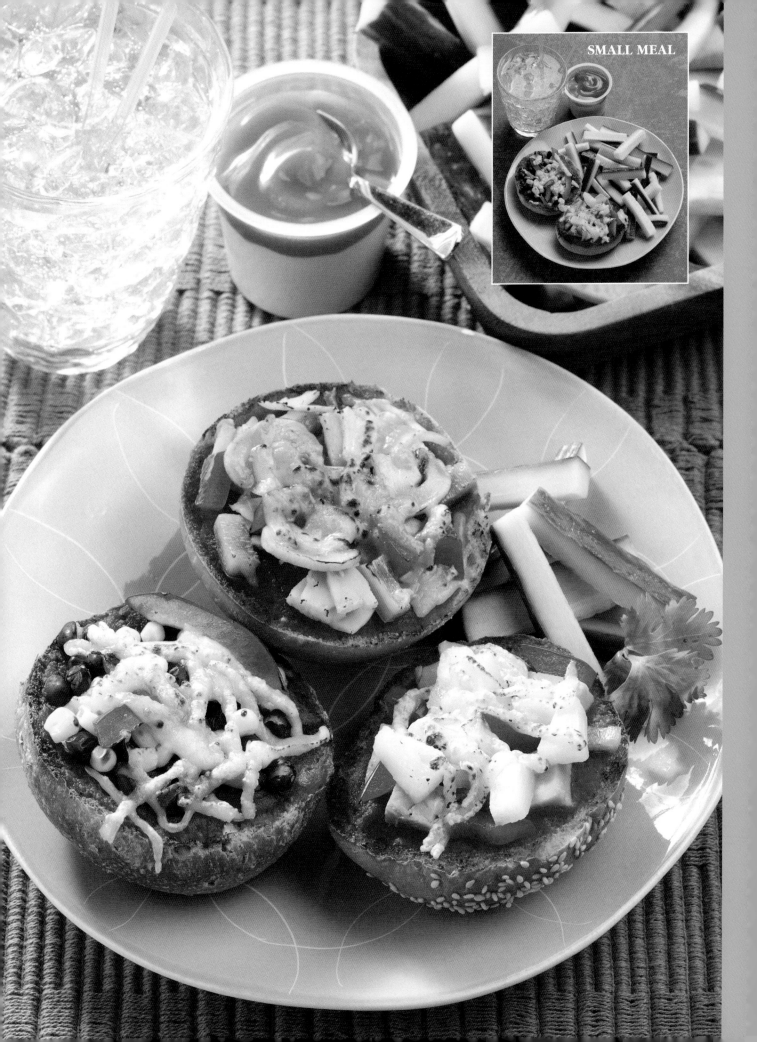

DINNER 1

Minute Steak & Potato

Is shortage of time one of your biggest challenges in making dinner? If so, this tasty, nutritious, quick meal is for you. Cook some potatoes, rice, or pasta to go along with it. Balance this meal out with some peas and carrots and sweet bell pepper on the side.

This meal is so good that sometimes you might want to serve it to guests, so I've added a wonderful trifle for dessert. You can make trifle the night before, so it's ready to eat the next day. An alternative to the trifle is a ½ cup (125 mL) of yogurt or pudding with one or two small plain cookies on the side.

Minute steak

Minute steak is outside or inside round steak that a butcher pounds until it's flattened. Also called tenderized frying steak, it cooks quickly, because it's a thin piece of meat.

Hamburger patties

You can also make this recipe with thin hamburger patties instead of minute steak. Cook your hamburger through (no pink color left) prior to adding the gravy.

Minute Steak

Makes 4 large servings (or 5 small)

1 small onion, sliced
2 tsp (10 mL) margarine or butter
1½ lb (750 g) of minute steak or hamburger patties (1 lb/500 g) for 4 small servings)
25 g package of fat-free Brown Gravy (look for the brand with lowest sodium)

Per large serving	
Calories	242
Carbohydrate	5 g
Fiber	0 g
Protein	39 g
Fat, total	6 g
Fat, saturated	2 g
Cholesterol	73 mg
Sodium	428 mg

1. In a large frying pan, melt the margarine or butter, then add the onions. Cook the onions until soft at medium heat.

2. Move the onions to the side, and add the meat to the pan and brown on both sides.

3. While the meat is cooking mix the contents of the gravy package with hot water in a glass measuring cup or bowl. Use the amount of water shown on the gravy package instructions (usually 1 cup/250 mL). Mix well with a whisk or fork.

4. Add the gravy to the pan with the onions and meat. Turn the temperature down to low-medium, cover with a lid, and simmer for 10–15 minutes.

Here, I've adapted my Aunt Mary Vivian's English Trifle to make it lighter and easier to make.

Lady Vivian's English Trifle

Makes 5 servings

¼ of an angel food cake

2 tbsp (30 mL) light raspberry or other fruit jam (labeled as less than 20 calories per tbsp/15 mL)

1 tbsp (15 mL) sherry

1 cup (250 mL) frozen raspberries, unsweetened (or other frozen berries), thawed and well drained (put in a sieve and let the juice drain out)

1 ready-to-eat no-sugar-added vanilla pudding (106 g)

½ cup (125 mL) whipping cream (unwhipped measure)

1½ tsp (7 mL) icing sugar

1 tbsp (15 mL) toasted sliced almonds

Per cup (250 mL)	
Calories	160
Carbohydrate	18 g
Fiber	2 g
Protein	2 g
Fat, total	9 g
Fat, saturated	5 g
Cholesterol	31 mg
Sodium	152 mg

Angel food cake

You can bake the angel food cake yourself using a boxed mix or from scratch (make it ahead so it has time to cool prior to making the trifle) or buy it ready-made from the bakery. Freeze the rest of the cake to make another trifle or other dessert later (such as angel food cake with fresh fruit).

Sherry

A dry sherry gives the trifle its distinctive flavor, but it still tastes scrumptious if you prefer not to add alcohol.

1. Cut the cake into pieces about 1 x 2-inch (2.5 x 5 cm). Place the pieces in a large bowl and add the jam. Mix gently with a spatula or spoon so that the jam coats the cake.

2. Drizzle the sherry over the cake.

3. Whip the cream until soft peaks form. Add the icing sugar at the end of the whipping.

4. Prepare the dessert in 5 individual dishes or in one large bowl. Make the following layers, starting from the bottom:
   – cake with jam and sherry
   – raspberries
   – pudding
   – whipped cream

5. Refrigerate for several hours so the flavors soak in.

6. Toast almonds by cooking at medium heat in a dry non-stick or cast iron frying pan, stirring regularly, until lightly browned. Prior to serving, garnish with the toasted almonds.

Your Dinner Menu	**Large Meal** (730 calories)	**Small Meal** (550 calories)
Minute Steak with gravy	large serving (¼ recipe)	small serving (⅕ recipe)
Potatoes with parsley	1½ medium	1 medium
Yellow or green beans	1–1½ cups (250–375 mL)	1–1½ cups (250–375 mL)
Bell pepper	¾ cup (175 mL)	¾ cup (175 mL)
English Trifle	1 serving	1 serving

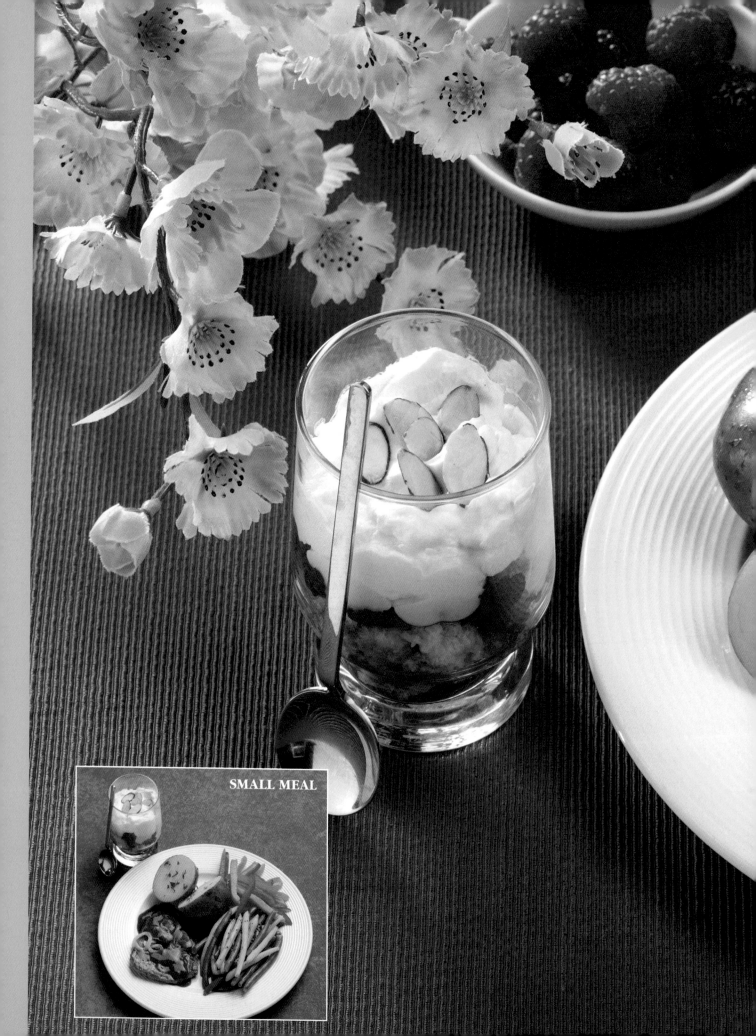

SMALL MEAL

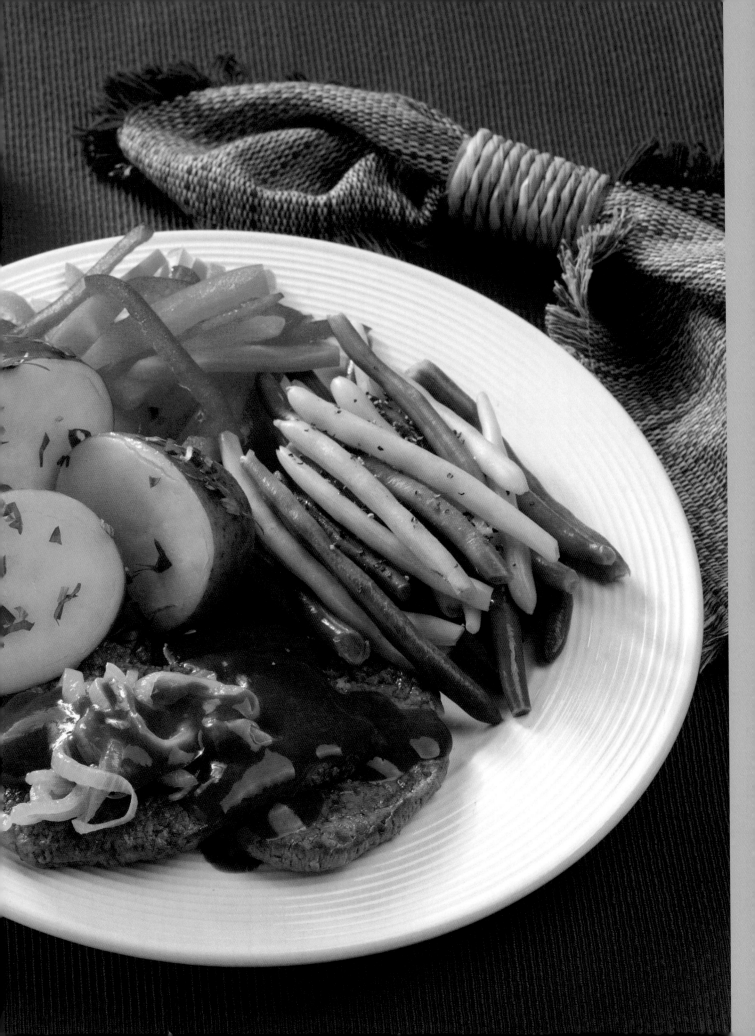

DINNER 2

Nuts and Bolts Stir Fry

If you want to make this meal vegetarian, you can add a few more nuts and omit the meat.

Do you ever buy a package of pork chops or chicken breasts and end up with one extra piece (perhaps a package of three but you are only cooking for two)? Instead of cooking up the extra piece of meat, keep the raw piece in your fridge for the next day – to make a stir fry. This stir fry only requires a small amount of meat (about an ounce per person) as the meat is complimented with vegetable protein (nuts). The "bolts" in this meal are the red pepper sticks!

For dessert with this meal, enjoy yummy Peach Cobbler.

Nuts and Bolts Stir Fry

Makes 4 large servings (or 5 small)

Use any combination of vegetables you have, such as asparagus, frozen mixed vegetables or cabbage.

2 medium carrots, peeled and sliced
2 stalks celery, sliced
30 sugar snap peas or 45 snow peas, cut in half (or ⅓ cup/75 mL frozen peas)
1 red pepper, cut into sticks
1 tsp (5 mL) vegetable oil
1 small onion, cut in small chunks
1 medium pork chop (or a 2-inch/5 cm piece of pork tenderloin) or 1 medium chicken breast, all fat trimmed off, sliced thinly (5 oz/150 g)
¼–½ tsp (1-2 mL) crushed (hot) red pepper (dried), or few dashes of hot pepper sauce (optional)
1 tbsp (15 mL) oyster sauce (or light soy sauce)
½ tsp (2 mL) of ground ginger
1 cup (250 mL) cashews, peanuts or almonds, salted and roasted
1 tbsp (15 mL) sesame seeds (toasted have the best flavor)

Brown rice

Brown rice raises your blood sugar a bit slower than white rice and is a good source of fiber. Prepare your rice without added salt.

Per large serving	
Calories	307
Carbohydrate	20 g
Fiber	4 g
Protein	15 g
Fat, total	20 g
Fat, saturated	4 g
Cholesterol	20 mg
Sodium	274 mg

1. Prepare your raw vegetables and place in a large bowl.

2. At medium heat, add the oil to a non-stick frying pan or heavy pot. Once hot, add your sliced meat and sear quickly until lightly browned. Add the onions and gently sauté.

3. Add the vegetables and the crushed hot pepper to your meat. Cook, uncovered, until lightly cooked.

4. Then, add the oyster sauce, ginger, nuts and sesame seeds and cook for another one or two minutes.

If you'd like, add a splash of milk or 1–2 tablespoons (15–30 mL) of light frozen whipped topping on your cobbler. It is also very good made with other canned fruit such as pears, apricots or fruit cocktail instead of peaches. However, this recipe does not work well with frozen fruit; a better topping for frozen fruit is a crumble.

This dessert can be replaced with a couple of plain cookies or ½ cup (125 mL) of ice cream or frozen yogurt or try a low-fat (0% or 1% MF) Greek yogurt.

Peach Cobbler

Makes 8 servings

Per serving	
Calories	135
Carbohydrate	27 g
Fiber	2 g
Protein	3 g
Fat, total	2 g
Fat, saturated	0 g
Cholesterol	23 mg
Sodium	140 mg

Preheat oven to 425°F (220°C).

3 14-oz (398 mL) cans sliced peaches,
    water or juice-packed, drained
⅛ tsp (0.5 mL) cinnamon
½ tsp (2 mL) almond extract
¾ cup (175 mL) flour
¼ cup (60 mL) sugar
1 tsp (5 mL) baking powder
¼ tsp (1 mL) salt
1 tbsp (15 mL) margarine or butter
⅓ cup (75 mL) skim milk
1 large egg

1. Place peaches in an un-greased 8 x 8-inch (20 x 20 cm) pan or casserole dish. Add the cinnamon and almond extract, and mix with the peaches.

2. In a medium-sized bowl, mix together flour, sugar, baking powder and salt.

3. With a fork, blend in the margarine to the flour mixture. Then add the milk and egg and continue to mix. Batter will be wet and gooey.

4. Spoon batter evenly over peaches.

5. Bake at 425°F (220°C) for 30 minutes or until lightly browned.

Your Dinner Menu	Large Meal (730 calories)	Small Meal (550 calories)
Nuts and Bolts Stir Fry	1 large serving (¼ recipe)	1 small serving (⅕ recipe)
Brown Rice	1 cup (250 mL)	⅔ cup (150 mL)
Milk	1 cup (250 mL)	1 cup (250 mL)
Peach Cobbler	1 serving	1 serving

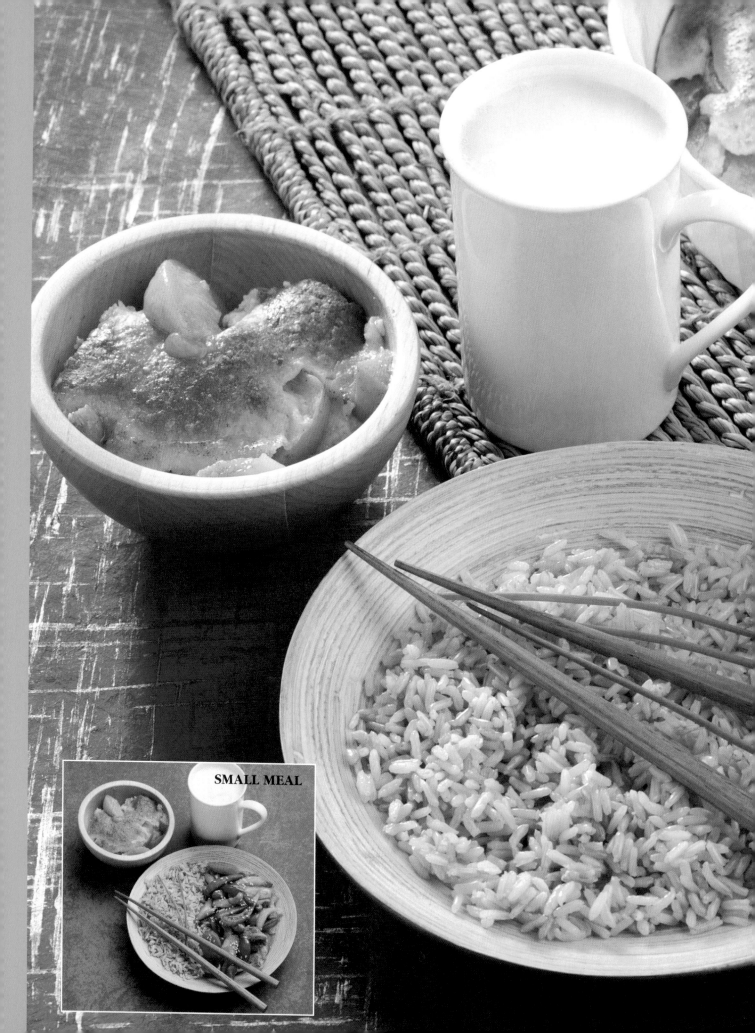

SMALL MEAL

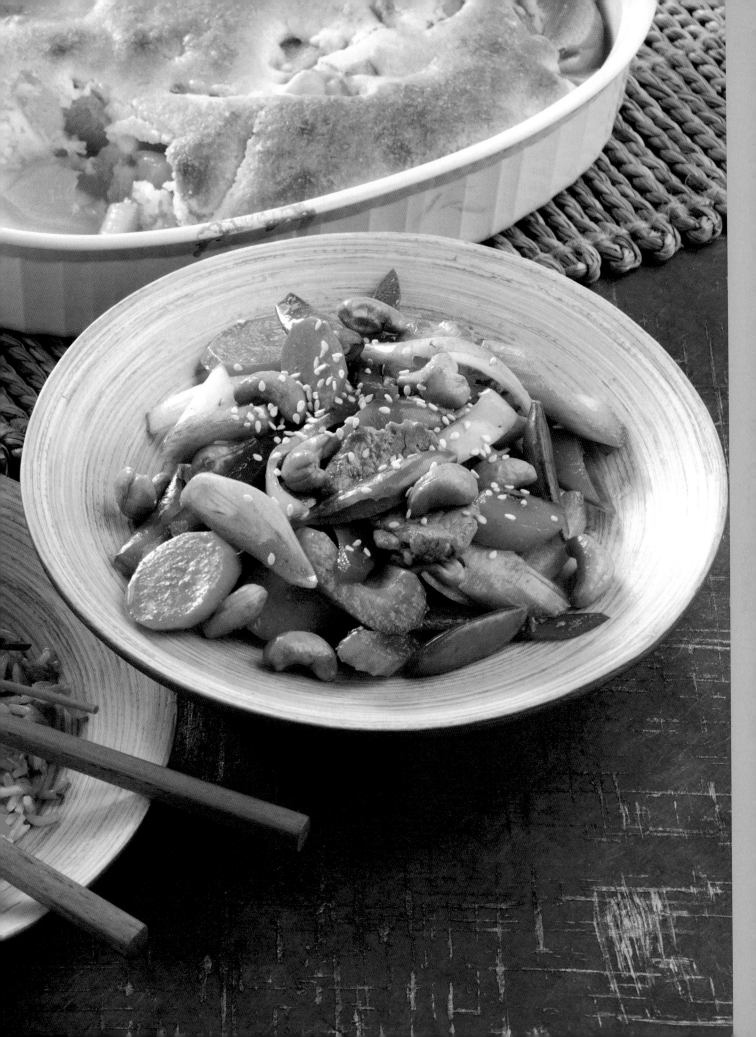

DINNER 3

Hot Chicken Salad

Enjoy Hot Chicken Salad with garlic bread and milk. Try Cinnamon Apple for dessert.

Hot Chicken Salad

For each salad serving:

2 cups (500 mL) of greens
½ carrot, thinly sliced
2 large radishes, thinly sliced
½ medium tomato, chopped or wedges
2 tbsp (30 mL) shredded cheese

Per serving	
Calories	98
Carbohydrate	9 g
Fiber	3 g
Protein	5 g
Fat, total	5 g
Fat, saturated	3 g
Cholesterol	15 mg
Sodium	125 mg

1. Make the Homemade Chicken Strips (recipe below) and place in the oven to bake.

2. While the chicken strips are cooking, prepare a large lettuce or spinach salad with tomatoes, carrots and radishes, or any combination of your favorite vegetables.

3. Remove the hot cooked Chicken Strips from the oven and put them on your salad (in strips or cut in pieces).

Homemade Chicken Strips

Makes 18 strips

½ cup (125 mL) bread crumbs
¼ cup (60 mL) dried parmesan cheese
½ tsp (2 mL) oregano
1½ tsp (7 mL) dried parsley
2–3 tbsp (30–45 mL) milk
3 large (or 4 small) chicken breasts,
   skinned and fat trimmed off (14 oz/420 g total)

Per strip	
Calories	44
Carbohydrate	2 g
Fiber	0 g
Protein	6 g
Fat, total	1 g
Fat, saturated	0 g
Cholesterol	15 mg
Sodium	56 mg

1. In a bowl (or plastic bag), combine the bread crumbs, parmesan cheese, oregano and parsley.

2. Pour the milk in another bowl.

3. On a cutting board, cut the chicken breasts into strips (six per each large chicken breast or four per each small chicken breast). Flatten each strip with your hand.

4. Dip each chicken strip into the milk. Then one at a time, dip in the crumbs to coat evenly.

5. Place on a greased baking sheet and bake in a 400°F (200°C) oven for 10 minutes then turn the strips over. Cook for another 5–10 minutes until chicken is white inside.

Add dandelion!

Wash some young dandelion leaves and roots. Add this to your salad. The leaves are a great source of vitamin C and the roots have soluble fiber. Remember, if someone sprays with lawn chemicals nearby, don't eat those dandelion plants!

***Homemade Chicken Strips** are low-fat and salt-free. If you are in rush you can use instead:*

- *a commercial coating mix on your chicken, or*

- *commercial frozen breaded chicken.*

These options will have more salt. The frozen breaded chicken will also have more fat. Consider reducing your portion of chicken strips slightly with these options.

Garlic Bread

Makes 1 slice (½ bun)

½ hot dog or hamburger bun,
   or 1 slice of bread
1 tsp (5 mL) margarine or butter
1/8 tsp (0.5 mL) garlic powder

1. In a small bowl, mix the margarine
   or butter with the garlic powder.

2. Toast your bread, and while hot,
   spread on the garlic margarine/butter.

Per slice	
Calories	106
Carbohydrate	13 g
Fiber	1 g
Protein	3 g
Fat, total	5 g
Fat, saturated	1 g
Cholesterol	0 mg
Sodium	153 mg

*For a meal variation,
substitute Garlic
Bread with Baked
Low-Fat Fries (See my
book **Diabetes Meals
for Good Health**.)*

Cinnamon Apple

Makes 2 servings

¼ tsp (1 mL) cinnamon mixed with
   1 tbsp (15 mL) sugar (or equivalent
   of a low-calorie sweetener)
2 small or 1 large apple, sliced

1. Add the cinnamon and sugar to the
   sliced apple in a microwavable bowl.

2. Microwave for about 30 seconds until
   apple is slightly tender.

3. Bake at 425°F (220°C) for 30 minutes
   or until lightly browned.

Per serving	
Calories	90
Carbohydrate	23 g
Fiber	2 g
Protein	0 g
Fat, total	0 g
Fat, saturated	0 g
Cholesterol	0 mg
Sodium	1 mg

*You can substitute
your own favorite fruit
for Cinnamon Apple.*

Your Dinner Menu	Large Meal (730 calories)	Small Meal (550 calories)
Hot Chicken Salad:		
Salad	1 serving	1 serving
Chicken strips	5 strips	3 strips
Light (low fat) salad dressing	1 tbsp (15 mL)	1 tbsp 15 mL)
Garlic Bread	1 bun or 2 slices of bread	½ bun or 1 slice of bread
Milk, skim or 1%	1 cup (250 mL)	1 cup (250 mL)
Cinnamon Apple	1 serving	1 serving

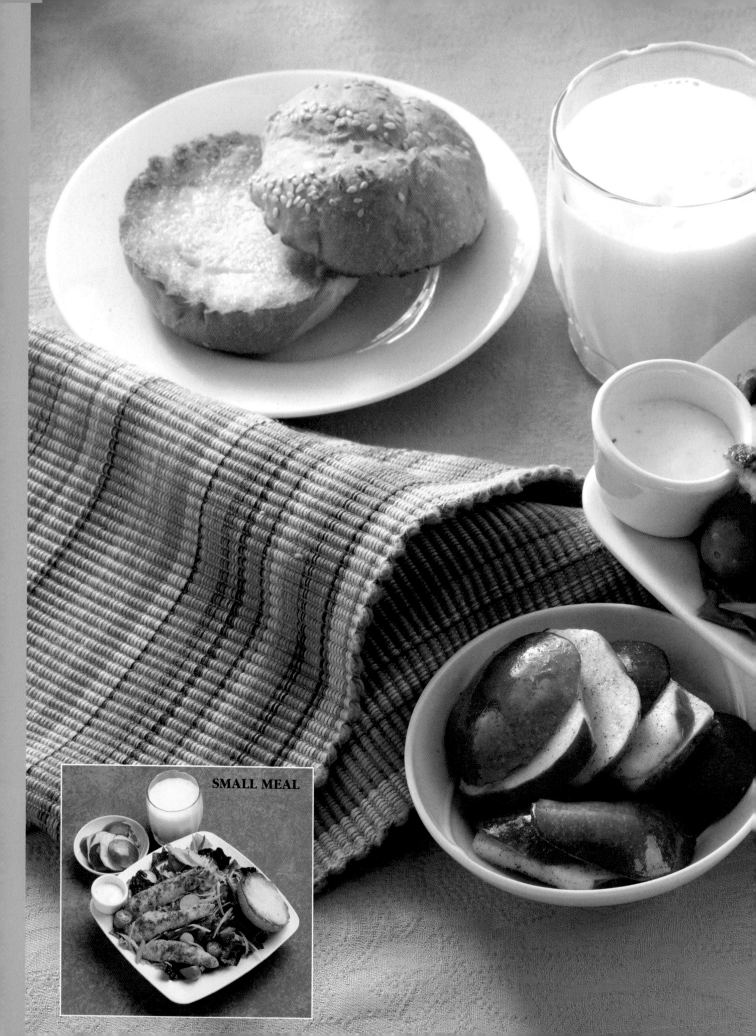

SMALL MEAL

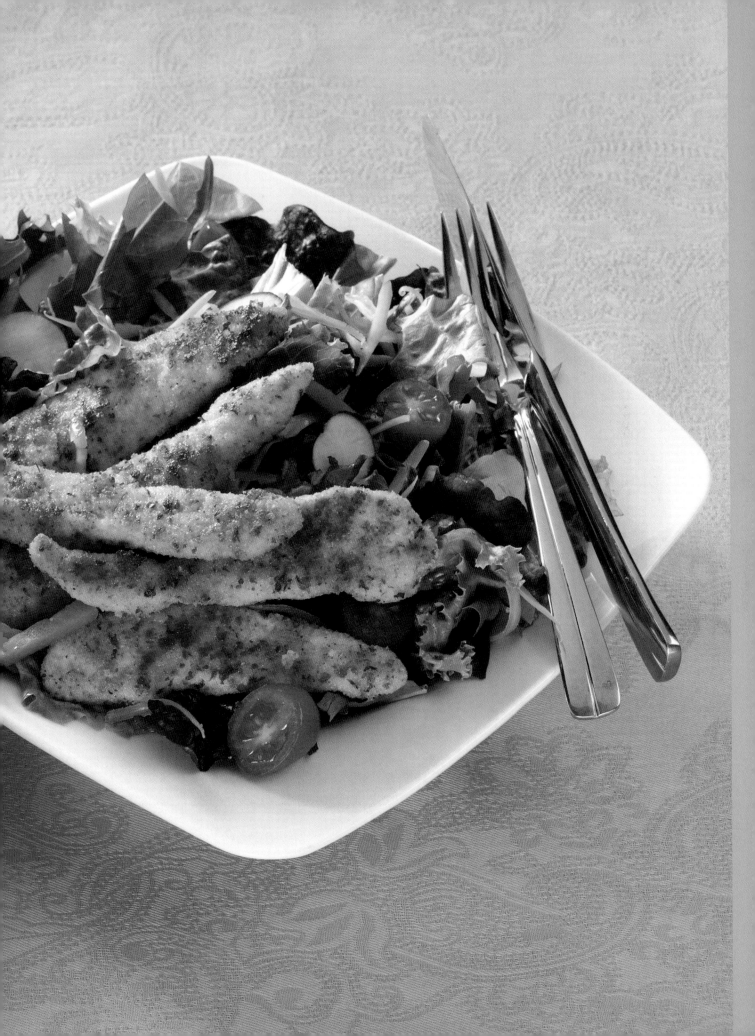

DINNER 4

Vegetarian Sauce & Pasta

My kids actually prefer this pasta sauce made with peanut butter and sunflower seeds to the traditional meat-based sauce (see Dinner 2 in my book *Diabetes Meals for Good Health*). Serve the sauce over corkscrew noodle (rotini pasta). For a change, try whole wheat macaroni or spaghetti. Add a salad on the side, and have fruit and yogurt for dessert.

Vegetarian Sauce

Makes about 10 cups

2 tsp (10 mL) oil
½ cup (125 mL) water
1 large onion, chopped
3 large cloves of garlic, finely chopped or minced
1 tsp (5 mL) oregano
¼ tsp (1 mL) each ground cloves and ground cinnamon
¼ tsp (1 mL) pepper
¼ tsp (1 mL) hot sauce (such as Tabasco)
28 ounce (796 mL) can diced tomatoes
half of a 28 ounce (796 mL) can of water
1 small tin (5½ oz/156 mL) tomato paste
3 large stalks of celery, chopped
1 large green pepper, chopped
1 small box (7 oz/200 g or 3 cups/750 mL) fresh mushrooms (or 10-oz (284 mL) can mushroom pieces, drained)
½ cup (125 mL) shelled, unsalted roasted sunflower seeds
½ cup (125 mL) crunchy peanut butter

Per cup (250 mL)	
Calories	168
Carbohydrate	15 g
Fiber	4 g
Protein	7 g
Fat, total	11 g
Fat, saturated	2 g
Cholesterol	0 mg
Sodium	197 mg

1. Place oil and water in a large heavy pot. Turn on heat to low-medium and add onion and garlic. Cook until soft, stirring occasionally. Add extra water if needed to keep moist.

2. Add the spices and hot sauce to the onions. Cook for 1 or 2 minutes.

3. Add the other ingredients to the pot and stir well.

4. Cover pot with a lid and cook for 45 minutes to an hour on low-medium heat. Adjust temperature so it is just a simmer. Stir every 10–15 minutes, so it doesn't stick. If too thick – add extra water. If too thin – take the lid off and cook uncovered for the last 15 minutes.

*This sauce has similar calories per cup (250 mL) as the Meat Sauce in Dinner 2 in my book **Diabetes Meals for Good Health**, so you can exchange with that meal.*

If you can't find roasted sunflower seeds, take blanched sunflower seeds and bake them on a shallow pan in a 350°F (180°C) oven for 5 minutes until lightly browned.

When cooking larger recipes, freeze extra food as soon as it cools. You'll have an easy meal for another day. You may want to freeze your cooking in single-meal containers.

Here's a delicious variation to a cabbage-based coleslaw. Cabbage, cauliflower and broccoli are all excellent cancer-fighting vegetables. The salad dressing can also be used on lettuce based salads.

Cauliflower and Broccoli Slaw

Makes 4 servings

1 cup (250 mL) cauliflower, chopped
1 cup (250 mL) broccoli, chopped
¼ cup (60 mL) Mayo Parmesan Salad
   Dressing
1 small red apple, cored and chopped
2 oz (60 g) (1 by 1-inch/2.5 by 2.5 cm slice
   from a 3-inch/7.5 cm block of cheese),
   cut in tiny cubes

Per serving	
Calories	90
Carbohydrate	10 g
Fiber	2 g
Protein	6 g
Fat, total	4 g
Fat, saturated	2 g
Cholesterol	11 mg
Sodium	268 mg

1. Combine ingredients.

Mayo Parmesan Salad Dressing

Makes ¼ cup (60 mL)

¼ cup (60 mL) fat free or light mayonnaise
1 tbsp (15 mL) parmesan cheese
1 tsp (5 mL) vinegar
1 tsp (5 mL) sugar
black pepper, to taste

Per tablespoon (15 mL)	
Calories	24
Carbohydrate	4 g
Fiber	0 g
Protein	1 g
Fat, total	1 g
Fat, saturated	0 g
Cholesterol	3 mg
Sodium	150 mg

1. Place all ingredients in a jar or container with a lid. Stir or whisk until smooth.

Your Dinner Menu	Large Meal (730 calories)	Small Meal (550 calories)
Vegetarian Pasta Sauce	1⅓ cup (325 mL)	1 cup (250 mL)
Rotini Pasta	1½ cups (375 mL)	1 cup (250 mL)
Cauliflower and Broccoli Slaw	1 serving	1 serving
Strawberries	1 cup (250 mL)	½ cup (125 mL)
Low-fat yogurt, no sugar added	¾ cup (175 mL)	¾ cup (175 mL)

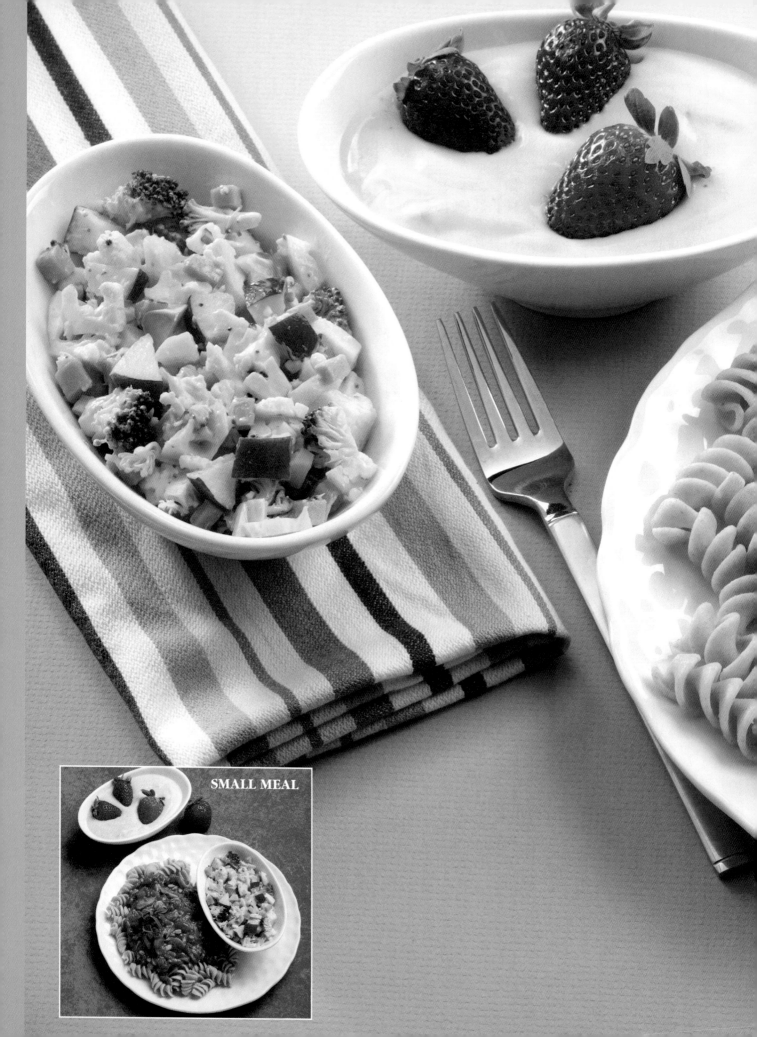

SMALL MEAL

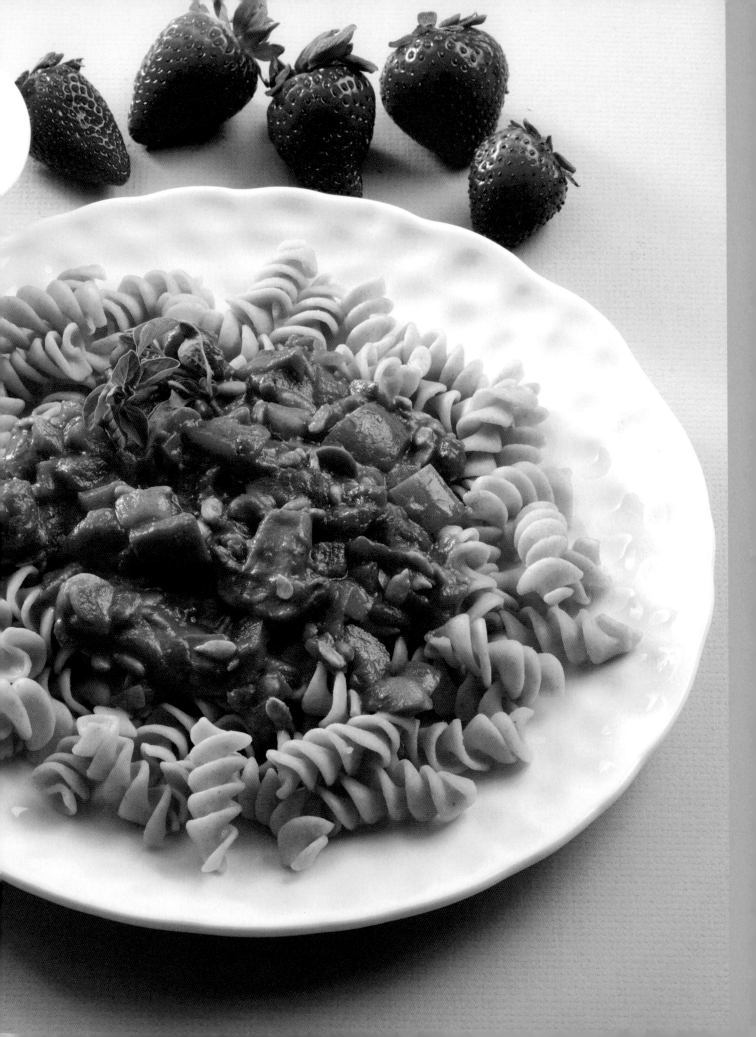

DINNER 5

Seafood Chowder

This chowder is an old time favorite from the island of Newfoundland, on the Canadian East Coast. Traditionally, fishing families made fresh chowder with whatever catch the fisherman brought home that day and served it with chunks of fresh hearty bread and butter. Enjoy this meal with green vegetables and for dessert, the delicious Lemon Zinger Pudding.

I adapted this recipe to use frozen fish and seafood, which is sometimes more readily available and less expensive than fresh. Using frozen fish, your soup will be cooked in half an hour. Depending on what quantities of fish and seafood you purchase, you may want to double the recipe to make a larger batch of soup. The soup is delicious the day you make it or next day. It also freezes well.

Seafood Chowder

Makes 8 cups (2 L)

1 tbsp (15 mL) of margarine or butter
1 medium onion, chopped
3 cups (750 mL) water
2 medium raw potatoes,
    peeled and diced
1 medium carrot, peeled and chopped
7 oz (200 g) frozen salmon (about two 2 x 3-inch/
    5 x 7.5 cm fillets)
7 oz (200 g) frozen white fish (about two 2 x 4-inch/
    5 x 10 cm fillets)
1 tsp (5 mL) dried parsley or flaked savory (not ground savory)
¼ tsp (1 mL) black pepper
7 oz (200 g) scallops
10 oz (300 g) shrimp (uncooked or cooked), about one shrimp ring, tails removed

Per cup (250 mL)	
Calories	173
Carbohydrate	9 g
Fiber	1 g
Protein	22 g
Fat, total	5 g
Fat, saturated	1 g
Cholesterol	105 mg
Sodium	180 mg

1. Place butter and onion in a large heavy pot. At low-medium heat, sauté onion in butter until soft.

2. Add water, potatoes, carrots, whole pieces of salmon and white fish, dried parsley and black pepper. Simmer uncovered at medium heat; stir occasionally. The fish will gently break into pieces as cooking. Cook until potatoes are tender and fish is cooked (no translucence), about 10–15 minutes.

3. Add the scallops and shrimp and continue simmering for another 5–10 minutes.

If you would like to use thawed or fresh seafood or fish, instead of frozen, simply reduce the cooking time by about 10 minutes. Add any fish juices to the chowder.

Yukon gold potatoes are nice in this recipe as they add a nice yellow color, but any potato will work!

If the shrimp you buy have the tails on, remove the tails before adding to the chowder. To easily remove the tails from frozen shrimp, first soak them in cold water for a few minutes.

Scallops add a wonderful flavor and texture, but unfortunately they are expensive. Instead, you can increase your portion of white fish or shrimp and omit the scallops.

Lemon Zinger Pudding

Makes 6 servings

Preheat oven to 350°F (180°C)

3 large egg whites
3 tbsp (45 mL) sugar
3 egg yolks
grated lemon peel from 1 lemon
    (2–3 tsp/10–15 mL)
¼ cup (60 mL) lemon juice (the juice
    from the lemon you just grated)
2 tbsp (30 mL) margarine or butter (softened)
¼ cup (60 mL) sifted all purpose flour
2 tbsp (30 mL) sucralose (e.g., Splenda)
1½ cups (375 mL) skim milk

Per serving	
Calories	140
Carbohydrate	15 g
Fiber	0 g
Protein	6 g
Fat, total	6 g
Fat, saturated	1 g
Cholesterol	96 mg
Sodium	95 mg

This pudding-cake is equally luscious warm or cold. The recipe includes part sugar and part low-calorie sweetener. If you replace the low-calorie sweetener (in the cake part of the recipe) with sugar, you will then add an extra 16 calories (4 g carbohydrate) per serving.

1. Place the egg whites in a medium-size glass mixing bowl. Place the egg yolks in a second medium mixing bowl. Add the sugar to the egg whites. Set the egg whites aside.

2. To the second mixing bowl with the egg yolks, add the lemon peel and juice, margarine, flour, sucralose and milk.

3. Using an electric mixer, beat the eat whites and sugar on high speed until soft peaks form.

4. Using the same beaters, beat the egg yolk mixture at medium speed, scraping the sides with a spatula. Beat until blended (it will be a bit lumpy).

5. Fold the egg whites into the egg yolk mixture, turning it gently with your spatula.

6. Pour the batter into an un-greased 8-inch (20 cm) square baking or casserole dish. Then, place this pan into another larger pan that is filled with about ½-inch (1 cm) of hot tap water. Make sure the water is below the level of the baking pan with the pudding.

7. Bake for 40 minutes, or until the top is lightly browned. Allow to sit in the pan with the water until the water has cooled, then remove the pudding dish.

Egg whites beat better if they are at room temperature. Take them out of the fridge when you start this recipe, and by the time you've completed step 2, the egg whites should be ready.

Cook the pudding in the oven inside a larger dish filled with some water. Cooking it this way allows this delicate pudding to cook without burning and to retain its lovely sauce.

Your Dinner Menu	**Large Meal** (730 calories)	**Small Meal** (550 calories)
Seafood Chowder	2 cups (500 mL)	1½ cups (375 mL)
Fresh bread	5 sticks (1½ thick slices)	3 sticks (1 thick slice)
Butter or margarine	2 tsp (10 mL)	1 tsp (5 mL)
Salad	1 large	1 large
Vinaigrette light salad dressing	1 tbsp (15 mL)	1 tbsp (15 mL)
Lemon Zinger Pudding	1 serving	1 serving

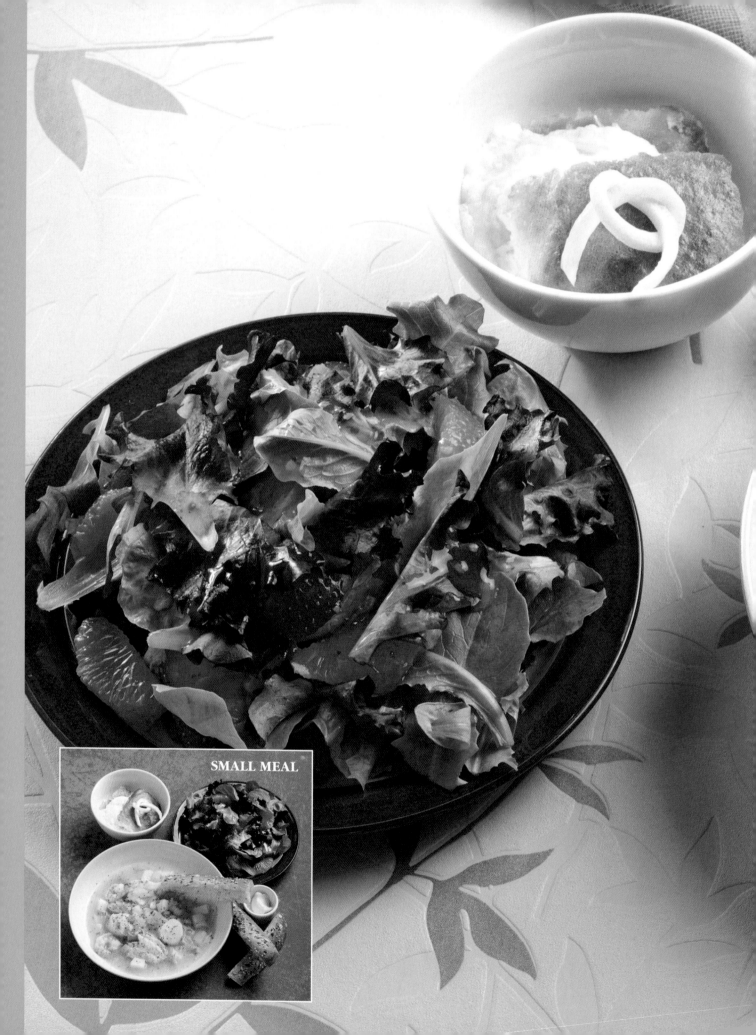

SMALL MEAL

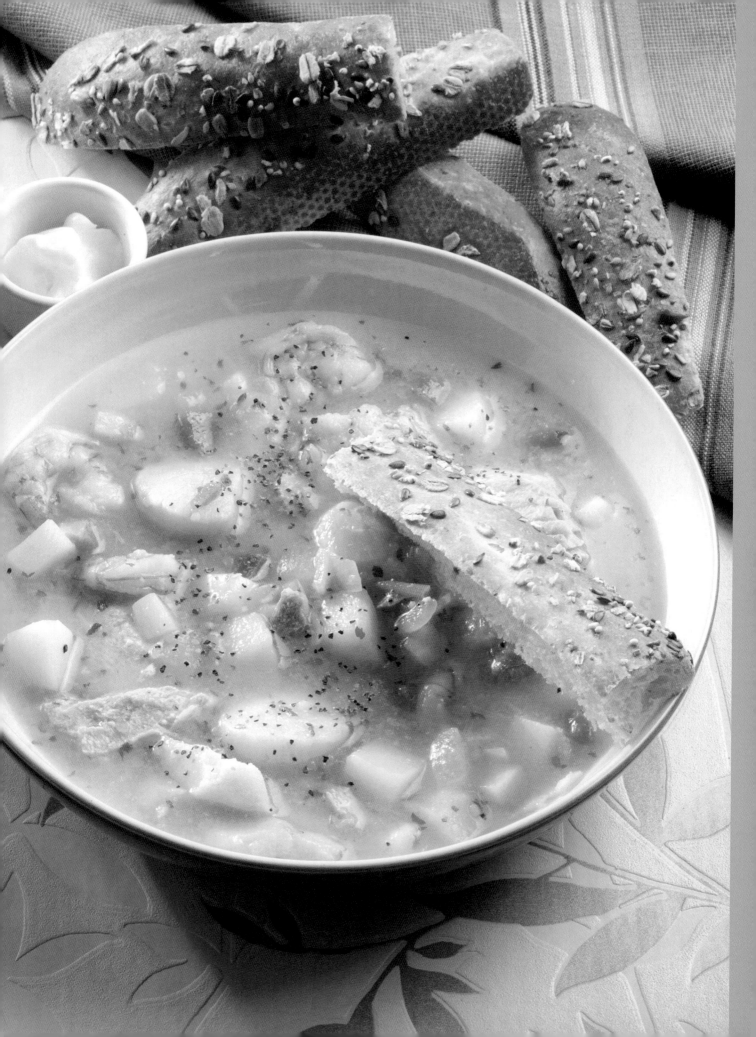

DINNER 6

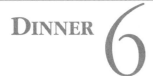

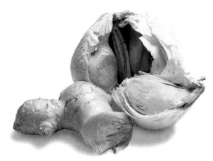

Chicken Curry & Rice

Make this curry the day ahead, for the best flavor. Curries thicken as they sit. This freezes well, so this is a large recipe and you can freeze the extra. If you are not freezing some, cut the recipe in half.

Easy Chicken Curry

Makes 6 large or 9 small servings

1 tbsp (15 mL) vegetable oil
¼ cup (60 mL) water
2 medium onions, chopped
6 cloves garlic, crushed
   or finely chopped
1 tbsp (15 mL) curry powder
2 tbsp (30 mL) garam masala
½ tsp (2 mL) salt (optional)
19 oz (540 mL) can of tomatoes (whole or chopped)
¼ cup (60 mL) packed fresh cilantro, finely chopped
1 cup (250 mL) unflavored low-fat yogurt
1 cup (250 mL) of chicken stock
   (1 package reduced salt bouillon + 1 cup/250 mL water)
18 skinned chicken drumsticks or thighs, skin removed
   (3½ lbs/1.7 kg weight with skin and bones or 3 lbs/1.5 kg
   weight with skin removed)
¼ cup (60 mL) fresh cilantro, roughly chopped, for topping

Per large serving	
Calories	352
Carbohydrate	14 g
Fiber	2 g
Protein	42 g
Fat, total	14 g
Fat, saturated	3 g
Cholesterol	145 mg
Sodium	581 mg

1. To a large heavy pot, heat the oil and water at low to medium. Add the onions and garlic to the pot. Cook until soft. Add the spices, stirring frequently, and cook for one or two minutes until the spices are well blended. Add a bit of water if too dry.

2. Add to the pot, the tomatoes, cilantro, yogurt and chicken stock. Blend together, then add the chicken pieces.

3. Cover the pot and simmer gently at low-medium heat. Stir periodically. Cook for 1–1½ hour, or until chicken is cooked. If too thick, add extra chicken stock or water if needed. If too thin, cook for the last 15–30 minutes without the lid.

4. After cooking, add chopped cilantro.

Do you like it hot?

This is a flavorful curry but is not spicy hot. If you like heat in your curry, add a teaspoon (5 mL) of chili powder or a few dashes of hot sauce.

Curry powder and garam masala are both fragrant Indian spice blends. Garam masala adds an important flavor to this recipe, but if it isn't available, replace it with curry powder (use 3 tbsp/45 mL in total) or an alternative Indian spice blend such as Korma or Biryani masala or vindaloo.

People often serve curries with a variety of condiments, such as mango chutney, pickles, marinated or curried vegetables, lentil dishes, dried coconut or fresh fruit. One condiment my parents enjoy with curry is a combination of chopped raw onions and tomatoes in an oil and vinegar mixture. I've chosen three easy side dishes with this curry. Raw grated carrots (1 carrot will shred into about 1 cup/250 mL of grated carrots), shredded coconut and sliced bananas.

Basmati rice is always nice with a curry – try a brown basmati. When cooked, the basmati rice grains have a wonderful flavor and don't stick together like many other rice. You can also use Converted white rice, long-grained white rice, or brown rice.

Fruit and Cheese Kebabs
Go light for dessert with fruit kebabs. Combine a variety of fruits and cheese on a wooden skewer in the amounts shown in the photograph. This equals about half a fresh fruit serving and half an ounce of cheese.

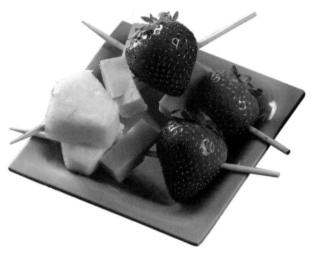

Your Dinner Menu	**Large Meal** (730 calories)	**Small Meal** (550 calories)
Chicken Curry	large serving (3 drumsticks plus sauce)	small serving (2 drumsticks plus sauce)
Rice, basmati	1 cup (250 mL)	⅔ cup (150 mL)
Sliced banana	½ small banana	½ small banana
Shredded coconut, unsweetened	1 tbsp (15 mL)	1 tbsp (15 mL)
Grated carrots	½ cup (125 mL)	½ cup (125 mL)
Fruit and Cheese Kebabs	3 small skewers	3 small skewers
Tea	1 cup (250 mL)	1 cup (250 mL)

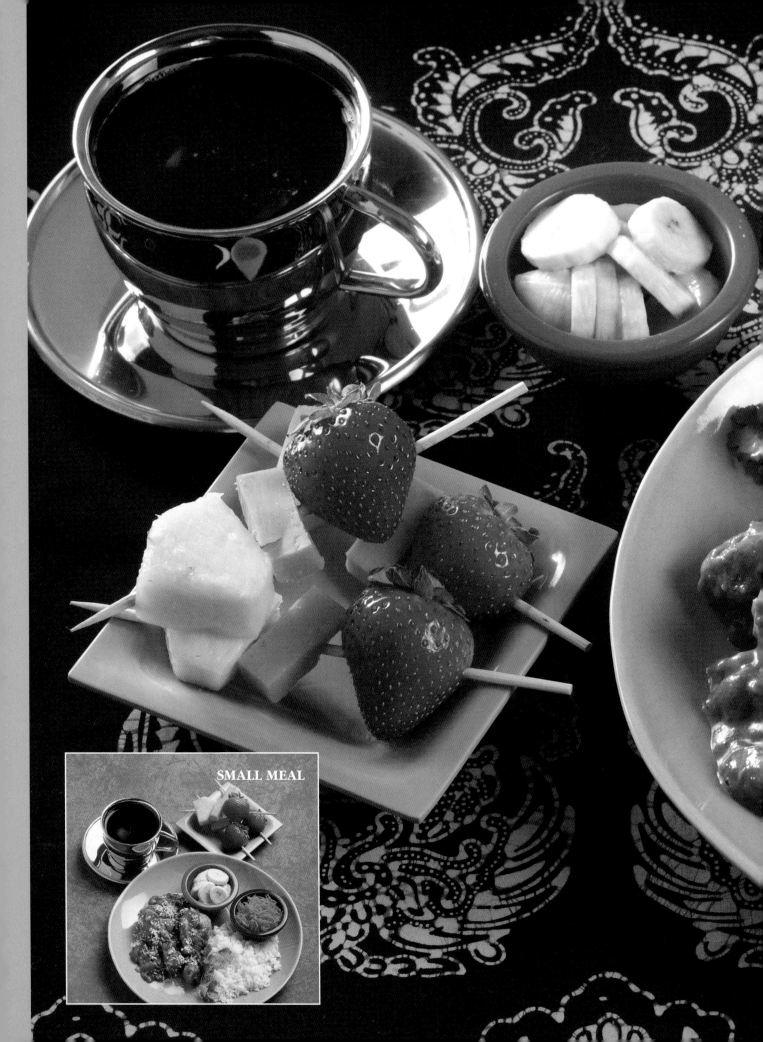

SMALL MEAL

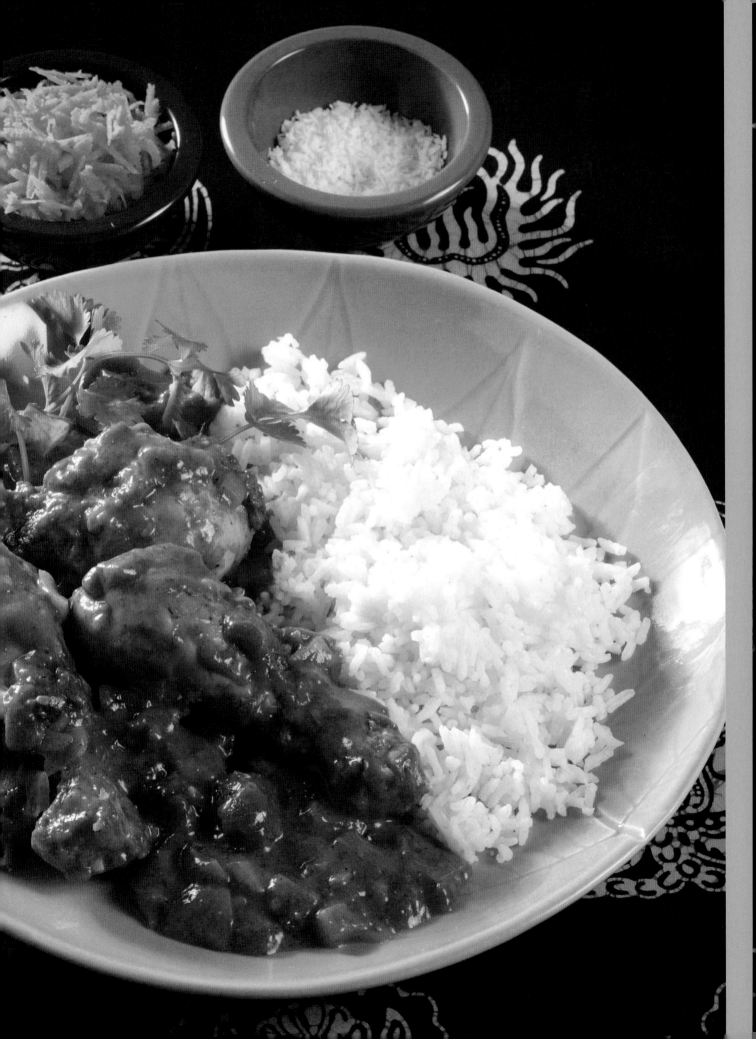

DINNER 7

Vegetable Omelet & Beans

What could be easier than eggs and beans for a satisfying meal? This omelet is easy to make but if you want an even easier meal you can turn the omelet into scrambled eggs, using all the same ingredients. The toast with honey or jam becomes your dessert with this meal.

Vegetable Omelet

Serves 1

If serving two, double the omelet recipe, and use a larger non-stick frying pan if needed.

1½ tsp (7 mL) margarine, oil or butter
½ small onion or 2 green onions including stems
1 cup (250 mL) finely chopped raw vegetables (such as celery, peppers, cauliflower, broccoli or mushrooms)
2 eggs
2 tbsp (30 mL) grated light cheese

Per omelet	
Calories	277
Carbohydrate	10 g
Fiber	2 g
Protein	18 g
Fat, total	19 g
Fat, saturated	6 g
Cholesterol	380 mg
Sodium	313 mg

1. In a small non-stick frying pan, sauté the onions and vegetables in the margarine or other fat at low-medium heat.

2. While the onions and vegetables are cooking, break the eggs into a small mixing bowl. Beat the eggs with a fork or whisk.

3. When the onions and vegetables are soft, transfer the mixture into a bowl and put to the side.

4. Pour the egg into the greased frying pan. Immediately tip the pan to even out the layer of egg. As the egg is cooking move any soft uncooked egg towards the edges of the pan, until all the egg is cooked.

5. Put the onion and vegetable mixture on one half of the omelet. Top with the grated cheese. Gently lift the other half of the omelet and fold on top. Lower the heat and cook it for another minute or two.

Beans, peas and lentils – an excellent choice!

Compared to animal sources of protein such as meat, fish or chicken, they are lower in saturated fat and a great source of fiber and they cost less. I suggest that you eat them at least once or twice a week. I add some drained, canned beans or lentils to make my leftovers go further, such as to a macaroni dish, spaghetti sauce or stew.

Here are some other ways to eat beans, peas and lentils:

- For lunch, make the Taco Soup on page 162, enjoy a split pea or black bean soup, or add beans or lentils to a vegetable soup to make a "meal in a bowl."

- Add cooked beans to a pizza (page 166), burrito or wrap.

- Add yellow lentils to a chicken curry (page 188). Then you can cut back on the chicken in your recipe.

More ideas from my cookbook *Diabetes Meals for Good Health:*

- Try Mexican Rice and Beans (pictured at right).

- Three of my dinner meals that help you cut back on meat by adding beans are: Chili con Carne, Tacos, and Beans and Wieners.

- Sun Burgers replace meat with romano beans, cheese and sunflower seeds.

- Curried Chickpeas and Potato Filling can be eaten as is or with a roti or tortilla shell.

- Santa Fe Salad, made with black beans, is delicious. You can make an easy bean salad with a can of rinsed and drained mixed beans, along with sliced peppers or cucumber and a vinaigrette dressing.

- For a snack, try hummus spread on crackers.

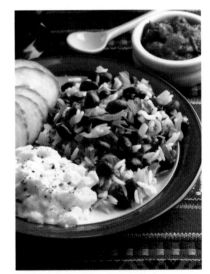

Mexican Rice and Beans from *Diabetes Meals for Good Health*, page 66.

Your Dinner Menu	**Large Meal** (730 calories)	**Small Meal** (550 calories)
Vegetable omelette	1 serving	1 serving
Baked beans	½ cup (125 mL)	¼ cup (60 mL)
Toast	2 slices	1 slice
Margarine or butter	2 tsp (10 mL)	1 tsp (5 mL)
Honey or jam	1–2 tsp (5–10 mL)	1–2 tsp (5–10 mL)
Mandarin oranges	2 small (or 1 medium)	2 small (or 1 medium)

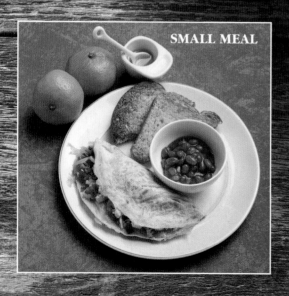

SMALL MEAL

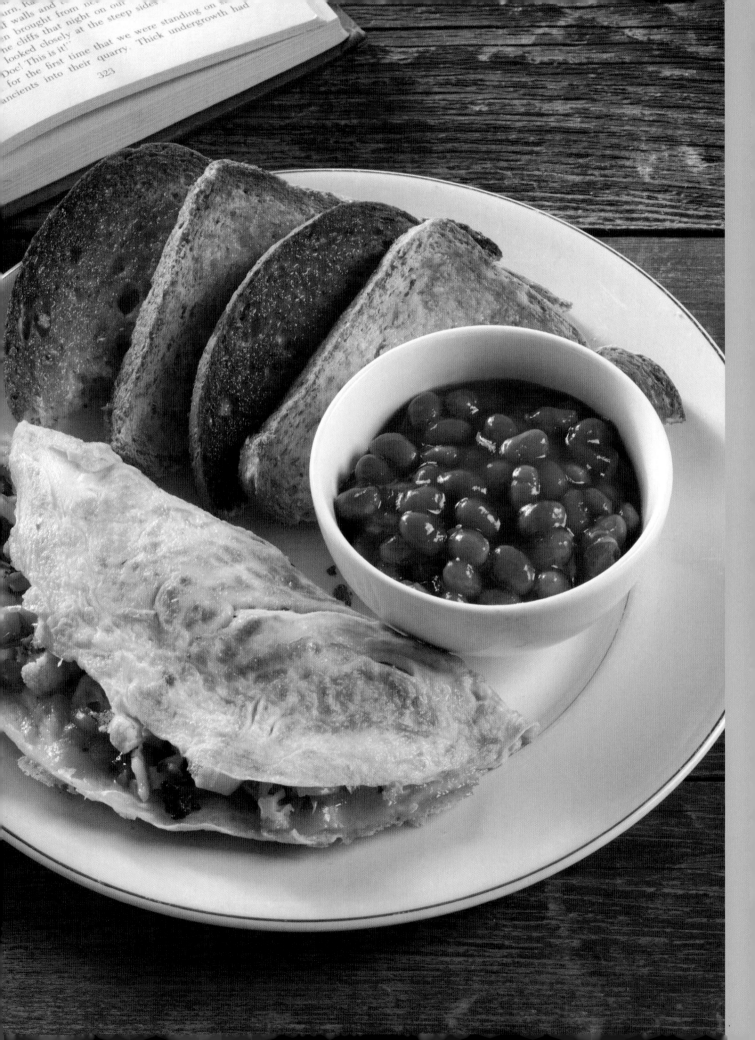

Snacks

In this section you will find photographs of four groups of snacks. The groups are low-calorie snacks, small snacks, medium snacks and large snacks. The calories for each snack within each group are about the same. The number of snacks you choose will depend on how many calories a day you want. Look at the chart on page 151 that shows the calories of the small and large meals, and different snacks.

Low Calorie (20 calories or less)

Small (50 calories)

Medium (100 calories)

Large (200 calories)

For most of us it's good to choose no more than three of the small, medium or large snacks a day.

Three small snacks add up to 150 calories, three medium snacks add up to 300 calories and three large snacks add up to 600 calories.

Do you want more snack ideas? My book **Diabetes Meals for Good Health** includes over 100 additional snack suggestions.

Low-calorie snacks or meal condiments

20 calories or less in each snack

Available carbohydrates in grams is marked in red.

1. 1–2 mini pickles 0
2. hot peppers 0
3. diet soft drinks, diet iced tea and packaged diet drink mixes 0
4. flavored waters (no sugar added) 0
5. pepper 0
6. water 0
7. herbal tea or other tea 0
8. diet gelatin (whipped Jell-O shown) 0
9. sugar-free Freezee 4 tsp (20 mL) 1
10. celery sticks, or broccoli or cauliflower bunch, or carrot, cucumber or zucchini sticks 2
11. coffee or chicory root coffee substitute 1
12. 1–2 mini limes 2
13. tomato 3
14. garlic 2
15. salt-free spice blends and a variety of other dried spices and herbs 0
16. 1 tsp herb paste 1
17. 1–2 sugar-free candies or mints 3
18. low-calorie sugar substitute 1
19. vanilla flavoring 0
20. fresh herbs 0

Small snacks

50 calories

Available carbohydrates in grams is marked in red.

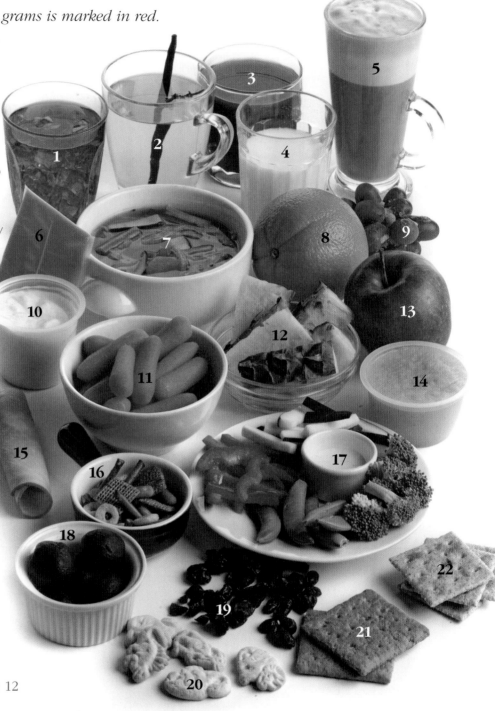

1. ⅓ cup (75 mL) cranberry cocktail (on ice) 12

2. hot apple cider (½ cup/ 125 mL apple juice, ½ cup/125 mL water plus vanilla or cinnamon stick) 15

3. 1 cup (250 mL) V8 juice 9

4. ⅔ cup (150 mL) low-fat milk 8

5. frothed hot coffee (⅔ cup/ 150 mL boiling water plus ⅔ cup/150 mL hot frothed low fat milk plus instant coffee) 8

6. ½ oz (15 g) cheese (1 slice) 1

7. 1½ cups (375 mL) vegetable soup (search "Weight Watcher Soup" on the internet for some easy and tasty recipes) 4

8. 1 orange 13

9. ½ cup (125 mL) frozen grapes 13

10. ½ cup (125 mL) no sugar added pudding 13

11. 13 baby carrots 8

12. 5 small pineapple spears 12

13. 1 small apple 13

14. ½ cup (125 mL) unsweetened applesauce 12

15. 1½ oz (45 g) slice of luncheon meat 0

16. 3 tbsp (45 mL) nuts and bolts 8

17. 1 cup (250 mL) raw vegetables with 1 tbsp (15 mL) light dressing 5

18. ½ cup (125 mL) pickled beets 11

19. 2 tbsp (30 mL) dried cranberries 9

20. 5 animal crackers 10

21. 2 Graham wafers 10

22. 4 whole wheat soda crackers 8

Medium snacks

100 calories

Available carbohydrates in grams is marked in red.

1. 100 calorie mini snack bag 18

2. ½ cup (125 mL) low-fat chocolate milk (with ice!) 12

3. Float (12 oz/355 mL of diet cola plus ½ cup/125 mL frozen yogurt) 11

4. 1 open-face sandwich (unbuttered) 12

5. 3 stone wheat crackers 14

6. ¾ cup (175 mL) low-fat yogurt (no sugar added) with pomegranate seeds 16

7. ¾ cup (175 mL) fat-free pistachio pudding 15

8. 2 donut "bits" 12

9. a ham and cheese slice (rolled) 3

10. 1 hard boiled egg 0

11. 1 medium pear 21

12. 1¼ cups (300 mL) blueberries 22

13. 1 piece of toast with 1 tsp (5 mL) margarine and diet jam 14

14. 1 small banana 21

15. 1 medium apple slice with a sprinkle of sugar and cinnamon 24

16. 14 almonds 1

17. 13 baked rice thin crackers 21

18. 100 calorie ice cream stick 18

19. 1½ cheese string sticks 1

20. 100 calorie granola bar 15

21. 1–2 celery sticks with 1 tbsp (15 mL) peanut butter or 3 tbsp (45 mL) light cream cheese 3

22. 2 3-inch (7.5 cm) crackers with ½ oz (15 g) cheese (try brie or blue cheese) 10

23. 2 tbsp (30 mL) roasted soybeans 5

24. 2 healthy lifestyle cookies 14

25. 7 oysters on 7 mini wheat crackers 8

199

Large snacks

200 calories

Available carbohydrates in grams is marked in red.

1. 1 cup (250 mL) of cream soup made with milk 15

2. Chef salad made with 2–3 oz (60–90 g) cheese and/or ham and 1 tbsp (15 mL) dressing 6

3. piece of thin crust cheese pizza 28

4. 1 cup (250 mL) cooked oatmeal with ½ cup (125 mL) low-fat milk 30

5. 5 cups (1.25 L) of popcorn (made with 1 tsp/5 mL of oil) 26

6. ¾ cup (175 mL) frozen yogurt in a cone 31

7. omelette (made with 1 egg plus 1 egg white, 1 oz/30 g of cheese, green onion and 1 tbsp/ 15 mL bacon bits) 3

8. 1 cup (250 mL) cereal (such as bran flakes) with ¾ cup (175 mL) milk 28

9. 1 cup (250 mL) fruit salad with ¾ cup (175 mL) no sugar added yogurt 36

10. 1 tomato and cheese sandwich (with 2 tsp/10 mL fat-free mayonnaise) 25

11. ½ 3-inch (7.5 cm) bagel with 1 tbsp (15 mL) light cream cheese 26

12. 1 chicken drumstick with a slice of bread and 1–2 tbsp (15–30 mL) cranberry sauce 18

13. 6 soda crackers with ¼ cup (60 mL) salmon or tuna mixed with 1 tsp (5 mL) fat-free mayonnaise 14

14. ¼ cup (60 mL) peanuts or other shelled nuts 3

15. ⅔ cup (150 mL) sunflower seeds in the shells 3

Eat This – Not That

Move from unhealthy to healthy choices using the charts on pages 202–216.

Each page shows four different versions of a food or drink.

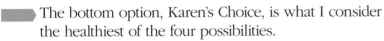 The option at the top of the page is the least healthy.

Generally, the bottom two choices are healthier than the top two choices.

The bottom option, Karen's Choice, is what I consider the healthiest of the four possibilities.

When shopping, read food labels before deciding what to buy. The following nutrients are listed for each food or drink:

- **Calories.** Compare the calories in the food items shown in the charts to your daily calorie needs – see page 151.

- **Carbohydrates ("Carbs").** Carbs include starch from foods such as rice, wheat or pasta, the natural sugars found in fruits, vegetables and milk, and added sugar. One teaspoon (5 mL) of added sugar equals 4 g of sugar. Labels list the amount of sugar separately under carbohydrate, but this still gives no indication of how much is added sugar and how much is natural sugar. If the product is a soft drink, you'll know that all of the sugar is added sugar.

- **Fiber.** Fiber is very good for you, especially when you have diabetes. Adults with diabetes should eat 25 to 50 g of fiber a day.

- **Fat.** One teaspoon (5 mL) of butter, margarine, lard or oil has 5 g of fat. Fat should make up no more than one-third of your daily calories.

  - A daily meal plan of 1,200 calories a day should include no more than about 9 teaspoons (45 g) of fat, including hidden fat.

  - A daily meal plan of 1,620 calories a day should include no more than about 13 teaspoons (65 g) of fat, including hidden fat.

  Limit saturated fats and try to avoid trans fats. See page 58 for information about healthy fats.

- **Sodium.** It is best to limit your total sodium intake to 2,300 mg a day (about 1 teaspoon/5 mL of salt). This is often a challenge: most food products have salt added, sometimes large amounts.

Choosing the "healthiest" option (Karen's Choice) was often challenging, because one food product might be lower in sugar or fat (which is good) but higher in sodium or lower in fiber (not so good).

The nutrients in the foods shown in the charts can differ among brands and sometimes between Canadian and American producers.

Caffeine content is listed only for food products that have more than 45 mg of caffeine. Because caffeine is an addictive drug, adults should limit it to 400 mg a day (300 mg if pregnant or breastfeeding). Children and teenagers should limit caffeine even more – or avoid it altogether.

Cold Cereal

1½ cups (375 mL) granola crunch with ¾ cup (175 mL) 2% milk

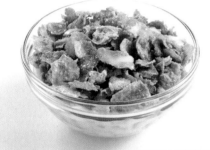

Calories	Carbs	Fiber	Fat	Sodium
710	97 g	9 g	30 g	203 mg

Granola is an excellent source of fiber and is lower in sodium than other cereal choices, but it is very high in calories, sugar and saturated fat. Limit your serving to ¼ to ⅓ cup (60 to 75 mL), or use it as a topping on plain cereal.

1½ cups (375 mL) frosted flakes with ¾ cup (175 mL) 1% milk

Calories	Carbs	Fiber	Fat	Sodium
279	57 g	1 g	2 g	359 mg

Frosted flakes are high in sugar — 6 tsp (30 mL) of sugar have been added to this serving. Sugar-coated cereals are best sprinkled on top of your corn flakes or bran flakes.

1½ cups (375 mL) corn flakes with ¾ cup (175 mL) skim milk

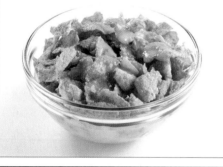

Calories	Carbs	Fiber	Fat	Sodium
208	41 g	1 g	0 g	347 mg

Corn flakes have lower carbs and sodium than the other cereal choices in this chart. This makes them a good choice. However, they have little fiber. You could boost the fiber with a sprinkle of natural bran or bran buds on top.

1½ cups (375 mL) bran flakes with ¾ cup (175 mL) skim milk

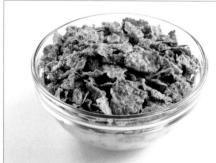

Calories	Carbs	Fiber	Fat	Sodium
209	44 g	6 g	1 g	467 mg

Bran flakes are my choice because they are an excellent source of fiber. Yet compared to frosted flakes and corn flakes, they are higher in sodium. If reducing sodium is your priority, choose the corn flakes.

KAREN'S CHOICE

FOOD FACT

Having a piece of fruit with your cereal adds healthy antioxidants and 2 to 5 g of fiber.

Restaurant Egg Breakfast

2 fried eggs, 2 slices of buttered white toast, 2 jams, 2 sausages, 1 cup (250 mL) hash browns, 1 tbsp (15 mL) ketchup, 20-oz (600 mL) coffee with 4 creamers (4 tbsp/60 mL) and 4 tsp (20 mL) sugar

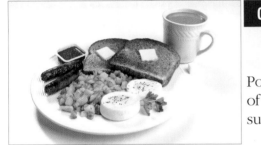

Calories	Carbs	Fiber	Fat	Sodium
1,147	123 g	6 g	62 g	1,194 mg

This "breakfast special" gives you a whole day's fat intake. Save this meal for special occasions. (Note: 1 package of jam = 2 tsp/10 mL and 1 creamer = 1 tbsp/15 mL) **Caffeine: 343 mg** (based on filter drip).

2 poached eggs, 2 slices of buttered brown toast, 1 jam, 2 sausages, ½ cup (125 mL) hash browns, 10-oz (300 mL) coffee with 2 tbsp (30 mL) whole milk and 1 tsp (5 mL) sugar

Calories	Carbs	Fiber	Fat	Sodium
705	66 g	6 g	39 g	886 mg

Poached eggs, less jam on your toast and just one mug of coffee are good changes. You will eat less fat and sugar at one meal. **Caffeine: 171 mg.**

2 poached eggs, 2 slices of buttered brown toast, 1 jam, 2 sausages, tomato slices, 10-oz (300 mL) coffee with 2 tbsp (30 mL) whole milk

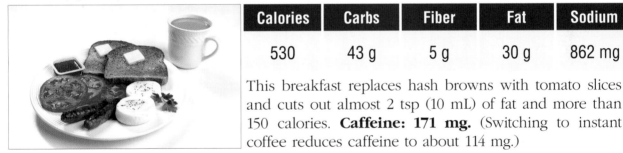

Calories	Carbs	Fiber	Fat	Sodium
530	43 g	5 g	30 g	862 mg

This breakfast replaces hash browns with tomato slices and cuts out almost 2 tsp (10 mL) of fat and more than 150 calories. **Caffeine: 171 mg.** (Switching to instant coffee reduces caffeine to about 114 mg.)

1 poached egg, 2 slices of unbuttered brown toast, 1 jam, tomato slices, 10-oz (300 mL) tea with 2 tbsp (30 mL) 2% milk

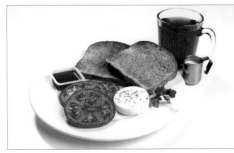

Calories	Carbs	Fiber	Fat	Sodium
286	42 g	5 g	8 g	480 mg

This is a trimmed-down, healthier breakfast. Choose a low-calorie sweetener for your tea (or coffee) if desired. **Caffeine: 59 mg.** (Decaf tea and most herbal teas have no caffeine.)

FOOD FACT Tea has almost three-quarters less caffeine than coffee. Plus, it is rich in antioxidants that may help keep your blood vessels healthy.

KAREN'S CHOICE

Bagel Breakfast

1 large (4-inch/10 cm or 102 g) bagel (unbuttered) with 3 tbsp (45 mL) cream cheese, 20-oz (600 mL) coffee with 4 creamers (4 tbsp/60 mL) and 4 tsp (20 mL) sugar

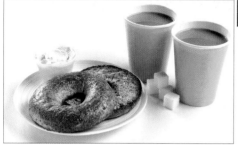

Calories	Carbs	Fiber	Fat	Sodium
640	81 g	3 g	28 g	751 mg

Bagels are a dense type of bread. One 4-inch (10 cm) bagel has the same number of carbs as 4 slices of bread. **Caffeine: 448 mg** (based on filter drip).

1 large (4-inch/10 cm or 102 g) bagel (unbuttered) with 1 tbsp (15 mL) cream cheese, 10-oz (300 mL) coffee with 2 creamers (2 tbsp/30 mL) and 2 tsp (10 mL) sugar

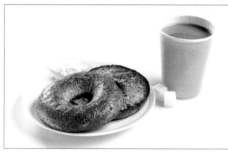

Calories	Carbs	Fiber	Fat	Sodium
445	70 g	3 g	12 g	647 mg

Simply cutting back on the size of your coffee makes a big difference in the amount of cream and sugar you'll use. Small changes are easier than big changes. **Caffeine: 224 mg.**

1 small (3-inch/7.5 cm or 53 g) bagel (unbuttered) with 1 tbsp (15 mL) light cream cheese, 10-oz (300 mL) decaf coffee with 2 tbsp (30 mL) 2% milk

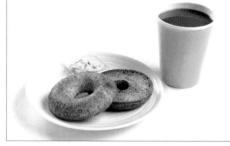

Calories	Carbs	Fiber	Fat	Sodium
206	33 g	1 g	4 g	367 mg

Here's a lighter choice! Not all coffee shops sell small bagels, but you can buy them at the grocery store, toast your bagel at home and add a smear of light cream cheese. **Caffeine: 4 mg.**

1 small (3-inch/7.5 cm or 53 g) bagel (unbuttered) with 1 tbsp (15 mL) sugar-free jam, 10-oz (300 mL) decaf coffee with 2 tbsp (30 mL) 2% milk

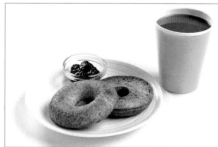

Calories	Carbs	Fiber	Fat	Sodium
192	37 g	1 g	1 g	323 mg

Switching from cream cheese to a sugar-free jam increases your carbs slightly but decreases total calories and fat. Low-calorie sweetener can be added to coffee or tea, if desired. **Caffeine: 4 mg.**

KAREN'S CHOICE

FOOD FACT Why does a bagel have a hole? Two reasons. The hole provides more even cooking and enabled traditional vendors to carry them on a string or stick.

Deli Sandwich

Rye bread, 2 thin large slices (2 oz/60 g) pastrami, 2 tsp (10 mL) mustard, 2 tsp (10 mL) butter, ¼ cup (60 mL) sauerkraut, 1 medium dill pickle

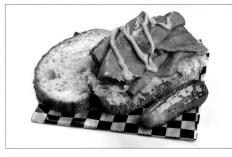

Calories	Carbs	Fiber	Fat	Sodium
330	35 g	6 g	14 g	2,101 mg

Did you notice the sodium? Save this sandwich for a special occasion only or choose one of the options below.

Rye bread, 1 thin slice (1 oz/30 g) pastrami, 2 tsp (10 mL) mustard, 2 tsp (10 mL) butter, 1 medium dill pickle

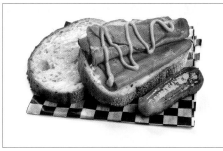

Calories	Carbs	Fiber	Fat	Sodium
286	33 g	5 g	12 g	1,515 mg

If you are buying a pastrami rye sandwich at a restaurant, ask the server to hold the sauerkraut. This helps reduce the sodium.

Rye bread, 1 thin slice (1 oz/30 g) pastrami, 2 tsp (10 mL) mustard, 1 medium dill pickle

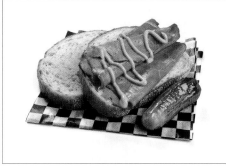

Calories	Carbs	Fiber	Fat	Sodium
218	33 g	5 g	4 g	1,461 mg

To cut calories and sodium further, ask for your bread to be unbuttered. If you use home-cooked sliced roast beef, turkey or chicken, the sodium is even further reduced.

Rye bread, 1 thin slice (1 oz/30 g) pastrami, 1 tsp (5 mL) mustard, lettuce, tomato, ½ medium dill pickle

Calories	Carbs	Fiber	Fat	Sodium
215	33 g	5 g	4 g	1,119 mg

This reduced-salt version still contains almost half of the suggested daily intake of sodium. So make sure not to have luncheon meat on a daily basis, or use your own home-cooked sliced roast beef, turkey or chicken.

KAREN'S CHOICE

FOOD FACT When buying bread, look for thinner or smaller slices that have about 70 to 80 calories per slice.

Cream Soup

Half of a 10-oz (284 mL) can of condensed cream of tomato soup, made with an equal amount of 3.3% (homogenized) milk, 3½-oz (100 g) tea biscuit with 2 tsp (10 mL) butter

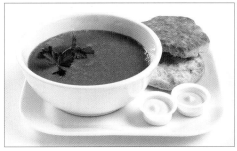

Calories	Carbs	Fiber	Fat	Sodium
617	76 g	3 g	30 g	2,031 mg

The extra fat in this meal comes from the whole milk in the soup and the butter on the biscuit.

Half of a 10-oz (284 mL) can of condensed cream of tomato soup, made with an equal amount of 2% milk, 3½-oz (100 g) tea biscuit with 1 tsp (5 mL) butter

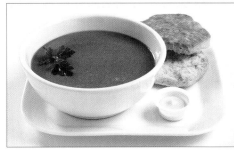

Calories	Carbs	Fiber	Fat	Sodium
568	76 g	3 g	24 g	2,006 mg

The switch to 2% milk cuts some calories and fat.

Half of a 10-oz (284 mL) can of condensed reduced-sodium cream of tomato soup, made with an equal amount of skim milk, 3½-oz (100 g) tea biscuit (unbuttered)

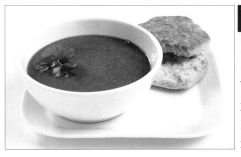

Calories	Carbs	Fiber	Fat	Sodium
523	77 g	2 g	19 g	1,679 mg

When you switch to skim milk, you reduce the calories and fat further. Choosing a reduced-sodium soup can cut salt by 20% to 30%, depending on the brand. Low-sodium varieties reduce the sodium even more, but are more difficult to find.

Half of a 10-oz (284 mL) can of condensed reduced-sodium cream of tomato soup, made with an equal amount of skim milk, 6 unsalted soda crackers, veggies

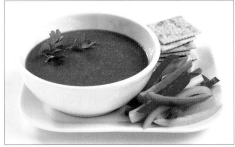

Calories	Carbs	Fiber	Fat	Sodium
262	47 g	3 g	5 g	805 mg

For an even lighter choice, switch to soda crackers and veggies on the side.

KAREN'S CHOICE

FOOD FACT Boil meat or poultry bones for a great soup stock. Add onions and herbs, vegetables and some barley, beans or noodles for a tasty low-salt soup.

Chicken Leg

1 drumstick and thigh, with skin, breaded and deep-fried

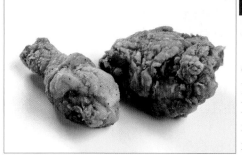

Calories	Carbs	Fiber	Fat	Sodium
360	12 g	0 g	21 g	368 mg

One piece of deep-fried chicken never hurt anyone. But eating fried chicken every day is a health risk. Fried chicken tends to be eaten with other high-fat foods, including fries, gravy and coleslaw laden with high-fat mayonnaise.

1 drumstick and thigh, with skin, coated with commercial crumb coating and baked

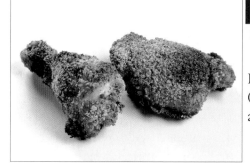

Calories	Carbs	Fiber	Fat	Sodium
286	4 g	0 g	19 g	234 mg

Here's a lower-fat homemade alternative using commercial crumb coating (such as Shake'n Bake™) for the chicken.

1 drumstick and thigh, skin removed, coated with commercial crumb coating and baked

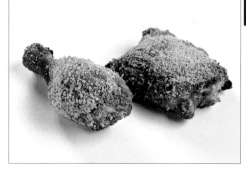

Calories	Carbs	Fiber	Fat	Sodium
173	4 g	0 g	7 g	217 mg

Remove the skin from the chicken and you remove 2¹⁄₂ tsp (12 mL) of fat for this serving. This is still a delicious alternative.

1 drumstick and thigh, skin removed, coated with salt-free spice blend and baked

Calories	Carbs	Fiber	Fat	Sodium
148	0 g	0 g	6 g	80 mg

This choice reduces the calories and sodium by using a commercial low-salt spice blend. Or try a homemade blend of oregano, thyme, paprika, black pepper and chili powder.

KAREN'S CHOICE

FOOD FACT — **By baking the chicken at home, you're not only making an awesome healthy change, but you're also saving money!**

Fast-Food Burger with All Toppings

Third-pound burger (4 oz/112 g cooked weight) with double cheese and bacon

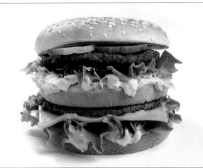

Calories	Carbs	Fiber	Fat	Sodium
780	53 g	3 g	44 g	1,990 mg

Restaurant burgers have layers of tasty ingredients, and that's reflected in the calories, fat and sodium. If you have fries and a drink with this burger, the fat and calories go up even higher.

Two single burgers (each burger = 1 oz/28 g cooked) with cheese and middle bun

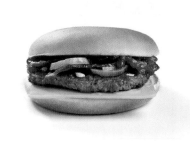

Calories	Carbs	Fiber	Fat	Sodium
540	44 g	3 g	29 g	1,020 mg

This is a reduction but still pretty loaded. Know what you are eating: check out the calories and nutrients of the fast-food item online before you go out to eat, or ask for the nutrient brochure at the restaurant.

Cheeseburger (1 oz/28 g cooked weight burger) with bacon

Calories	Carbs	Fiber	Fat	Sodium
340	34 g	2 g	15 g	910 mg

This option has significantly less calories, fat and sodium. It's a good alternative and still tastes great!

Cheeseburger (1 oz/28 g cooked weight burger)

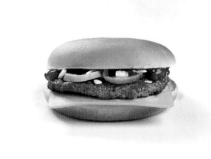

Calories	Carbs	Fiber	Fat	Sodium
300	33 g	2 g	12 g	750 mg

Of the four options here, this is the best choice when you're eating at a fast-food restaurant. Instead of choosing the meal deal, order individual items from the menu. Ask for a small fries or a salad on the side, and have milk instead of a soft drink.

KAREN'S CHOICE

FOOD FACT

It may seem like a waste not to get the meal deal, but remember: all those extra calories go to *your* waist.

Restaurant Pizza

3 pieces of thick-crust 12-inch (30 cm) deluxe pizza (with 6 pieces per pizza)

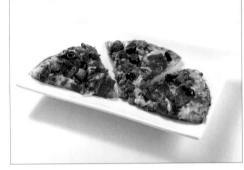

Calories	Carbs	Fiber	Fat	Sodium
1,659	143 g	7 g	87 g	3,474 mg

This option has the same number of calories as a large breakfast, lunch and dinner meal in this book combined – all in just three pieces of pizza! This serving has a whopping 1¹/₂ tsp (7 mL) of salt and more than a day's worth of fat.

3 pieces of thin-crust 12-inch (30 cm) deluxe pizza (with 6 pieces per pizza)

Calories	Carbs	Fiber	Fat	Sodium
1,346	91 g	7 g	81 g	2,757 mg

Cut carbs significantly by switching to thin-crust pizza. To cut calories, fat and sodium, choose a pizza with fewer toppings.

2 pieces of thick-crust 12-inch (30 cm) pizza with two toppings, salad with a light dressing

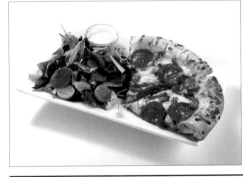

Calories	Carbs	Fiber	Fat	Sodium
944	95 g	4 g	46 g	2,114 mg

To help fill you up, drink water and have a salad or a half plate of your favorite cooked vegetables with your pizza.

2 pieces of thin-crust 12-inch (30 cm) pizza with two toppings, salad with a light dressing

Calories	Carbs	Fiber	Fat	Sodium
782	65 g	4 g	44 g	1,742 mg

Add some extra vegetables to your pizza. Some of my favorite toppings are onions, asparagus, peppers, mushrooms, fresh tomatoes, sun-dried tomatoes and zucchini. Even this choice is salty, so it's best to not choose it every week.

FOOD FACT **Slowing down your eating can help you eat less. Eat some vegetables or salad before your pizza, and drink water before and with your meal.**

KAREN'S CHOICE

Ready-to-Serve Noodles

Noodles in a bowl, chicken flavor (110 g dry weight)

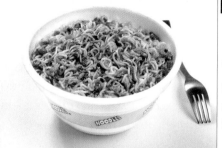

Calories	Carbs	Fiber	Fat	Sodium
481	70 g	3 g	17 g	2,278 mg

This product has a shocking amount of salt. Studies show that people with diabetes are not able to get rid of excess sodium as efficiently as people without diabetes. Eating too much sodium can worsen high blood pressure.

Noodles in a cup, chicken flavor (64 g dry weight)

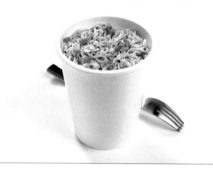

Calories	Carbs	Fiber	Fat	Sodium
280	41 g	2 g	10 g	1,325 mg

The cup serving is smaller than the bowl and so has less sodium. However, this serving is still high in sodium.

Noodles in a cup, chicken flavor (64 g dry weight), made with half the spice mix

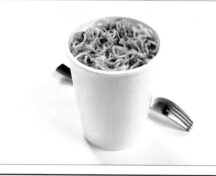

Calories	Carbs	Fiber	Fat	Sodium
274	39 g	1 g	10 g	776 mg

Here's an easy change to cut the salt in half: only add half the package of spice mix!

Noodles in a cup (64 g dry weight) without the chicken flavor mix, made instead with 1 tsp (5 mL) salt-free spice blend (or fresh herbs and/or chili or black pepper)

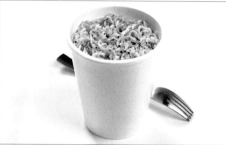

Calories	Carbs	Fiber	Fat	Sodium
268	37 g	1 g	10 g	226 mg

Are you ready to replace the whole package of spice mix with a low-salt seasoning or some tasty fresh herbs? You'll still enjoy the noodles, and you'll no longer have to worry about all that added salt.

KAREN'S CHOICE

FOOD FACT A noodle bowl is the carb equivalent of about 5 slices of bread and a noodle cup is equivalent to almost 3 slices of bread.

Potatoes

1 large serving (6 oz/175 g) fast-food french fries

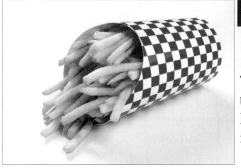

Calories	Carbs	Fiber	Fat	Sodium
560	74 g	6 g	27 g	430 mg

The total fat in a serving of french fries is a concern if they're eaten regularly or daily. Also of concern is that fat heated to a high temperature in a deep-fryer changes into an unhealthy type of fat.

1 large serving (6 oz/175 g) baked frozen french fries, unsalted

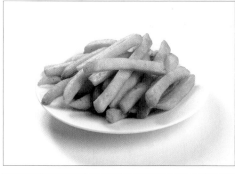

Calories	Carbs	Fiber	Fat	Sodium
350	55 g	6 g	13 g	53 mg

Bake these lower-fat fries at home and serve them as part of a meal.

1 large baked potato with no added fat, with 2 tbsp (30 mL) fat-free sour cream, 1 tsp (5 mL) butter or margarine, and chopped green onion

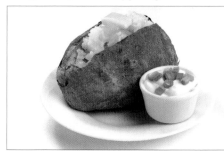

Calories	Carbs	Fiber	Fat	Sodium
298	61 g	5 g	4 g	92 mg

As an alternative to fries, try a baked potato. The carbs are a bit higher in this choice because of the toppings.

1 large potato, cut into sticks, tossed in 1 tsp (5 mL) oil and baked

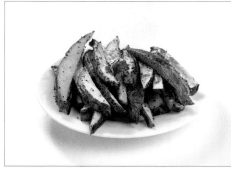

Calories	Carbs	Fiber	Fat	Sodium
276	55 g	5 g	5 g	17 mg

This is a delicious and easy way to make home-baked fries. To spice them up, sprinkle on flavorings such as dried dillweed, chili powder or a commercial salt-free spice blend.

FOOD FACT — **Potatoes are an excellent source of vitamin C and potassium.**

KAREN'S CHOICE

Caesar Salad

Restaurant Caesar salad: 4 cups (1 L) romaine lettuce, ¼ cup (60 mL) Caesar salad dressing, ¼ cup (60 mL) croutons and 2 tbsp (30 mL) Parmesan cheese, plus 2 pieces of garlic bread

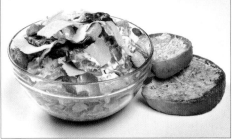

Calories	Carbs	Fiber	Fat	Sodium
798	58 g	8 g	57 g	1,564 mg

Many are surprised that a large Caesar salad from a restaurant has as many calories as a large burger. The reason is that Caesar salad dressing is mostly oil and is high in fat. Topped off with the garlic bread, this salad is not light!

Restaurant Caesar salad: 4 cups (1 L) romaine lettuce, ¼ cup (60 mL) Caesar salad dressing, ¼ cup (60 mL) croutons and 2 tbsp (30 mL) Parmesan cheese

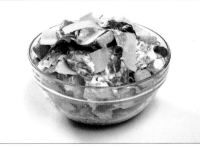

Calories	Carbs	Fiber	Fat	Sodium
442	16 g	5 g	40 g	967 mg

To avoid the extra calories, ask the waiter not to bring out the garlic bread.

Restaurant Caesar salad: 4 cups (1 L) romaine lettuce, 2 tbsp (30 mL) Caesar salad dressing, ¼ cup (60 mL) croutons and 1 tbsp (15 mL) Parmesan cheese

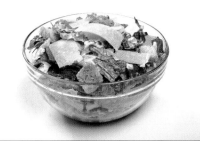

Calories	Carbs	Fiber	Fat	Sodium
263	15 g	5 g	21 g	554 mg

Ask for a small amount of salad dressing on the side and limit your serving of dressing to 2 tbsp (30 mL). Some restaurants have an option for a light salad dressing.

Homemade Caesar salad: 4 cups (1 L) romaine lettuce, 1 tbsp (15 mL) light Caesar salad dressing, ¼ cup (60 mL) croutons and 1 tbsp (15 mL) Parmesan cheese

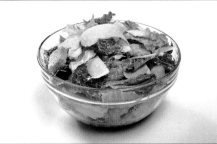

Calories	Carbs	Fiber	Fat	Sodium
125	17 g	5 g	5 g	400 mg

Simple and fast to prepare at home, this light salad choice makes a terrific appetizer or meal accompaniment. Light salad dressing is higher in salt, so you might want to have regular salad dressing instead.

KAREN'S CHOICE

FOOD FACT

Dark green lettuce, such as romaine, is rich in folate, which is helpful for your blood cholesterol.

Yogurt

¾ cup (175 mL) 6% fruit yogurt, sweetened with sugar

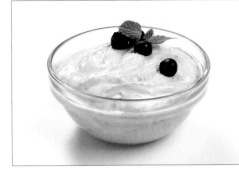

Calories	Carbs	Fiber	Fat	Sodium
240	29 g	0 g	11 g	98 mg

This high-fat yogurt has double the fat of a homogenized milk. Some other yogurts have extra fermenting bacteria added and are labeled as better for you. But look at the label, because they may be made with a higher-fat milk or extra sugar. They may not be the right choice for you.

¾ cup (175 mL) 3% frozen yogurt

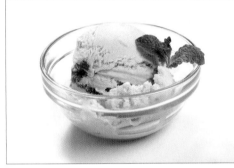

Calories	Carbs	Fiber	Fat	Sodium
150	29 g	0 g	3 g	90 mg

Frozen yogurt is a nice dessert choice and has fewer calories than the high-fat yogurt above. It has similar calories to a 2% sweetened fruit yogurt.

¾ cup (175 mL) fat-free (0% fat) fruit yogurt, sweetened with sugar

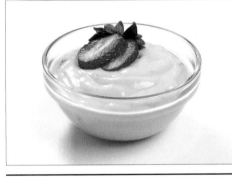

Calories	Carbs	Fiber	Fat	Sodium
173	35 g	0 g	0 g	107 mg

This is a better choice because there's no fat, but there is still added sugar.

¾ cup (175 mL) fat-free (0% fat) fruit yogurt, sweetened with a low-calorie sweetener, plus ½ cup (125 mL) blueberries or other fresh or frozen fruit

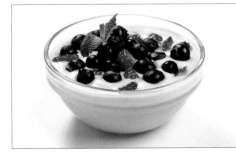

Calories	Carbs	Fiber	Fat	Sodium
128	24 g	2 g	0 g	109 mg

By choosing a fat-free yogurt sweetened with a low-calorie sweetener, you avoid extra fat and added sugar. Like all yogurts, it contains natural sugar (carbohydrate) from the milk.

KAREN'S CHOICE

FOOD FACT

Yogurt is perhaps the oldest fermented milk product. There are records of its use dating back 2,500 years!

Muffin or Donut

Large blueberry bran muffin (128 g)

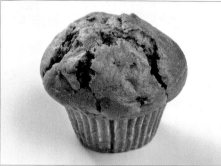

Calories	Carbs	Fiber	Fat	Sodium
380	58 g	5 g	15 g	530 mg

A common misconception is that coffee shop muffins (especially low-fat ones) are healthier than donuts. This is false because the muffins are made so large, they end up having more sugar and fat than standard-size donuts.

Cake donut (60 g) or cream-filled donut (89 g)

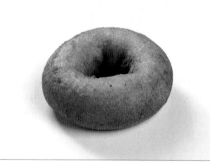

Calories	Carbs	Fiber	Fat	Sodium
253	30 g	1 g	14 g	328 mg

Many coffee shops have the nutrient information of their muffins, donuts and other foods and drinks listed online. If you eat at one regularly, compare the nutrient listings.

3 donut "holes" (50 to 55 g total)

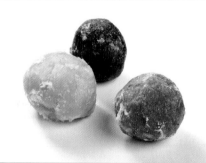

Calories	Carbs	Fiber	Fat	Sodium
219	26 g	1 g	12 g	284 mg

For a lighter donut choice with your coffee or tea, choose two or three donut "holes."

Homemade Bran Muffin

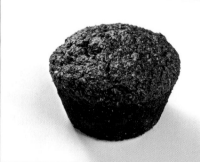

Calories	Carbs	Fiber	Fat	Sodium
144	29 g	4 g	3 g	234 mg

This high-fiber muffin is made from a commercial low-fat muffin mix, or you can make it from scratch using the recipe found on page 58 of *Diabetes Meals for Good Health*. Although this choice appears to have more carbs than the 3 donut holes, the available carb is less.

KAREN'S CHOICE

FOOD FACT

The size of the muffin determines the total amount of sugar and fat. Bigger muffins can have similar amounts of sugar and fat as donuts.

Apple Dessert

1 piece of homemade double-crust apple pie (⅙th of a 9-inch/23 cm pie), made with 5 apples

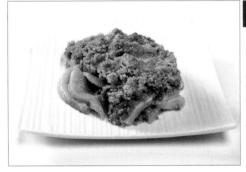

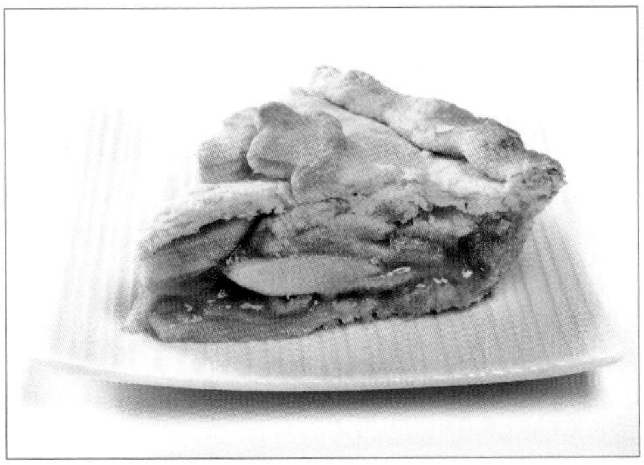

Calories	Carbs	Fiber	Fat	Sodium
556	71 g	3 g	29 g	517 mg

Enjoy apple pie just occasionally. Once you add a double crust to a pie, it's like adding 4 slices of buttered bread to your fruit filling. Ice cream on top of your pie will add more sugar and fat.

¾ cup (175 mL) traditional apple crisp (⅙ of recipe, see below)

Calories	Carbs	Fiber	Fat	Sodium
314	55 g	2 g	11 g	378 mg

Recipe includes 5 apples, ¾ cup (175 mL) flour, 1 cup (250 mL) brown sugar, ¾ tsp (3 mL) salt, 1 tsp (5 mL) ground cinnamon and ⅓ cup (75 mL) butter or margarine. Using a topping rather than a crust cuts the calories and fat.

¾ cup (175 mL) healthier apple crisp (⅙ of recipe, see below)

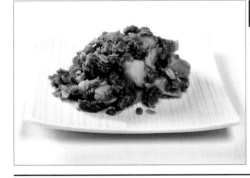

Calories	Carbs	Fiber	Fat	Sodium
224	37 g	3 g	9 g	62 mg

Recipe includes 5 apples, ¼ cup (60 mL) whole wheat flour, ½ cup (125 mL) rolled oats, ½ cup (125 mL) brown sugar, 1 tsp (5 mL) ground cinnamon and ¼ cup (60 mL) butter or margarine. If you want, you could replace some of the brown sugar with a low-calorie sweetener.

1 Baked Apple (recipe can be found on page 165 of *Diabetes Meals for Good Health*)

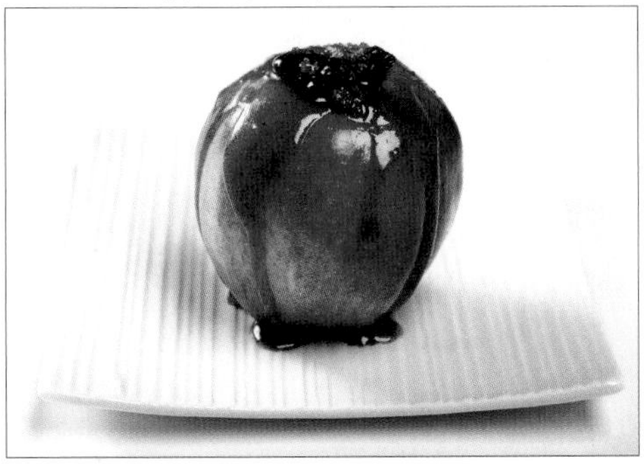

Calories	Carbs	Fiber	Fat	Sodium
141	32 g	3 g	3 g	23 mg

Recipe includes 2 medium apples, 1 tsp (5 mL) butter or margarine, 1 tbsp (15 mL) of brown sugar, ¼ tsp (1 mL) cinnamon, ¼ tsp (1 mL) lemon juice, 1 tbsp (15 mL) raisins, and a pinch of nutmeg (if desired). Makes 2 baked apples.

KAREN'S CHOICE

FOOD FACT — Adding cinnamon to desserts and cereals helps replace some of the sweetening, so you don't need to add as much sugar.

215

Popcorn

Large buttered movie theater popcorn (20 cups/5 L with 6 pumps of butter, equal to 3 tbsp/45 mL)

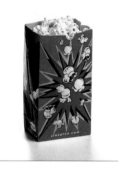

Calories	Carbs	Fiber	Fat	Sodium
1,405	126 g	22 g	96 g	2,190 mg

The amount of fat and salt in this super-sized serving might be enough to scare you or make you cry, if the movie doesn't.

Small buttered movie theater popcorn (7 cups/1.75 L with 3 pumps of butter, equal to 1½ tbsp/22 mL)

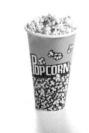

Calories	Carbs	Fiber	Fat	Sodium
538	44 g	8 g	39 g	803 mg

Studies have been done where people were given very stale popcorn at a movie theater, and they still ate it all. If you want to eat less, buy a smaller serving.

4 cups (1 L) home-popped popcorn, made with 1 tsp (5 mL) oil for ¼ cup (60 mL) kernels, plus 3 shakes of salt (¹⁄₁₆ tsp/0.25 mL)

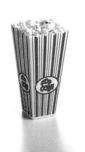

Calories	Carbs	Fiber	Fat	Sodium
164	24 g	4 g	6 g	147 mg

A better choice. It contains about half the fat and sodium of the same amount of movie theater popcorn. Try peanut oil for a great flavor! Electric popcorn makers with motorized stirring rods make yummy popcorn with little oil.

4 cups (1 L) air-popped popcorn

Calories	Carbs	Fiber	Fat	Sodium
122	25 g	4 g	1 g	1 mg

Popcorn can be air-popped with an electric air popper or a microwave popcorn popper.

KAREN'S CHOICE

FOOD FACT Popcorn is believed to have been discovered by Native Americans over 5,000 years ago when corn was being cooked over the open fire.

2. Being Active

2

A prescription for exercise   **218**

Getting started   **219**

Ten benefits of regular exercise   **221**

Low-impact aerobic exercise   **223**

Walking and treadmills   224

Biking and exercise bikes   228

Swimming or water exercise   230

Aerobics and dancing   232

Other home or gym exercise equipment   234

If you have arthritis – ten exercise tips   237

Staying flexible   **238**

Flexibility exercises   239

Strengthening exercises   **240**

Arm and upper body exercises   242

Stomach and lower body exercises   243

Ten tips for a healthy back   244

A fitness plan for you   **246**

Fitness plan 1 (least active)   247

Fitness plan 2 (active)   250

Fitness plan 3 (most active)   252

Managing setbacks   254

Precautions   **255**

If you have a heart problem – ten precautions   255

Warning signs to stop exercising   258

Keeping your eyes healthy when exercising   259

Keeping your feet healthy when exercising   260

Low and high blood sugar when exercising   262

A Prescription for Exercise

You've been really tired the last two months and your blood sugar is higher than usual. You go to see your doctor and she gives you two possible answers.

Answer One
Doctor: "Here's a prescription. Take this pill twice a day, and it will help with your blood sugar and tiredness that you have told me about."

You: "Yes, thank you, Doctor."

When you say yes:
1) You trust your doctor.
2) You are willing to try something to feel better.
3) It sounds easy.
4) You can start right away.

Answer Two
Doctor: "The best prescription for these health issues you have told me about would be to go for a walk every day."

You: "Well no, I can't walk. I don't have time to walk during the day. Anyways, it's too cold outside, my knees hurt and I just don't have the energy."

When you say no: You still trust your doctor and would like to try something to feel better, but, walking is more of a challenge. It will require a change to your daily routine.

Nearly half of North Americans don't exercise. Inactivity is as harmful as smoking. Yet far more people are inactive than smokers.

- If you answer "yes" to the pills and "no" to the walk, you are like many others. We all wish that doctors will find a pill that will make us better without too much change on our part.

- Yet, when you say "yes" to the pills, it shows you are willing to change and that you are thinking of your future. You want to be in control of your diabetes.

- If you answer "yes" to the walk, then you recognize that exercise can be one of the most powerful medicines that we have for good health.

Exercise – A powerful medicine for good health.

This chapter will help you find ways to include exercise as part of your prescription for good health. You can choose a fitness plan that will be easy and comfortable for you. An exercise plan will give you energy, not take it away.

Getting Started

Like anything in life, change is a process and takes time. In this chapter you will read how others have overcome their barriers to exercise and become active. You can too.

One step at a time

Increase exercise gradually. You should always be able to do the "Talk Test." This means you can talk comfortably when exercising. If you are overweight or older, avoid high-impact and intense exercise such as jogging or skipping rope. These put excessive pressure on your back and joints and can injure your feet. Read more information on the risk of high-impact exercises and other Precautions (on pages 255–262).

You can avoid sore muscles by warming up or cooling down before and after exercise. One easy way to warm up and cool down is to begin and end your exercise session at a slower pace. For example, walk slowly for the first few minutes, then increase your pace to a comfortable level; then walk slowly again for the last few minutes of your walk.

First, move more at home and work

Even small changes in how we live can make a difference. Start with replacing some sedentary activities with active activities. Take walks at home or at work, use stairs instead of the elevator, park or get off buses further away from buildings and walk. Consider gardening, fishing, house cleaning, playing pool and doing hobbies. Little things add up. People who move a little all day long burn more calories than people who sit a lot.

Second, take longer walks or do other aerobic exercise

A variety of aerobic exercises are outlined on pages 233–237. Replacing just a half hour of television time every day with a walk or other aerobic exercise can help fight against weight gain.

Third, do strengthening and flexibility exercises

Strengthening and flexibility are part of your walk, bike or swim, but you may now be ready to do some specific exercises for optimum overall fitness for your age. See pages 238–245.

Watching television, using computers or video games and commuting are activities that occupy more and more of our lives. Yet these activities burn virtually no calories. They contribute significantly to the rise of obesity.

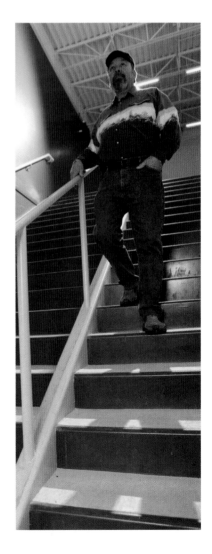

Fourth, choose a Fitness Plan

This will help you put all these things together, manage set backs and help motivate you. You will find three different Fitness Plans on pages 246–254. Fitness Plan 1 includes exercises while seated and short walks. Fitness Plan 2 starts off with 15–30 minute walks, while Fitness Plan 3 includes longer walks or other aerobic exercise. The body is an amazing machine, and almost everyone can gradually increase their fitness level.

If you plan to do exercises more vigorous than brisk walking, talk to your doctor. Also see Precautions.

How many steps should you take each day?

- If you are elderly or in poor health, you may only be doing a few hundred steps a day. Building up to 1,000 or 2,000 steps would be an achievement.

- 2,000 steps are about equal to walking a mile (1,250 steps equals a kilometer).

- If you already do 2,000 steps a day, then try to add an extra 1,000 steps to your day over a period of a month.

- For improved health, it may take several months to build up to 5,000.

- 10,000 steps a day is considered ideal for many.

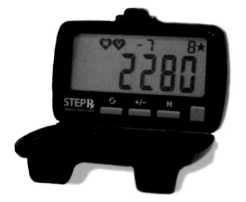

Wearing a pedometer helps you learn how many steps you take each day.

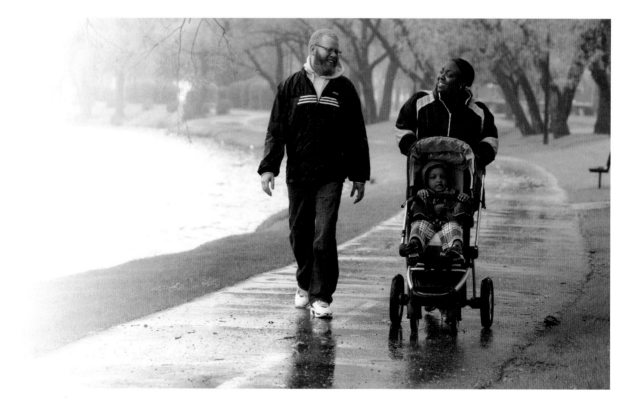

Ten Benefits of Regular Exercise

1. *Reduces blood sugar*

- Exercise helps insulin work better. If you are overweight, walking can help you lose body fat. Then insulin does an even better job of lowering your blood sugar.

- When you exercise, your muscles need fuel (sugar). Insulin goes to work and moves sugar out of your blood and into your muscles.

- When you take a short walk, you use a small amount of blood sugar. You use more blood sugar if you walk farther.

Exercise helps your body's insulin work better for 12 to 24 hours.

Improving your blood sugar means fewer diabetes complications.

2. *Strengthens your blood vessels and heart*

Your heart pumps faster when you exercise. This helps move the blood around your body. This improves circulation and reduces swelling in your hands and feet. Regular exercise improves your blood pressure, cholesterol and immunity, and helps prevent heart attacks and strokes.

3. *Helps you breathe easier*

Exercise will improve your breathing. That's because it strengthens the heart's ability to pump oxygen. If you have asthma or emphysema, this is especially important.

4. *Reduces your body fat*

Exercise helps you change fat into muscle. You feel toned. Exercise also boosts your metabolism so you burn more calories. This can help you lose weight or maintain weight loss.

No matter what your body size, large or small, exercise is crucial for a healthy long life.

5. *Helps digestion and reduces constipation*

Your stomach and bowels are large muscles. Exercise and increased blood flow helps them work better.

6. *Reduces your risk for certain cancers*

Studies show that exercise helps reduce cancer, including colon and breast cancer. Exercise reduces constipation and so waste and toxins leave the body more quickly. This reduces the risk of colon cancer. Exercise can help reduce excess weight which decreases certain hormones, like estrogen. This can then reduce the risk of breast cancer.

7. *Strengthens your muscles and bones*

As your muscles get stronger, you will have more energy. Exercise in your youth builds strong bones. As you get older, exercise helps maintain these strong bones and reduces osteoporosis and hip fractures.

8. *Reduces lower back pain*

Exercise gives you better posture and balance. It keeps your back muscles and joints strong and flexible.

9. *Helps you sleep better*

The exertion tires you out. Exercise also calms your body and mind (in part through the release of hormones such as serotonin), helping you fall asleep easier and sleep longer.

10. *Reduces stress*

Exercise releases "happy hormones" into your blood. This helps you relax and is good for your brain because it helps you think more clearly. Walking away from stressful situations gives you time to think about solutions and positive plans for the future.

What are your reasons to exercise? Think about it.

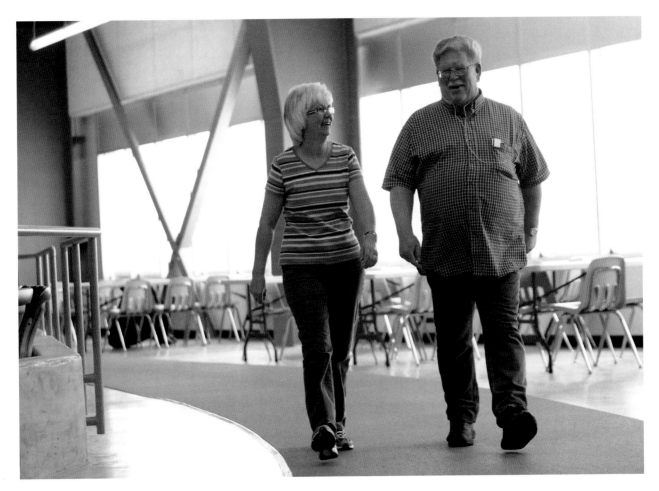

Low-Impact Aerobic Exercise

What is low-impact aerobic exercise?

Aerobic exercise involves continuous movement of your legs and arms, for example, walking or swimming. When you do aerobic exercise your heart rate will rise and stay above your heart's resting level. Oxygen flows through your blood vessels to your organs, muscles and your brain. You'll feel your heart beating faster, and your breathing is a bit deeper. You may feel warm and start to sweat. To do productive exercise, you don't need to overwork your heart; you just need a gradual increase.

Low impact means the exercise increases your heart rate (is aerobic) but doesn't cause sudden jarring that stresses the joints, bones and muscles. Walking is one of the best low-impact exercises. Walking doesn't put excess stress on your joints and feet, and there is just enough impact to strengthen your bones. Swimming is very low impact as the water buoys your body weight. Biking on a smooth surface is also low impact because the bicycle seat carries your upper body weight.

This chapter will focus on the most common aerobic exercises among adults with diabetes, including:

- Walking (or using a treadmill)
- Biking (or using a stationary bike)
- Swimming
- Dancing, aerobics and weight training
- Exercise using other exercise equipment

Other aerobic exercises include:

- golfing, when walking the course and carrying your clubs
- walking up and down stairs
- raking leaves and heavy gardening (hoeing and digging)
- wheeling yourself in a manual wheelchair
- cross-country skiing or snowshoeing
- rollerblading, ice skating, or road or ice hockey
- rowing, canoeing, hiking or rock climbing

> ### Recommended amount of exercise
> The Canadian and American Diabetes Associations recommend at least 150 minutes of walking or aerobic exercise a week. This is about 20–25 minutes a day or 30 minutes five days a week. *This is less than 3% of your awake day.*

> ### High intensity "start and stop" exercise
> *This includes snow shovelling, chopping wood with an axe, heavy carpentry, tennis or badminton. These can be strenuous. Take rests as needed – pace yourself.*
>
> *If you have diabetes eye damage, called retinopathy, take precautions when doing these exercises. See page 40–41 and 259.*

Studies have found that dog owners do almost twice as much walking each week as compared to those who did not own a dog.

Consider joining a walking group or hiking club.

Wear shoes that support and cushion your feet and have good traction. Boots should keep your feet warm in the winter. See pages 290–293 for more information on footwear.

Walking and treadmills

Walking is the #1 exercise choice because:

- It is low cost – just you and your walking shoes.
- You can do it anywhere: in a parking lot, apartment hallway, indoor track, down a city street or country road, or in a mall.
- You can walk alone, with a friend or family member, or with your dog (or offer to walk a neighbor's dog).
- You can listen to music as you walk, enjoy the sounds of nature, or partake in a bustling city.
- Walking is a lifelong activity.

Is safety a concern for you when walking?

- If possible, walk with someone else. If walking alone, only walk in open, well-lit areas and vary your route.
- If you prefer walks on your own, tell someone where you're taking a walk and when you'll be back.
- If you walk in the dark, wear a reflective safety vest (available at hardware stores) so vehicles can see you.
- If you do choose to wear earphones, keep the volume low so you can still hear noises around you.

If you get pain or cramping in your lower legs when walking:

This is often due to decreased blood flow (poor circulation) to the muscles in your legs. This means that as you walk, your lower leg muscles are short of oxygen. This is a common sign of Peripheral Arterial Disease (PAD). Talk to your doctor if you have these symptoms. If you have PAD, you likely also have blocked vessels in other parts of your body.

If you have PAD-related pain, it's still important to exercise daily. Try this:

1. "Stop and go." This means walk for 2 minutes, then slow down or stop (or sit down if you can) for 1 minute. Then walk 2 minutes and stop for 1 minute, and so on. This allows time for the oxygen to get to your muscles. With regularly doing this, you may be able to gradually increase the "go" portion to 3 minutes, then 4 minutes, and so on.

2. Limit or avoid walking up hills or prolonged stair stepping as this can make the pain worse. Consider trying swimming, cycling, walking slowly on a treadmill, using an elliptical trainer, or doing chair exercises instead.

3. Do ankle rotations (see page 239) once or twice a day to help improve blood flow to your lower legs.

Paulette's story

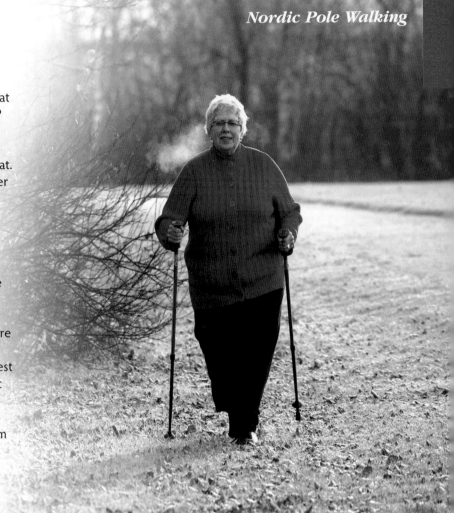

Nordic Pole Walking

I'm 71 years old, and exercise is more important than ever. Really, it's common sense, if you don't use it you lose it. There are people who are a lot older than me that are in very good shape, and why are they? They're exercising, they're walking, and maybe they're doing some weights three times a week. I think walking poles are great. They are designed to help you walk further and faster and it takes the pressure off all your joints. So when a person is heavier especially, it's helpful. Some people walk with a cane, but this is better because you have two poles. And if a person has back problems, some do, it seems to help there too. The poles also help you strengthen your arms and upper body. It's a plus in every way. I did a fair bit of research before buying my poles. I like the ones designed so that your palm side of your hand can rest on the top of the pole, plus it's ergonomic so your fingers fit around the handles real well, so I preferred that. They cost about $100 instead of $60 or $30, but I like them better. There are many people who say "I can't walk" but if they had these poles, they could.

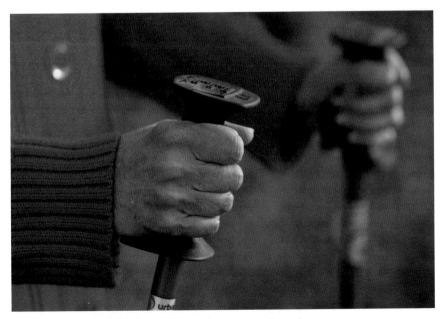

The poles should be adjusted to your height.

The tips of the poles are cushioned with rubber plugs for summer walking, with an option for spikes for the winter.

225

John's story

Becoming active is very difficult for me because I am so busy. My commute to work takes over an hour each way. I work in a hectic office. There's never time for a break. I do quite a bit of volunteering, and of course, there is always work to do at home and in the yard. When I finally get some time to myself, I need to relax. Watching TV is my way of relaxing.

When I found out I had diabetes, my doctor referred me to a diabetes center. I went there, but I felt really angry when they told me I should walk everyday. I felt the diabetes workers and my doctor didn't understand what my life was like. Exercise was just one more thing to have to cope with. I'm an "all or nothing" kind of guy, and so it was either get really active or not at all.

So I kept on doing what I had always done. After a few months, I started feeling even more tired. I had a hard time reading because my vision was often blurry. I thought it was probably my diabetes so I went back to see my doctor again. Sure enough my sugars were up. He gave me a diabetes pill this time but said I needed to become more active, or the sugars would go up again. He said if I could fit in even some short walks, that would help. He said to break my exercise into 10 or 15 minute blocks.

Let me tell you, I was scared about losing my vision. I thought about what my doctor said and realized I had to make some changes. This is what I did. I started to take a 15 minute walk at my lunch break. If I had a meeting at lunch, then I took a 15 minute walk in the afternoon. The first few weeks I missed quite a few walks, but I was doing more than before. It took me about a month before I was walking at least three days a week. What I found was that on the days I walked I wasn't as tired. I actually got more done, especially in the late afternoon. Now three months have passed. I still don't get for my walk some days, but if the weather is nice, I try and go a little longer. Plus, I try to walk on the weekend.

For me, getting active paid off. I now know it's possible to fit exercise into your life, even into a busy life like mine. I'm not having any more blurry vision. I feel better. In the end, that's probably most important.

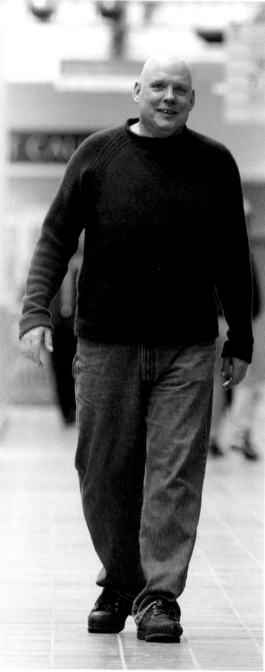

Other ways to fit walking into a busy schedule:

- You don't need hours – only minutes. Walking just 8 minutes sometime after each meal adds up to about 25 minutes a day. This meets the American and Canadian Diabetes Associations' recommendation for 150 minutes of aerobic exercise a week.

- Consider cutting out even a half hour of television or screen time to take a walk.

If the weather is bad or you'd rather walk indoors, consider using a treadmill.

A treadmill usually has a belt powered by electricity. The treadmill sets the pace and challenges you to keep up. The most useful treadmill features are setting the speed, length of time, and elevation. Then you can get a consistent workout. Start off and end your session at a slower pace. Slowing down your pace for the last 5 minutes helps prevent dizziness when you step off the machine.

Safety strap and pulse rate monitor

Wear a safety strap so the machine will stop if you fall off. If you have a heart condition, use a treadmill with a heart rate monitor. This is an important safety feature. Use the guidelines provided by your doctor, or with the treadmill or on page 256.

A manual treadmill works without electricity. You need to work harder to get the walking belt moving which can put too much strain on your knees. Generally, a better option is an electrical treadmill.

A treadmill takes up space so people often put it in an out-of-the-way place like a storage room or basement. It easily gets forgotten. If the treadmill is easy to see and in a nice environment near music or a TV, you are more likely to use it.

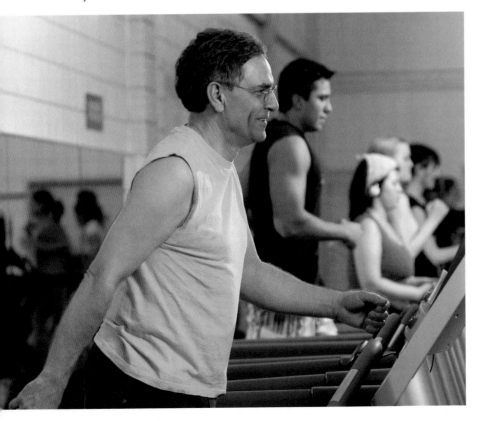

A more expensive treadmill will generally have:

- *A bigger motor, usually 2 or more horsepower (if you are a heavier person this is a good feature)*

- *A quieter motor (works at less than 4,000 RPMs)*

- *a walking belt that is long enough for most people to walk a full stride (usually at least 54 inches/ 135 cm).*

- *a longer warranty (usually 5–10 years on the motor)*

- *special features such as the ability to program walking speeds and times*

- *option for moveable handle bars for upper body strengthening*

Before buying home exercise equipment, try it out for fit and comfort.

It is best not to hang on to the treadmill handles. Swing your arms, as you do when you walk. Then you'll burn more calories and improve your balance. Use the handles if you feel unsteady or need to relieve some weight off your knees.

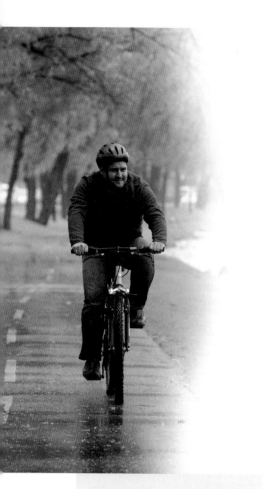

Biking and exercise bikes

Outdoor biking

Warm up and cool down: Start off and end your ride at a slow pace.

To increase calorie burning and further reduce your blood sugar: Bike up hills, for longer, or at a higher speed or resistance (higher gear). Also, combine biking with some walking.

For safety: Wear a helmet. Ring your bell when you pass walkers. Carry water for longer bike rides. If biking at night, it's a good idea to wear a fluorescent vest and to have a light at the front and back of your bike.

Proper positioning: Keep your elbows slightly bent for better shock absorption. Try to shift your hand positions often to prevent strain. Set the height of your bike seat so that when you peddle, you extend your legs almost completely.

Go for comfort: For extra comfort, consider replacing the standard seat with a wide seat. A recumbent bike (with a chair-like seat and back support) may be more comfortable. Recumbent bikes are also easier to climb on and off and are good if your balance is poor.

Stationary exercise bike

- *Look for the same features on a stationary bike as on a street bike, such as a wide padded seat or a recumbent position for sitting.*

- *Put your stationary bike in front of your television as a reminder to get on it! Make it convenient for yourself.*

- *On some more expensive stationary bikes, there are movable handlebars. These provide upper body exercise while you are peddling.*

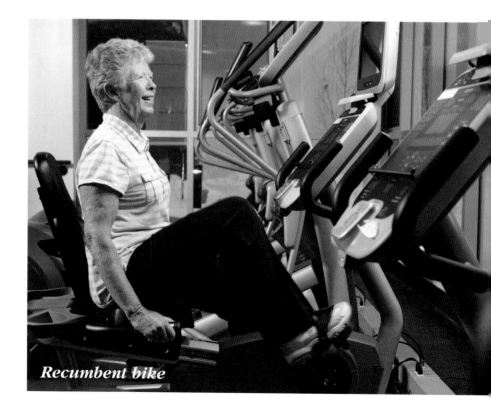

Recumbent bike

Milly's exercise plan

I wasn't really a very well person. I felt my weight limited me from doing a lot. I have a small apartment and I mostly stayed in. Home Care came into my home twice a week to help me with my bath. My favorite place was my lazy chair in the living room. My next favorite was my kitchen chair. I liked to look out of the window, watch TV, read my book, and visit with my granddaughter. But then my eyes started getting worse, and I couldn't even see my feet very well. I developed a problem on one of my toes. It became infected, but I didn't realize it at first. The nurse who now comes to trim my toenails told me I had very little circulation in my feet. I needed to do some exercise or next time I might lose my toe. I bought myself a mini exerciser. I started doing a couple of minutes in the morning after breakfast. I find time passes faster if I peddle while watching TV. Each day I tried to do a bit more. Now after a month I can do almost 10 minutes at a time. Usually I peddle after supper too. Also, I put the exerciser up on my table and turn the peddles with my arms. As I'm peddling I can look out the window and see what is happening outside. The funny thing is that since I started doing all this for my feet, it has helped me in many other ways. I never thought I would be a very active person again, but I'm finding I can do more about my home, and can get out a bit more. So far, I haven't had any more problems with my toes and I have less swelling in my feet and legs. Mostly I just feel better.

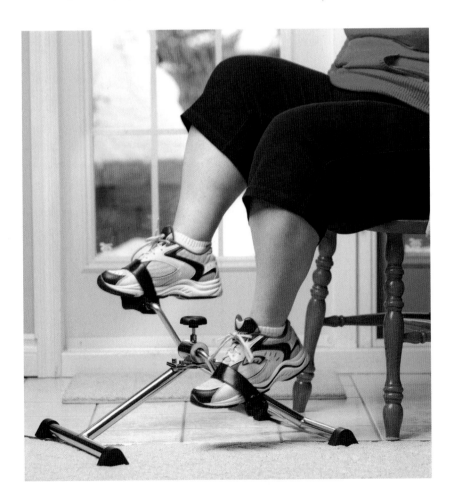

Mini exerciser

This takes up less space than a bike. You can peddle it while sitting in your favorite chair. Do you have smooth flooring rather than carpet? If so, you may want to put your mini exerciser against the wall so it doesn't move ahead as you are cycling. Some mini exercisers sold have adjustable heights. This is useful if you are shorter, so you can easily reach the pedals. A mini exerciser is a cheaper option than an exercise bike and you can buy one at a catalogue order store or medical supply store.

229

Swimming and water exercise

Swimming laps: Over time, increase your laps and vary your strokes.

Build strength: Water gives good resistance which helps build strength and endurance.

Get flexible: Swimming involves long strokes that increase flexibility. When swimming, kick from your hips, not your knees, for greatest benefit. You may find your range of motion is larger in water than on land (for example, you can swing your legs higher).

If you can't swim:

- Use a kickboard and kick your way down the pool. Make sure there is a lifeguard on duty.

- Some pools offer special exercise programs for people in wheelchairs that allow for muscle movement and exercise.

- Walk or jog in shoulder or waist deep water:
  – Walking in deeper water reduces the weight on sore hips, knees, ankles and feet.
  – Keep your feet flat on the bottom of the pool rather than walking on your toes.
  – Keep your body straight, rather than leaning forward.
  – Swing your arms, keeping them close to your body.
  – Walk forward, backward, or sideways taking side steps.
  – Join an aquafit class (water exercises with an instructor).

Aquafit (exercise in water) in a class with an instructor may motivate you. These are routines done in a shallow pool or in deeper water. In deeper water you can wear a flotation vest. This helps keep your body straight as you walk in the water.

Aquafit tips

- *Wear water shoes (also called "aqua socks") to cushion and protect your feet.*

- *Aquasize in a group with others and an instructor can help motivate you.*

- *Have fun!*

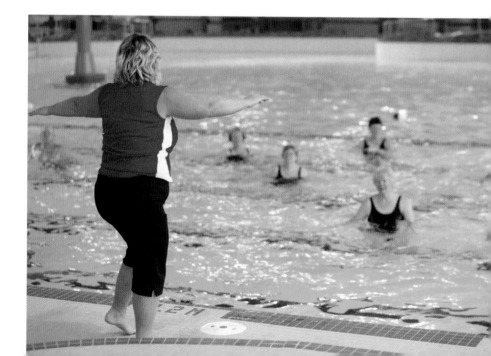

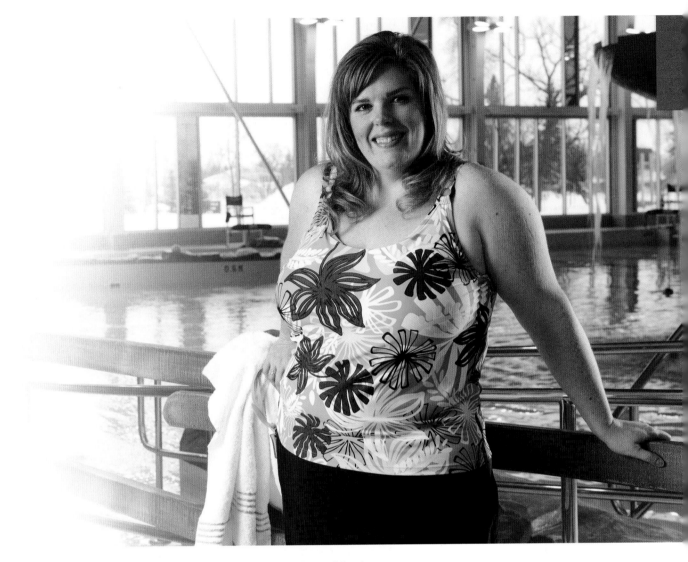

What to wear in the pool? There are many styles of bathing suits for different body sizes. On the internet search "modest swimwear," "plus size swimwear," or "UV protective swimwear" for some great styles with discreet coverage.

Tips for women – choose:

- shirt-like tops and skirt-like bottoms or leggings
- bright color at the chest and a darker color below
- up and down patterns or stripes to make your hips look smaller

Tips for men – choose:

- dark solid colors with option of vertical strips on the side
- bold graphics or funky patterns or colors attract the eye so there is less focus on your body
- longer, short-style bathing suits
- a t-shirt or tank top is allowed at many pools

Prevent injuries:

- *Give yourself room to exercise so you don't bang into anything.*

- *A cool home temperature will be more comfortable and safe.*

- *Start slowly. Don't feel you have to keep up with the program until you're ready.*

- *Some tiredness and muscle stretching is expected but if any move really hurts, don't do it. You may not be ready for it yet, or it may be wrong for you.*

- *To reduce the impact on your ankles, legs and knees: Exercise or dance on an exercise mat, carpet or softer floor rather than tile or cement. To protect the bottoms of your feet, wear a pair of shoes with good support.*

- *Always keep knees slightly bent, avoiding straight leg sit-ups, or raising both legs at once. Avoid deep knee bends.*

- *Stand tall (like someone is pulling a string at the top of your head).*

- *Breathe deeply.*

Aerobics and dancing

Start off at home

- March on the spot or dance at home to your favorite music. Try chair dancing, see page 248. Take one or several song breaks during the day. This improves circulation to your feet and brain.

- Follow along with an aerobic or dance DVD (or video). Check local TV channels for home exercises.

- Exercise or play sports along with a TV home game using a wireless remote (such as Wii).

- Equipment for home exercises may include:
  - a set of weights
  - rubber exercise bands for stretching and strengthening
  - a small towel for stretching
  - a foam exercise mat (such as a kids' play mat or "anti-fatigue" mat)
  - a small step (to step up on as you exercise)

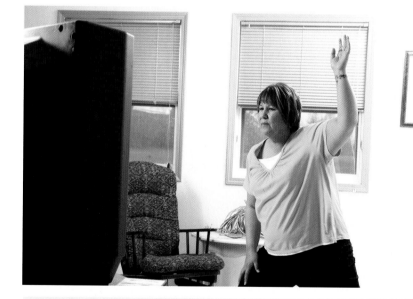

Sylvia's story:

After I developed diabetes, I did two things that helped my blood sugar. First, I kept careful food records. And second, I used my Leslie Sansone walking DVD every day. In the privacy of my own home, I do my exercises. No one sees me do this or sees me sweating. The DVD I bought had three levels to it. I started with the easiest level and I really struggled with this. It wasn't easy. Over a period of three months I was surprised that I could manage the second level and finally, the most advanced level. I was a large woman but I lost weight and my doctor is really pleased with my blood sugars.

When you're ready, go to a class or gym

- Try square dancing, country line dancing, belly dancing, or ball room dancing. Try an ethnic traditional dance or a seniors' dance night.

- With a friend, or on your own, join an exercise class. Most community centers and gyms have different aerobics classes.

- Personal gym trainers can set up an exercise program that is right for you. A trainer coaches and encourages you on a regular basis. Hiring a certified fitness instructor for even one or two sessions is a great investment for getting started right.

- Exercise programs (such as Curves for women or SilverSneakers in the USA for men or women) are popular, too. This is a great option for doing a set of controlled exercises.

Questions to ask when using an exercise or dance DVD or attending a class:

- Are the instructors certified in their field?

- Is low-impact exercise a priority?

- Does the instructor encourage you to monitor your heart rate during the class?

- Is the difficulty level suitable? Some exercise programs go from beginner to moderate to advanced, as well as classes for different ages. You can move up a level as you become stronger.

- Are the moves easy, with clear instructions and safety precautions? For example, are there tips on how to protect your back or knees?

- Is there a warm up and cool down?

Wayne's story:

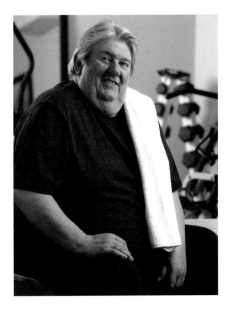

If you've never been overweight, you don't understand the physical and mental toll it has on your life. It's hard for heavier people to listen to someone who hasn't been through what we've been through. Going to the gym can be terrifying because whether people think bad things about you or not, you think they do. However, if you are heavy and struggle with fear of exercising in front of people, understand that most of them are happy to see you there, and get excited for you and your choice to lose weight (this I've learned from experience). For me, I started exercising on my own for a few months, until I worked up the strength and courage, to go to a gym. At first I felt like people were looking at me, but maybe it was just because I was new. After a while, I kind of belonged. Everyone is working towards their own goals. You are worth it. You will never succeed until you believe that about yourself.

Other home or gym exercise equipment

Some people find that if they do their exercise at the same time each day or evening, this makes it a habit – a good habit! Remember, even 5 minutes, 3 times a day, can add up to 15 minutes a day, and can make a difference.

- For your comfort, it's best to try out a piece of equipment before you buy it. Go to a fitness store or consider a one day pass at a fitness club to try out various machines.

- Read reviews about exercise gear online or in magazines. Youtube.com is a good place to watch online videos of how people use these tools for working out.

- If cost is the bottom line, an exercise bike costs less than an electronic treadmill. Find good deals on exercise equipment at second hand stores, ads in the paper or online, and at yard sales.

When used properly and in good condition, the exercise equipment mentioned here is safe. Even so, please note the cautions listed.

Deciding what to buy:

- Treadmills and exercise bikes are the most common exercise equipment. See pages 224–229. These are safe and excellent options. A bike (or mini exerciser) is easier to move into your home, while a treadmill is heavy and takes up space.

- Ellipticals, ski machines, stair steppers, rowing machines and weight machines are also good options for use at home or at a gym. See pages 234–236.

Caution

Mini trampolines or full-sized trampolines used without supervision can result in a fall with a serious neck or head injury.

Weight loss with no exercise?

Vibrator belts and chi machines won't help you lose weight, but they may help reduce stress by relaxing you, and this might bring down your blood sugar for a short time.

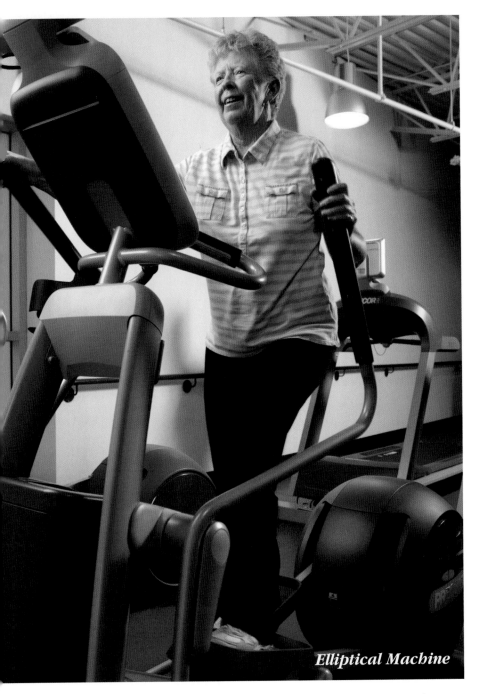

Elliptical Machine

The elliptical machine is easy on your joints. It combines upper and lower body muscle work, so you burn more calories. Your feet never leave the pedals. You can pedal forwards and backwards. It's described like "running in mid-air" making it very low-impact. It's quieter and uses less electricity than a treadmill.

A cross-country ski machine feels like the gliding motion of cross-country skiing. It also combines upper and lower body muscle work. The machine should have adjustable poles for greatest comfort. There should be a smooth leg sliding action and independent arm-lever motion.

Stair steppers in gyms are usually designed to exercise your legs yet be easy on your joints, like ellipticals. They often have movable handles for upper body strengthening.

Home stair steppers are available without handles. These home versions are light and easy to store, but can be hard on sore, arthritic knees. Look for a smooth stepping action, solid frame, and an adjustment for your height. The pedals should be parallel to the floor when stepping. Home steppers are also available with arm handles which provide support and balance. Some steppers are available with movable handles.

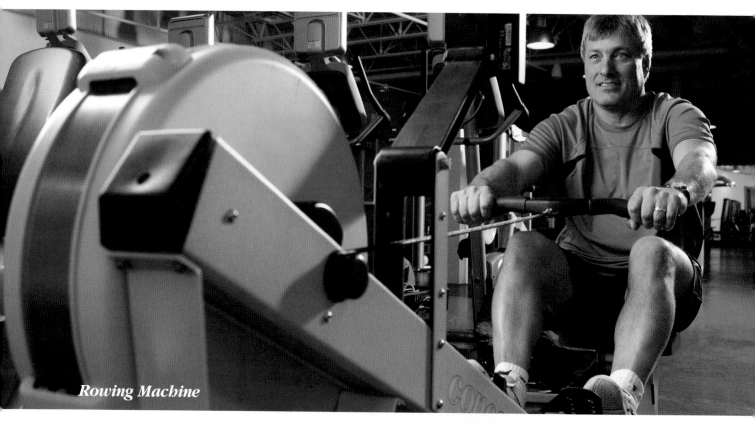

Rowing Machine

A rowing machine also provides a full body workout with low-impact. Look for a smooth oar action. For example, a cable rower with a fly wheel. This is a good option if you have foot or balance problems, or lower leg weakness.

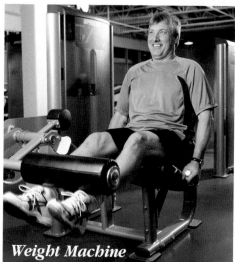

Weight Machine

Weight lifting, using machines or free weights burns sugar and calories, and builds muscle. With a weight machine, the weights attach to the machine rather than free dumbbells.

Caution

Rowing machines: When rowing, keep your back in a straight position. Don't bend so far forward that when you pull back you use your lower back instead of your legs (this stresses your back). Remember to breathe deeply while rowing.

Weight lifting: To avoid injury, use proper technique, increase weights slowly, and breathe properly (never hold your breath when lifting). Go to a reputable gym or sports store for training sessions before doing this alone. Don't use weights you can't comfortably manage. Do not use heavy free weights without supervision. If you have retinopathy or poorly controlled high blood pressure, don't lift weights over your head. This increases the pressure at the back of your eyes. See pages 40–41 and 259.

If you have arthritis in your hips, knees or ankles – ten exercise tips

Good diabetes control is very important in managing arthritis. This is because when blood sugar is high over many years this can cause changes to muscles and bones. These changes further aggravate joint pain and stiffness, especially in hands, feet and shoulders.

1. **Take your pain medications** regularly, as prescribed.

2. **Choose the right time to walk,** when your pain is less and you feel most relaxed.

3. **Limit your walks** (for example, to just 5–10 minutes) but consider walking several times a day.

4. **A good pair of walking shoes** will support your feet as well as provide cushioning for your knees, see page 290–293. You may benefit from a rigid or semi rigid orthotic in your shoe – talk to your foot specialist or doctor. If you have an option to walk on a soft surface such as a rubber track, this will be easier on your knees than a concrete side-walk.

5. **Even a small weight loss helps** to decrease the weight on your hips, knees and ankles, and lessen joint pain.

6. **Use heat before and cold after.** Before you exercise put a hot cloth on your joint. This will warm it up and help make your tissues and joints less stiff. After you exercise, apply a cold cloth (or ice inside a cold cloth) for 5–10 minutes. At the same time, elevate your knees if comfortable. This will reduce pain, inflammation, swelling and muscle spasms.

7. **Low-impact exercises.** These are the kindest to your joints. They include swimming, biking, elliptical trainer, chair exercises, walking or Tai Chi (a slow paced traditional Chinese exercise). On a bike, start with a low resistance, so you peddle easily, and build up gradually. A recumbent bike further reduces knee strain. You may be able to manage smaller amounts of bicycling or walking pain-free or with less pain. When walking, weight on the knees is reduced with the use of a shopping cart, walker or walking poles, or when walking in water.

8. **Avoid exercises where you squat or do deep knee bends.**

9. **Rest your knees.** When standing for a long time (for example, doing dishes, or standing at a work bench) raise one foot on a small block to relieve pressure off that knee. After 5 or 10 minutes, switch legs.

10. **Don't overdo it.** When your knees say rest, sit or lie down.

Arthritis Association

If there is an arthritis support group in your community, they may be able to provide you with exercise ideas or an exercise DVD. Also, ask your doctor for a referral to a physiotherapist or exercise specialist for individualized recommendations.

Being active helps arthritis in two ways:

1. *Keeps your muscles and joints as movable and strong as possible.*

2. *Improves your blood sugar.*

After exercise, some mild soreness is normal, but if you develop joint pain that lasts two hours or more, cut back. Consult your doctor if needed.

237

Staying Flexible

Flexibility refers to the ability of your muscles to stretch. Flexibility gives you a better range of motion. Stretching improves your body's circulation and posture. It also helps to warm up and relax muscles. Do these exercises before your walk or aerobic exercise, or combined with strength training.

Common flexibility exercises are:

- stretching to tie up your shoe or put on your coat
- stretching up to the top shelf

Easy exercises at home: See the next page for some examples.

Exercises with good stretching include:

- swimming which involves stretching
- swinging your arms while you are walking
- dancing
- bowling
- Tai Chi, yoga and pilates. It's a good idea to take a class to learn how to do these properly.

Suggestions when doing flexibility exercises:

- Take it slowly and gently: If you push your muscles to be too flexible too soon, you will injure small muscles and have inflammation and pain; this can increase your blood sugar.
- Be safe. The exercises shown in this book are safe for you as a person with diabetes, however not all exercises found in books, on the internet or on DVDs are safe.
- Here are two examples of unsafe exercises:
  - Neck rotation: Turning your head in a complete circle puts too much stress on your neck. A safer neck exercise is to lean your ear into your shoulder, or to tuck your chin into your chest.
  - Forced or bouncy stretching: Do not overstretch. If you are forcing a joint beyond its normal range of motion this can be dangerous. For instance, having someone help to stretch your arm further than you normally stretch. Another example is if you are desperately trying to touch your toes (even though you haven't done it in 50 years!). This can tear muscles, ligaments and tendons.

Remember, exercise should never be painful. Stretch your muscles slowly and gradually.

Stretches should be done smoothly and held for about 10 seconds.

Flexibility exercises

Neck stretch

Sit in a chair and relax your arms and shoulders. Start with your head to one side. Slowly lower your head forward and move it across your chest in a smooth semi-circle to the other side and then back. Do three times.

Ankle rotations

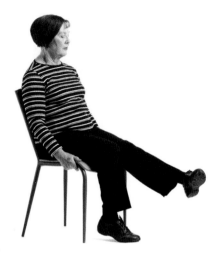

Sit in a chair. Extend one leg. Make complete circles from your ankles. Repeat with the other foot. Do ten rotations.

Calf stretch

Stand with your hands resting against a wall. Place one leg forward and the other leg straight back. Point toes straight ahead and keep both heels on the floor. Lean forward, keeping back knee straight. Hold. Return to starting position, relax. Repeat 5 times with alternate legs.

A variation of this exercise can be done sitting with one leg up on a chair, knee slightly bent. Lean forward and hold the stretch.

Seated hamstring stretch

Sit up straight on the edge of your chair. Straighten out one leg (but don't lock your knee) with your heel on the floor. Pull your toes back as much as you can. Keep your back straight and lean forward from your hips. You will feel a stretch in the back of your legs; the hamstring is the muscle at the back of your thigh. Hold. Return to starting position, relax. Repeat 5 times with alternate legs.

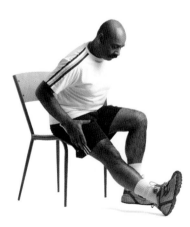

Strengthening Exercises

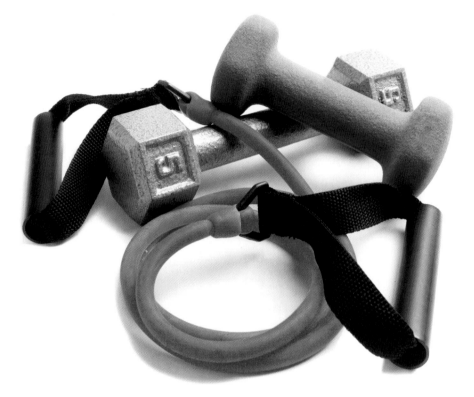

Making your body stronger and more flexible is a part of walking, biking, swimming and all aerobic exercise. Boosting the strength of your muscles and bones is important. Here are some specific exercises that make you stronger.

Common strengthening exercises are:

- Lifting weights to strengthen arm and shoulder muscles.

- Stretch bands for upper and lower body strengthening. Bands are an alternative to lifting weights, but sometimes take a bit more coordination. The thicker or shorter the band, the more strength you need to stretch it. To learn proper and safe use of stretch bands, consult an exerciser trainer at a gym, or watch a youtube video by a qualified instructor (search "resistance band demo").

- Stomach tucks to strengthen and tone the abdomen.

- Back exercises to further strengthen your abdominal and back muscles.

- Climbing stairs and doing leg lifts with weight machines to strengthen the legs.

- A complete weight lifting and strength training workout at a gym.

Do you wonder if sex is good exercise?

If you enjoy sex, then the answer is yes! The aerobic benefit is on average about equal to climbing two flights of stairs. But there's more – regular sex keeps you flexible and strengthens muscles inside and out.

Strengthening exercises make your muscles stronger. Then your insulin works better, and this can help bring down your blood sugar.

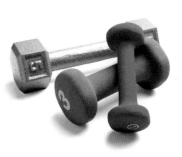

Suggestions when doing strengthening exercises:

- **Keep the exercise smooth and slow.**

- **Avoid jerky movements and lifting above your head,** especially if you have poorly controlled high blood pressure or advanced retinopathy, see page 40–41 and 259.

- **Remember to breathe** while you are exercising, otherwise your blood pressure could go up. Breathe in through your nose when lifting weights. Breathe out through your mouth when bringing weights down.

- **Do one set at a time and rest in between:** A common set is lifting a weight 10 times. As you become stronger, you may want to increase to two sets. For example, lift the weight 10 times (one set) then rest 1–2 minutes, and then do another set.

- **In general, to increase your strength, you need to fatigue your muscles.** Therefore, choose a weight that you have a hard time lifting ten times. Increase your repetitions and when you are ready, move to a heavier weight. For example: start with a 2 lb (1 kg) weight for two sets. Then after a few weeks, lift a 5 lb (2.5 kg) weight for one set, increasing to 2 sets when you feel ready.

- **When you start doing strengthening exercises, it's normal to feel mild muscle stiffness lasting one day.** If this stiffness lasts longer, then reduce your weights or your number of sets.

- **If you feel pain or discomfort,** stop the exercise. If you have acute (severe) pain in a joint, an exercise often needs to be adapted.

How often should I do this?

- *To maintain strength:* Twice a week, do one or more sets.

- *To build muscles:* Three times a week, do one or more sets.

Doing exercises properly helps prevent injury

If you are unsure how to do an exercise, try to meet with a fitness specialist at a gym.

At all ages, it's possible to become more fit and reverse the natural loss of muscle tone. People in their 80's and 90's can maintain or increase their strength through weight training. Bone and muscle strength helps reduce the risk of falls as you age.

Arm and upper body exercises

These exercises don't take long to do. For example, one or two sets can fit into the time of the television ads of your favorite show. If sitting, sit straight up and have your feet flat on the floor. If standing, place your feet shoulder width apart and slightly bend your knees.

You can do one arm at a time or both together. Do these exercises slowly for the greatest benefit.

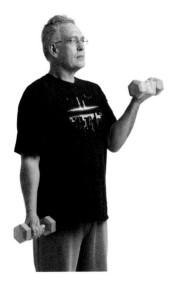

Biceps Curl

Hold the weight in your hand with palm-up and *slowly* curl your arm up to your shoulder bending at the elbow. *Slowly* return to extended position and repeat with alternate arms or do both arms together.

Arm Roll

Holding a weight, extend your arms straight out slightly below your shoulder height. Move your hands in slow, controlled small circles. Moving your hands in larger circles and lifting a heavier weight will increase strengthening. Repeat with alternate arms or do both together.

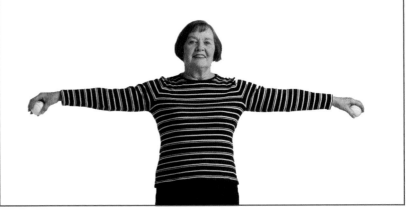

Arm Chair Pushup

Sit in an office chair or other chair with arms. Put your hands on the arms and lift your bottom off the chair and hold for a few seconds. Even lifting slightly, exercises your arms. Over time, work up to lifting for 10 seconds.

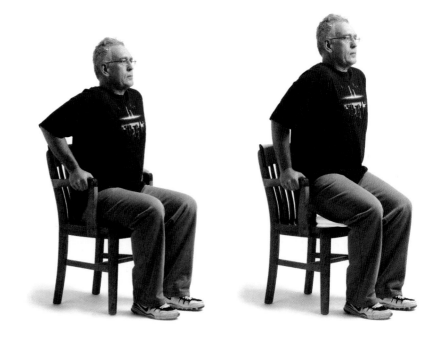

Stomach and lower body exercises

For all three of these exercises, remember to:

- Keep breathing – do not hold your breath
- Hold your exercise for 2–3 seconds. Over time, work up to a 10-second hold.

Exercise that strengthens your waist also strengthens your lower back.

Stomach tucks - easy alternatives to sit ups

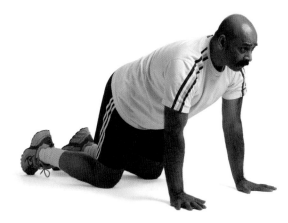

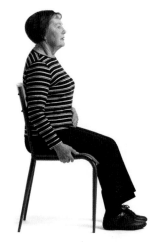

Stomach tuck - option 1

- Go on your hands and knees.
- Keep your back straight, parallel to the floor. Don't move your back.
- Hold in your stomach, then relax.

Stomach tuck - option 2

- Sit upright against the back of a chair.
- Draw in your belly button.
- Hold in your stomach, then relax.

Wall squat

This exercise helps strengthen your back, abdomen, buttocks and thighs. It's a great exercise if you sit a lot. Stand with your back flat against a wall (including the back of your head). Keep your tummy tucked in. Keep your feet flat on the floor and about two feet out from the wall. Bend your knees slightly and slide down the wall. Going down a few inches is a good start, and over time work up to a deeper squat. Your knees shouldn't extend beyond your ankles. Hold. Slowly return to starting position and repeat.

The best exercise for your legs is walking, biking or swimming. Chair leg exercises are shown on pages 248–249.

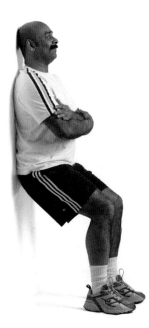

Talk to your doctor or physiotherapist about back exercises.

If a health professional treats you for a back injury, please follow the exercises that he or she recommends.

Lift carefully

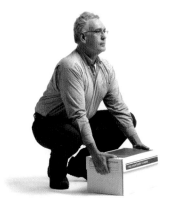

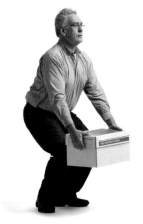

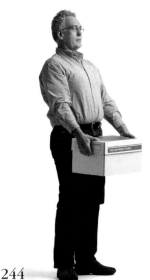

Ten tips for a healthy back

1. **Do simple back exercises.** Exercises help keep your back strong allowing you to stay active. See page 245.

2. **A daily walk.** This helps strengthen the muscles that support your back. If you lose some extra weight around your waist, even 5–10 lbs (2.5–4.5 kg), this can help relieve pressure off your back.

3. **Stand and sit tall.** When you walk, keep your back straight and chin up, relax your shoulders, and tighten your stomach muscles. This helps maintain good posture. Sitting posture is also important. If you work at a computer, look straight ahead at the screen, not up or down. Keep your knees level with or slightly higher than your hips. Your elbows should be at a 45° angle from your body. To relieve back strain take short breaks (walk or move around or do the two back exercises).

4. **Use a support, if needed, when walking.** Using a walker, walking stick, cane, or Nordic walking poles (see page 225) reduces the weight on your back. Also, lean on a shopping cart while walking in a mall or store. As your back gets stronger, you may no longer need support.

5. **Take the pressure off your back while standing.** Slightly bend your knees or rest one foot up on a small step.

6. **Avoid arching backwards.** Also, when doing exercises while lying or sitting, always keep the knees bent or slightly bent. And, don't raise both legs at one time.

7. **Lift carefully.** Before lifting, place your feet at shoulder width. Bend your knees, keep your back straight and hold the object close to your body as you lift it. Don't twist your back. Use a push cart or wheelbarrow to move heavy things. Get help as needed.

8. **Lower back massage.** Ask a friend or family member to gently massage your back, or go to a licensed massage therapist.

9. **Good sleeping position.** If you like to sleep on your back, place a pillow under your knees. If you like to sleep on your side, lie with your knees bent with a pillow between them. This helps reduce twisting of your back. A good mattress also helps.

10. **Take pain pills as prescribed.** Use appropriate pain pills. Plan your exercise for the time of day that you feel your best.

Back exercises

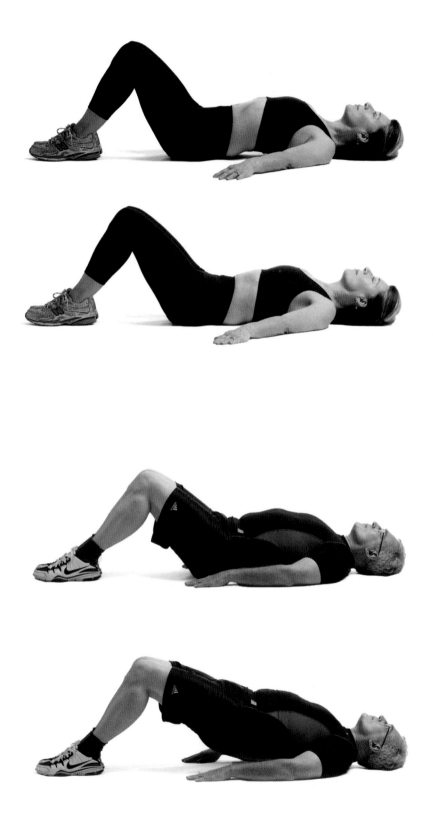

Do these exercises daily or several times a week.

Pelvic Tilt – stretches your back:

- *Lie on the floor or on a hard mattress. Lie on your back with your knees bent.*

- *Keep your feet flat on the floor and your arms at your sides.*

- *Tighten your tummy to press your lower back against the floor (or bed). Hold 5 seconds, then relax.*

- *Repeat five to ten times.*

The Bridge – strengthens your back:

Start in the same position as the Pelvic Tilt.

- *Part your knees slightly.*

- *Slowly lift your hips upwards so your weight is on your feet and shoulder blades. Even lifting just an inch or two is beneficial.*

- *Keep your stomach tight and your abdomen in line with your thighs. Hold for five seconds and return to the starting position. Relax.*

- *Repeat five to ten times.*

245

A Fitness Plan for You

How much walking or aerobic exercise do you do right now (in addition to your usual daily activities)? Based on your present amount of exercise, choose one of the three fitness plans below.

Each fitness plan increases in difficulty over an eight week period. At the end of eight weeks, you may be ready to move to the next level. Make daily walking (or other aerobic exercise) a priority. Add in the strengthening and flexibility exercises as you are able.

Amount of exercise I do right now:

My exercise is limited. On average, I do less than 15 minutes of walking or other aerobic exercise each day.

Other considerations

- I have limited my exercise in the past because of arthritis, muscle pain, shortness of breath, or my weight.
- I have poor balance.
- I have had a stroke or partial leg amputation.
- I use a wheelchair or walker sometimes or all the time.

→ **Fitness Plan 1**
Least Active
(pages 247–249)

I am relatively fit. I want to maintain or increase my fitness. On average, I do 15 to 25 minutes of walking or other aerobic exercise every day.

→ **Fitness Plan 2**
Active
(pages 250–251)

I am fit and I want to stay this way! On average, I do 30 minutes or more of walking or other aerobic exercise every day.

→ **Fitness Plan 3**
Most Active
(pages 252–253)

Fitness levels not included in this book:

- If you have partial or full paralysis: Consult a physiotherapist or exercise specialist.
- If you are a runner, or train for marathons, triathlons or competitive sports: Consult your doctor, diabetes educator, or sport specialist. A specialist who is knowledgeable about diabetes can advise you. It's important to learn about risks, ways to avoid injury, and your need for fluid, carbohydrates and calories.

Fitness Plan 1 (Least Active)

This plan includes short walks and exercises you can do while sitting in a chair. See Chair Exercises on pages 248–249. As needed, use a cane or walker, or walk with a companion for support. Even if you are not as mobile as you used to be, there are still ways to become stronger, and more flexible and to improve your circulation. This decreases your risk of diabetes complications.

In eight weeks, you can increase your exercise from 5 minutes to 20 minutes a day. This exercise is in addition to your usual daily activities.

Over the next eight weeks, gradually increase the intensity (speed) of your aerobic exercise.

Week	Number of minutes a day of walking or chair exercises	Strengthening & flexibility
One & Two	**5 minutes** (as one session or two 2½-minute sessions)	**Twice a week:** • Do 5 bicep curls each arm, using a 1 lb (0.5 kg) weight.
Three & Four	**10 minutes** (as one session or two 5-minute sessions)	**Twice a week:** • Do 10 bicep curls each arm, using a 1 lb (0.5 kg) weight. • Add in 5 stomach tucks.
Five & Six	**15 minutes** (as one session or two or three shorter sessions)	**Twice a week:** • Do 10 bicep curls and 10 tricep curls each arm, using a 1 lb (0.5 kg) weight. Increase to a 2 lb (1 kg) weight if able. • Add 5 stomach tucks. **Once a week:** • Add in one set of flexibility exercises.
Seven & Eight	**20 minutes** (As one session or two or three shorter sessions). Make a small increase in your intensity if you are able. Consider joining a swimming program, or getting home exercise equipment such as a mini exerciser or recumbent bicycle.	**Two to three times a week:** • Do 10 bicep curls, 10 tricep curls and 10 arm rolls each arm, using a 1, 2 or 5 lb (0.5, 1 or 2.5 kg) weight. • Also add 5–10 stomach tucks. • Fit in one set of flexibility exercises. • Do daily back exercises if needed.

Many standing exercises can be adapted to do while sitting. For example, the bicep curl and arm roll on page 242. Other seated exercises are shown on page 239, 242 and 243.

Chair Exercises

Here are a few exercises especially designed for strengthening. For all of these exercises, sit up straight, hold in your tummy and push your bottom to the back of your chair. This helps protect your back.

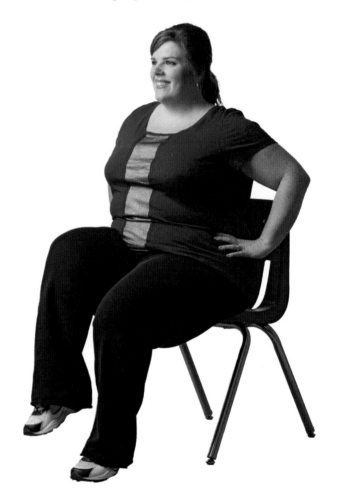

Leg walk

Place your hands on your hips with your feet flat on the floor. Raise one foot about 6 inches (15 cm) off the floor. Return foot to the floor and repeat with the other foot. Alternate left and right legs in a rhythmic manner. Walk for several minutes, and increase your time as you are able.

Heather's story:

Chair dancing is good for anyone who is having a problem with their feet or their legs. If you can't properly walk outside, it's a new concept in aerobic fitness. It's important to be in a really comfortable chair with good back support, which I have in front of my computer. Put on some peppy music of some sort, I like *Mamma Mia*, because it's got a good beat, but you can pick the one you want. If I pick 4 or 5 songs, that's 15 minutes, and it goes very fast when you're going to the music.

Then you take your feet and go up and down, and back and forth. Let's say the left foot five times, the right foot five times, go sideways five times, and then you go backwards. And then you can just take your leg and lift your foot up to straighten out your leg, up and down five times. You know what they say "do what you are comfortable with." If you can do it ten times, fine. I prefer to do each foot five times. Then go all the way around, doing each five times, and then do them all again. And while you are sitting, put your arms in front and go back and forth. Put your arms above your head and make scissors, or make circles out to the side. Anything that is some form of movement is good.

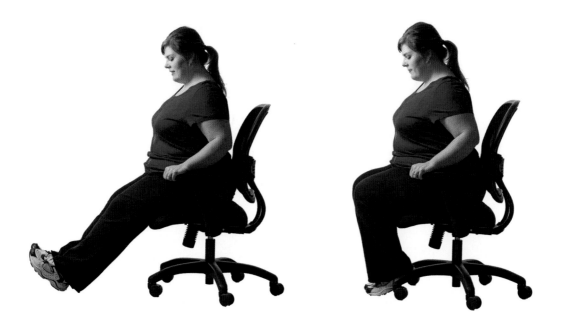

Moving chair exercises

Sit in an office chair or wheelchair. With your feet flat on the floor, pull yourself forward or backwards.

You are never too old or too large to start moving.
The key is to find the right kind and amount of exercise for you. Even a small amount of exercise can make a big difference. People of all ages, including older adults, can become stronger and healthier by becoming more active.

Darrel's story:

I am 53 years old and I had a stroke four years ago. The stroke left me in a wheelchair and affected the left side of my body. I've had diabetes for more than ten years.

I ended up in an institution and they told me I would never go home. I was very discouraged at first but then I didn't believe that I'd have to stay there. I started moving a little bit of my limbs at a time. Then I would say, if I could move for 5 minutes, then I could move 10 minutes. I had a therapist at the beginning but then I started going it by myself, because the therapist only allowed so much time to work with me. I got home, and I started moving around in my kitchen. My kitchen is what got me well, believe it or not. I started moving. I started bending. I started lifting pots. I started standing, you know, trying to get things out of the cabinet, because nobody was here to get them. So I started doing things like that and then I said wow, what a workout! And then I tried again and again and again. I started to appreciate my kitchen. I started loving my kitchen. I wanted to love the food that I eat. I was able to start cooking with one hand and enjoying the food that I prepared. I didn't want to enjoy food as much as before, but I wanted to enjoy what I did eat.

Now, I am walking 50 feet (15 m). I can sit in a regular chair when I have a visitor. I can stand a little bit longer. I use a walker. Now I have a therapist again and they are showing me how to walk a limited space without the walker. I don't really like the walker, but I have it for support. The leg and arm on my left side can work a little bit, maybe about 80%. I move my muscles more as I start thinking positively. I'm able to do a lot more and that has helped me out a whole lot.

Fitness Plan 2 (Active)

Start off slowly and gradually increase the amount of exercise that you do.

In eight weeks, you can increase your aerobic exercise from 15 to 45 minutes a day. This exercise is in addition to your usual daily activities.

Over the eight weeks, gradually increase the intensity (speed) of your aerobic exercise.

Week	Number of minutes a day of walking or other aerobic exercise (such as biking or swimming)	Strengthening & flexibility
One & Two	**15 minutes** Warm up and cool down by walking slowly for the first and last few minutes of your walk or other aerobic exercise.	**Twice a week:** • Do 10 bicep and 10 tricep curls each arm using a 1 lb (0.5 kg) or 2 lb (1 kg) weight.
Three & Four	**25 minutes of aerobic exercise** (as one or two sessions)	**Twice a week:** • Do 10 bicep and tricep curls each arm using a 2 lb (1 kg) weight. • Add in 5 stomach tucks and wall squats.
Five & Six	**35 minutes** (as one or two sessions) To burn more calories, increase your pace a bit. If walking, swing or pump your arms.	**Twice a week:** • Do 10 bicep curls, tricep curls and arm rolls each arm using a 2 lb (1 kg) weight. • Do 5 stomach tucks and wall squats. **Once a week:** • Add in one set of flexibility exercises.
Seven & Eight	**45 minutes** (As one session, or break into two or three shorter sessions to total 45 minutes). If you want, try swimming, biking, tennis, skating, curling, dancing or golf. You may want to get yourself an exercise DVD or enroll in an exercise class. Consider going to a gym for a complete training program designed for you. Keep it interesting! Challenge yourself if you're ready for it.	**Three times a week:** • Do 10 bicep curls, tricep curls and arm rolls each arms using a 2 or 5 lb (1 or 2.5 kg) weight. • Do 5–10 stomach tucks and wall squats. • Add in one set of flexibility exercises. • Do daily back exercises if needed.

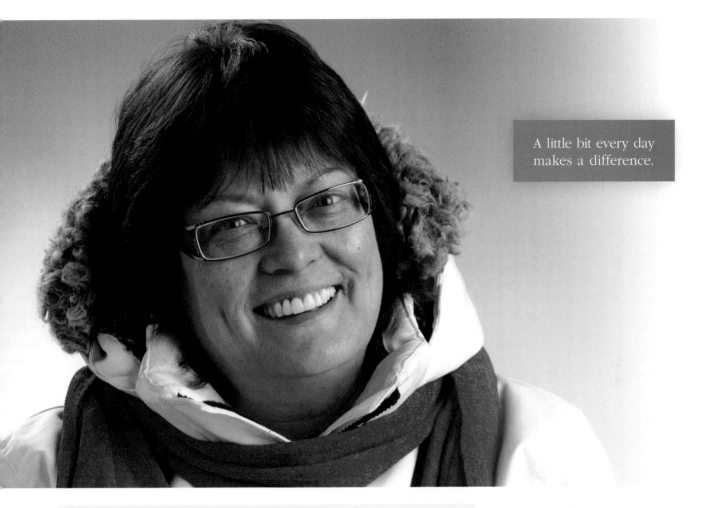

A little bit every day makes a difference.

Mary-Lou's story:

I find walking is the most convenient for me. I walk outdoors or use my treadmill.

Beating the weather was my biggest barrier. It was either too cold or too hot! I decided rather than let the weather beat me, I'd beat it!

When it's cold I dress in layers, including a big hood on my jacket and padded pants. I tend to have cold hands and feet so I wear warm mitts and lined boots that give me enough room to wiggle my toes and comfortably fit over a pair of warm socks. I wear a pair of non-slip grips that fit over my shoes or boots. Mine have small cables that provide grip on the snow or ice. They work great.

In the summer when it's hot out, and I'm walking, I carry a water bottle with me. This way I can walk further without getting so thirsty. I love the sun, but I know too much is not good for me. If it's hot, I cover up with a hat and light clothing, and wear sunscreen. Mostly, I go for my walk early in the morning or in the evening when it's cooler. My whole family is into making me healthier! My daughter gave me a neck wrap. I put it in my freezer ahead of time, and wrap it around my neck when I go out for a walk on hot days. This helps keep me cool.

I don't go out on really cold or really hot days. Instead, I use my treadmill, or walk in the mall.

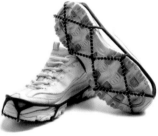

Shoe grips for winter walking

To prevent falling, try shoe grips, a walking stick with a spike on the bottom, or a pair of ski poles or Nordic walking poles (see page 225).

251

Fitness Plan 3 (Most Active)

As with Fitness Plan 1 and 2, start off slowly and gradually increase the amount of exercise that you do.

In eight weeks, you can increase your aerobic exercise from 30 minutes to 60 minutes a day. This exercise is in addition to your usual daily activities.

Over the eight weeks, gradually increase the intensity (speed) of your aerobic exercise.

Remember, when doing strengthening exercises, take a one to two minute break between sets of 10.

Week	Number of minutes a day of walking or other aerobic exercise (such as biking or swimming)	Strengthening & flexibility
One & Two	**30 minutes** Warm up and cool down by walking slowly for the first few and last few minutes of your walk or aerobic exercise. To burn more calories, increase your pace. If walking, swing or pump your arms.	**Twice a week:** • 10 bicep curls, 10 tricep curls and 10 arm rolls each arm using a 2 lb (1 kg) weight. • 10 stomach tucks and wall squats.
Three & Four	**40 minutes** (as one session or two 20-minute sessions) Try a different aerobic exercise to add variety to your workout.	**Twice a week:** • Increase weights to 5 lbs (2.5 kg) and continue with upper and lower body exercises. • Add in a set of flexibility exercises.
Five & Six	**50 minutes** (as one session, or two 25-minute sessions)	**Three times a week:** • Continue with above but increase it to three times a week.
Seven & Eight	**60 minutes** (As one session, or two 30-minute, or three 20-minute sessions). You are so fit now! You may want to try something new – some tennis or golf, or go dancing or canoeing. Maybe get yourself an exercise DVD or enroll in an exercise class. Consider going to a gym for a complete training program designed for you. Challenge yourself if you're ready for it.	**Three times a week:** • Continue with above but increase to two sets of each. • Consider enrolling at a gym for extra strengthening and stretching, and for a weight program designed for you. • An exercise specialist could recommend more types of exercises and stretches.

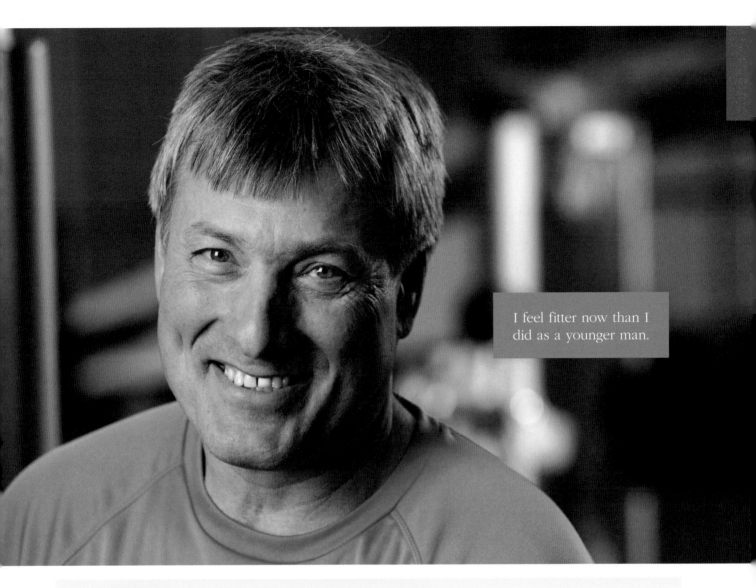

I feel fitter now than I did as a younger man.

Derek's story

I am a lawyer and I have spent many years at university. Yet with all that education, I knew very little about nutrition and fitness. I always thought that I ate a balanced diet and kept busy but over the years I gained weight, bit by bit. I was diagnosed with diabetes five years ago. At that time, I weighed 220 lbs (100 kg).

My wife bought me your book *Meals for Good Health*. It consolidated a lot of basic nutrition information that I did not know, especially about calories and portions. I found it very easy to follow. It provided the road map. I lost 30 pounds (14 kg) over a one year period. I have kept my weight at this level ever since.

At the beginning when I started to lose weight, I deliberately did not do the thirty minutes a day of walking you recommended in your book. I wanted to isolate the weight loss arising from reduced calorie intake from weight loss arising from exercise. In other words, I wanted to know for sure that the weight loss happened because I followed the portions in your book. Once I could see I was losing weight from eating less, I started adding in exercise.

First, I started walking. Losing some weight gave me the confidence to join a gym. I started a combination of fast walking on the treadmill, using the elliptical trainer, and doing some weight training for my legs and arms. I am now able to do forty minutes on the treadmill and rowing machine – and I wasn't even doing that as a young man! I feel a lot fitter. That has led me to take up other things that I hadn't done in years. For example, my wife and I have taken up golfing and we walk with our clubs, we don't take the golf cart.

253

Managing setbacks

Setbacks happen. You may be ill, get bored, have an injury or a personal crisis. This could cause you to stop doing your Fitness Plan. If you've had a setback and stopped doing exercise, here are some tips to get back on track.

Don't delay. If you've missed a few days or a week, try to get back to your usual schedule.

Don't double up. Don't do two days of exercise in one day.

Go back to an earlier level if needed. If you missed a few weeks, go back to an earlier week level in your Fitness Plan. Then work your way back up.

Consider a walking buddy. If you're having a hard time exercising alone, would a walking partner motivate you?

Choose a time to exercise. The best time to exercise is the time you'll do it! Most people do well with a routine, so choosing a regular time (whether it's morning, afternoon or evening) is often helpful. An hour or two after you've eaten is a good time to exercise. At this point, you've digested most of your food and turned it into sugar. Your blood sugar is usually up, and exercise will help bring it down.

Log your exercise. Keeping a log of your exercise can help motivate you. Use one check for ten minutes of continuous aerobic exercise such as walking. If you skip exercising, use a calendar or journal to record why. See if you can find solutions to avoid any future setbacks.

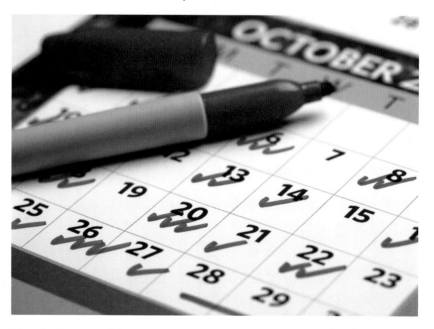

Remind yourself to exercise! Put notes on your bathroom mirror, TV remote or computer.

Precautions

If you have a heart problem – ten precautions

1. **Avoid or limit high-intensity and high impact activities.** High intensity exercise includes strenuous weight lifting or heavy snow shoveling. If shoveling a heavy wet snow fall, don't lift the snow above your head, and do the shoveling for short periods of time over several days. Ask for help from healthy relatives or neighbors, or hire help.

   High-impact exercises include jogging or sprinting. These can damage joints (see page 260). They can also cause blood pressure to go up, sometimes to a dangerous level.

2. **Monitor your heart rate.** Here are three different ways to monitor your heart rate.

   The "Talk Test"

   This means that if at any time during your exercise you can't talk in a normal voice, you are pushing too hard – slow down. Listen to your body.

   Take your own pulse

   Another way is to take your own pulse.

   Use your first two or three fingers (not your thumb) to gently press on your pulse at either your wrist or neck. Count for just 10 seconds and then multiply by 6 to get your number of beats in a minute. See Target Heart Rate chart on page 256. Practice so you can do this quickly, as your heart starts slowing down as soon as you stop exercising.

   Use a monitor

   Use an electronic monitor on a treadmill or other piece of exercise equipment.

   Use the Target Heart Rate as a guide for what your pulse should be. See page 256.

Please ask your doctor "Have I been diagnosed with a heart problem?"

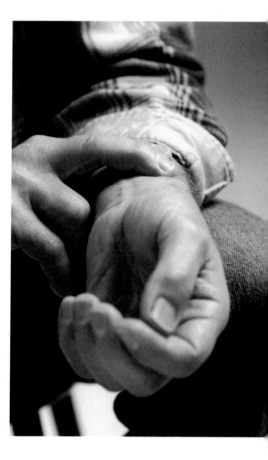

255

Target Heart Rates are only a guide. If you feel discomfort, slow down below the lower limit. If you are pregnant keep slightly below the upper numbers. Some heart conditions and medications (such as beta blockers for high blood pressure) can change your heart rate. Ask your doctor what is a safe Target Heart Rate for you.

Target Heart Rate

Depending on your age, there is a Target Heart Rate for you that includes a range of two numbers. It's good to exercise with your heart beating somewhere between the two numbers. At first, you may exercise at a lower pace than your Target Heart Rate. Gradually build up your stamina. After a while, you may be able to comfortably exercise closer to your upper number. But don't go above your upper number, or you'll be overworking your heart.

Age	Target Heart Rate	
	Beats per 10 seconds	Beats per minute
20–30	23–28	140–170
31–40	22–27	130–160
41–50	20–25	120–150
51–60	18–23	110–140
61–70	16–21	100–130
Over 70	15–20	90–100

3. **Avoid bending your head lower than your heart,** especially right after exercising. For example, raise your foot up on a chair to take off your shoes rather than bending down.

4. **Don't exercise right after eating a heavy meal or drinking alcohol.** After you eat, your blood diverts to digest food in your stomach. Exercise can then overwork your heart. Alcohol can speed up your heart rate. Alcohol also increases your risk for low blood sugar if you are on insulin or certain diabetes pills.

5. **Don't exercise in hot environments,** or sit for long periods in saunas or whirlpools. The heart has to work extra hard to cool you down when you're hot.

6. **Drink water when exercising.** Drink water before and after your walk. When your blood sugar is high, water is especially important so you don't get dehydrated.

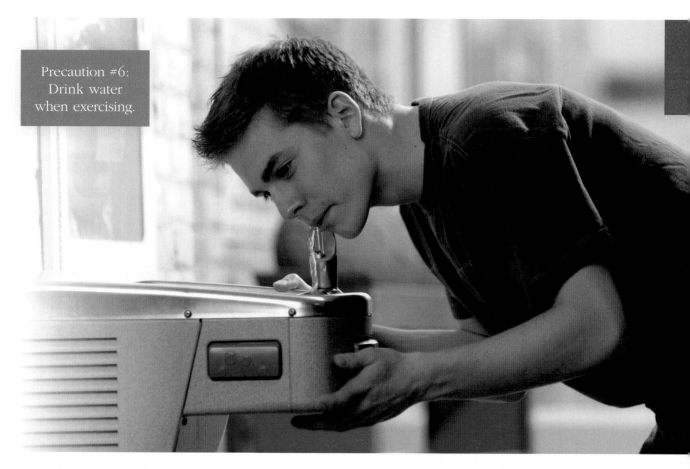

Precaution #6:
Drink water
when exercising.

7. **Breathe deeply** while exercising to increase the amount of oxygen in your blood.

8. **Warm up before vigorous exercise.** Cool down afterwards.

9. **Take heart medications** as prescribed by your doctor. Use prescribed drugs, like nitroglycerine, as recommended.

10. **Your doctor may order an ECG (electrocardiogram) stress test.** This is a test that measures your heart's health. An ECG can expose an undiagnosed problem such as a partially blocked blood vessel leading to the heart that could make exercise dangerous. An ECG stress test also measures blood pressure, heart rate and heart rhythm. A medical professional supervises you while doing this test. It helps give your doctor answers as to what exercise you should or shouldn't do.

Your doctor may order an ECG stress test if you:

- are at high risk for heart disease, and
- were previously inactive, and
- wish to do an exercise program more vigorous than brisk walking.

Diabetes and overheating

If you have had diabetes for a long time you may notice that you don't sweat as much as you used to. This is because the sweat glands are stimulated by nerves, and diabetes can damage nerves. Sweating is the body's natural way of cooling down. With less cooling, it's really important to drink water and not get overheated.

If you've recently had a heart attack:

- Doctors recommend an activity program for almost all heart patients. Talk to your doctor.

- The goal is to help heal your heart through a very structured exercise program that gradually increases how much you do. It often includes walking, and use of a treadmill or bicycle.

- In your community, there may be an exercise facility for people who have had a heart attack. Their programs usually include a physician or other health professional nearby and safety precautions in place.

Regular exercise should never cause serious pain or distress. Slowly increasing amounts of exercise helps avoid or decrease soreness and fatigue. Also avoid exercising right after you eat. If you do get a sore muscle or cramp, massage and stretch it gently.

Certain signs mean you should stop exercising right away and seek medical help. Also, see "Warning Signs of Heart Attack and Stroke" on page 28.

Warning Signs
Stop Exercising
Immediately seek medical help if you have

- Chest pain or tightness in chest if severe or persists more than two minutes.

- Pain in arm or jaw.

- Difficulty breathing or you can't talk.

- Profuse sweating.

- Severe joint or muscle pain.

- Pain at the back of your calf that suddenly worsens or becomes severe.

- An irregular heartbeat.

- You feel faint, dizzy, or nauseated.

- Someone notices you are very pale or "off" color.

- Extreme fatigue.

Keeping your eyes healthy when exercising

It's important to exercise as it helps improve blood sugar and circulation to your eyes. However, if you have diabetes retinopathy (see pages 40–41) there are certain exercises and activities that should be avoided. The kind of exercise that you need to avoid or limit will depend on the stage of your retinopathy. Talk to your eye doctor and ask if you need to limit any exercises.

If you have a mild non-proliferative retinopathy, you may not need to restrict any exercises. With a more severe amount of non-proliferative retinopathy and definitely with proliferative retinopathy, there are restrictions. Exercise restrictions for retinopathy mostly apply to exercise that increases your blood pressure, are high impact or cause jarring, or involve holding your breath. These exercises could worsen your retinopathy or lead to severe eye complications such as a detached retina.

Here are some examples of activities that your eye doctor may suggest you limit or avoid if you have retinopathy:

- All high impact exercise (such as running or jumping).
- Exercises that involve blows such as boxing or karate or jolts, such as tennis or contact sports like hockey.
- Activities that involve a sudden change in pressure such as sky diving, under water diving or bungee jumping.
- Strenuous exercise at altitudes higher than 5,000 feet (1500 m).
- Lifting of heavy weights.
- Lifting any weights above your head.
- Strenuous shovelling, for example, of heavy, wet snow where you lift the shovel above your waist or are pushing hard.
- Dropping your head below your waist (unless recommended to do this by your eye doctor following eye surgery).
- Holding your breath while exercising.
- Strenuous trumpet playing.

For advice, please talk to your eye doctor.

Have you had laser eye treatments or eye surgery?
If so, carefully follow your doctor's exercise restrictions both before and after surgery.

When walking outdoors in the sunshine, wear sunglasses to protect your eyes from ultraviolet light.

Keeping your feet healthy when exercising

For more information on footcare, see pages 282–295.

- Avoid high-impact exercise or activities that cause damage or injury to your feet.

- Wear shoes that protect your feet.

- Look after your feet properly and check them everyday.

- After exercise, check your feet for any red or warm spots. This might be a sign of an infection underneath your skin.

- Follow your doctor's recommendations if you have an open sore or ulcer on your foot. In some cases you may need to stay off your feet until it heals. Chair exercises or biking (if you use an unaffected part of your foot) may be an option. If you have an open sore, you should not go swimming.

Why to avoid high-impact exercise:

Walking is a low-impact exercise

Walking – the force on each foot is about one and a half times your weight.

When you walk, one foot is always on the ground. Each foot lands with a force one and a half times your weight. For a 200 lb (90 kg) person, the force on each foot would be 300 lbs (135 kg).

Low-impact exercise reduces your chance of injury.

Jogging is a high-impact exercise

Jogging – the force on each foot is about three times your weight.

When you jog, both feet are off the ground together. Therefore, each foot lands with a force of three or more times the weight of your body. For a 200 lb (90 kg) person, the force would be at least 600 lbs (270 kg).

That's a lot of weight on the bottom of your feet, or on a worn or older joint.

Talk to your doctor or exercise specialist if you wish to run, or do marathons. This high-impact exercise will increase your risks for injury, especially if you:

- are older

- are overweight

- have any diabetes complications such as foot problems or retinopathy, or

- have other health conditions such as high blood pressure

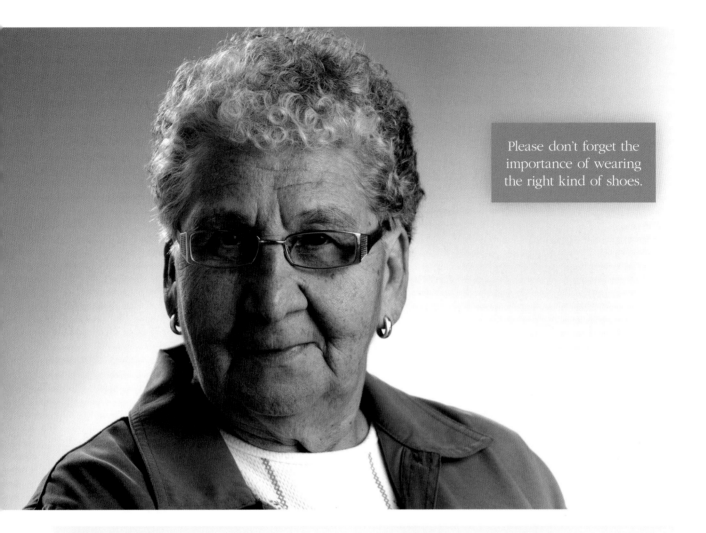

Please don't forget the importance of wearing the right kind of shoes.

Elsie's story:

Nearly one in every four people has sugar diabetes in my community. I have seen many people suffer because of the sugar. Now so many young people have this disease. When my doctor told me that I had diabetes, I knew I wanted to do something right away. I am an elder (a spiritual leader) here. People look up to me. I talked to the dietitian that comes up to our community twice a month. She helped me learn what I should and shouldn't be eating. I drank a lot of soft drinks so this is the first thing I got rid of and replaced with diet drinks. I made other changes too. One thing I did was I started walking. I walked a lot. Over a period of 6 months I had got myself up to walking almost 1 hour every day. My blood sugars were a lot better and I felt better too. That is the good news.

The bad news is something else. I didn't know about proper foot care. I wasn't checking my feet at all. I wasn't wearing a proper pair of shoes. I walked so much that my shoes wore out. There was a hole in one of them. I didn't know this because I had lost the feeling on the bottom of my foot. No one told me that this could happen with diabetes. There are so many things I didn't know about diabetes.

That hole in the bottom of my shoe caused a rubbing on my foot. I got a bad sore there. By the time I got to the clinic, the sore was worse and went all the way to my bone. It got infected. Eventually it turned into gangrene and to tell a long story short, I lost first my foot and then my leg to below my knee. Now I wear an artificial leg. Looking after my diabetes is now more difficult because I can't walk as much.

I am telling my story so you don't make the same mistake I did. Exercise is very, very important to fight diabetes. I still believe it, but please do the exercise safely. I could have prevented all of my foot problems if I had just known about checking my feet and the importance of wearing the right kind of shoes.

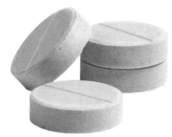

glucose tablets

How much exercise can I do when my blood sugars are high?

When your blood sugar is consistently 16 mmol or more (300 mg/dl), follow the Fitness Plan 1 or 2, breaking exercise up into smaller sessions if needed.

The most important thing is to take steps to bring down your blood sugar. You may need to reduce your food portions. You may also need some extra diabetes pills or injected insulin. Talk to your doctor or diabetes educator right away.

Low blood sugar when exercising

A low blood sugar is when your blood sugar goes below 4 mmol/L (75 mg/dL). You may feel shaky and dizzy. Treat this by eating 3–5 glucose tablets or 1 tablespoon (15 mL) of sugar. Low blood sugar can happen when you exercise if you are on insulin or certain diabetes pills. For complete information about low blood sugar signs, symptoms, causes, prevention, treatment and safety guidelines, see pages 331–338.

High blood sugar when exercising

You may be surprised to learn that exercise can cause either low blood sugar or high blood sugar.

In type 2 diabetes, there are two main reasons why exercise can cause blood sugar to go up:

1. Your body is warm and you may be thirsty or a bit dehydrated right after you finish exercising. This causes your blood sugar to go up. After you drink some water and rest, it usually will come down in about half an hour or less. Wait at least half an hour after exercise before testing your blood sugar, unless you think your blood sugar is low.

2. You have high blood sugar staying at about 16 mmol/L (300 mg/dL) or higher for days, weeks or months. This means that you are short of insulin or your insulin is not working properly. If you do strenuous or prolonged exercise such as long walks or heavy weight lifting, your blood sugar may actually get worse rather than go down.

Here's why:
Although you have lots of sugar in your blood – it can't get to your exercising muscles due to a shortage of insulin. Your muscles send a message to your brain that they need sugar. Then your body responds by sending more sugar to your blood from your liver stores. This extra sugar still can't be moved into your muscles because of the shortage of insulin. The sugar then builds up in your blood. The result is that your blood sugar actually goes up.

3. Becoming a Non-Smoker

Why You Should Stop Smoking   **264**

Ten Steps to Stop Smoking   **267**

1.	Prepare	267
2.	Set a quit date	269
3.	Choose "cold turkey" or reduce slowly	270
4.	Consider quit-smoking aids	271
5.	Time to quit	274
6.	Control cravings	275
7.	Prevent weight gain	277
8.	Tips for other changes	279
9.	Manage slips	280
10.	Enjoy being a non-smoker	280

3

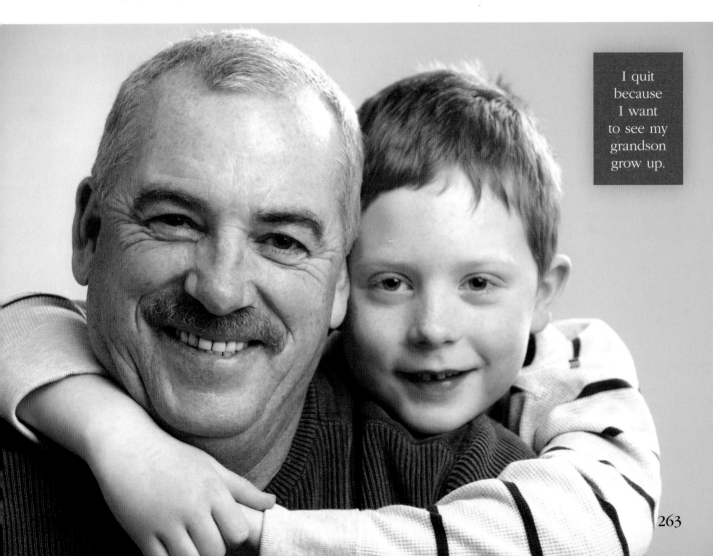

I quit because I want to see my grandson grow up.

Who is a smoker?

Smoking includes cigarettes, cigars or a pipe. Smokeless tobacco and chewing tobacco also contain nicotine. All of these cause health problems, and quitting requires similar steps.

The benefits of quitting smoking start right away

No matter how long you have been smoking, the benefits of quitting start within the first hour. Right away, there's an improvement of your blood pressure and pulse. After the first day the carbon monoxide clears out of your body. In just a couple of days you'll have more energy and less shortness of breath. In a few weeks your body has better circulation. In a few months, your lung function will improve by about ten percent. One year after you quit, your risk of heart attack will be half of that of a smoker with diabetes and your risk for a foot amputation will be one third less. This is amazing!

Most smokers would like to be non-smokers. You may have quit many times and then returned to smoking. This chapter will help you stop smoking for good!

You will learn why quitting smoking is so important for a person with diabetes. And you will learn ten steps to stop smoking.

When the time is right for you, join the millions of smokers who quit smoking to become non-smokers.

Why You Should Stop Smoking

There are many reasons to quit smoking – but which ones are most important to you?

You want to feel better
You will have less shortness of breath, have more energy and feel younger. You will get fewer colds and lung infections. You will feel clean and fresh, food will taste better, and your skin will feel softer.

You want to stay as healthy as possible
Smoking (nicotine, carbon monoxide and toxins) has three major health effects on your body.

1. **Cancer**. You may already know that smoking is the main cause of lung cancer, but smoking also contributes to cancers that affect the mouth, throat, pancreas, colon, rectum, kidney, bladder and cervix.

2. **Breathing difficulties**. Smoking can cause a variety of breathing problems such as bronchitis or emphysema.

3. **Heart attack and stroke**. Smoking damages and narrows blood vessels throughout your body, and increases blood pressure.

Smoking and diabetes together worsen complications

When you have diabetes and you smoke, you are more likely to have certain diabetes complications compared to the person with diabetes who does not smoke. This is because both nicotine and high blood sugar narrow and damage blood vessels and decrease the flow of oxygen in your body. They also both decrease your body's ability to use insulin properly and cause insulin to work less effectively.

For example, these diabetes complications occur more frequently in the person who smokes:

- Heart attack and stroke
- Gangrene and amputations to the lower leg or foot
- Kidney problems
- Vision loss (retinopathy)
- Nerve damage
- Erectile dysfunction
- Gum disease

You want to save money

Smoking costs a lot of money! If you're on a limited budget, imagine having that money to spend on healthy food and fitness opportunities.

You want to be a good example for your family

- You can reduce the risk of smoking in your family. Studies show that children are more likely to smoke if one or both of their parents smoke.
- If you are pregnant, you want to have the healthiest baby possible.
- By not smoking in the home, workplace and vehicles, you eliminate the danger of second-hand smoke.
- Make your home a safe one! Becoming a non-smoker will reduce the risk of a fire in your house. Smoking is the largest cause of home fire fatalities.

It's never too late to quit smoking.

There are now more ex-smokers than smokers (in Canada and the USA). Others have done it – so can you.

Marg's quit smoking story

I am 80 years old. My best friend and I started smoking at the age of 15. We all did it – surreptitiously. We smoked while on the school grounds and also we used to get on the street car at noon, go downtown to the bus depot and sit in the ladies rest room at the bus depot, have our lunch and smoke. It was a very grungy place but it was a secret place.

Of course my mother eventually caught me. She was very disappointed and she told me how bad it was for my health and she hoped that I would quit. I was about 18 by this time.

I continued to smoke after I married and until I became pregnant with my first child. For the reason that I did not want to harm my baby, it seemed easy to quit. Nevertheless, I did start again when my child was about 9 months old. My husband was a continuing smoker.

My next quitting time was pregnancy again. I am not sure when I started smoking again. In my defense, I did not smoke while breastfeeding or holding babies. However there was second hand smoke all around. We were not aware of the dangers of second hand smoke in those days.

With my third pregnancy I also quit smoking and again started months later after the baby's birth.

I do not remember that it was difficult to quit when I had such an important reason.

Later, to quit just for myself with no real impending reason it was not easy. Over 30 or so years, I tried, at least seven times to quit. I tried nicotine gum, I tried cold turkey, I joined the Seventh Day Adventists no smoking program, I tried total relaxation and I tried over-kill (smoking cigarette after cigarette one after the other till you felt sick – it was supposed to turn you off smoking). I would quit for a while and then start again. My husband smoked all this time.

One fine day we both decided to quit smoking. We finished off the cigarettes that we had (ten or so) and then quit cold turkey. We had each other and there was no smoking or cigarettes in the house. Doing it together was what I needed and also what my husband needed. We did not quit for any special health reasons we quit because we knew and had known for years that it was a very stupid thing to do.

I guess the story here is that one has to be honestly motivated to quit. Your own health or the health of loved ones or finally recognizing how very ignorant and wasteful it is. Also, it is a very expensive habit, and for my husband and I we smoked over 2 packs a day, and quitting, allowed us to save money and then do things in our retirement that we might not have been able to afford. I don't remember that it was extremely difficult but then it is a long time ago – 35 years now. We have never, not for one second, ever regretted giving up that filthy habit. Unfortunately my husband developed emphysema and it is very sad to watch him struggling to get his breath with the smallest effort. If only we had not smoked or had quit earlier.

Quit-smoking aids such as nicotine patches and toll-free quit phone lines were not available when Marg was trying to quit smoking. These might have helped her and her husband quit smoking sooner.

Ten Steps to Stop Smoking

1. Prepare

If you are like most smokers, you began smoking as a teenager. Often due to peer pressure, or to show independence or to feel adult. There are those who "try it" but who never become smokers. Others become addicted almost at the first puff. Smoking is an addictive habit.

Smoking is now a long-time companion for you. It provides you with stimulation, and is a convenient tool to handle stress and cravings. If you prepare, saying goodbye is less difficult. Becoming a non-smoker is more than just quitting. It's a process of learning new healthier habits. To be a non-smoker is a hard journey – but it is worth it.

Before you quit, think about the following questions:

What are *your* reasons to quit?
Your reasons are the best ones. Make a list.

What are your smoking triggers?
Triggers are times or things that make you want to smoke. Examples of triggers are drinking coffee or alcohol, watching TV, playing cards or bingo, driving, coping with a crisis or finishing a meal.

How will you manage your smoking triggers?
One way is to develop new healthier habits and relieve stress by going for a walk, drinking water, deep breathing and a hobby that keeps your mind and hands busy. You will find many useful tips to help you deal with smoking triggers throughout these Ten Steps.

Set up support

Studies show that you are more likely to succeed if you have at least one person (friend, family or professional) who will listen to you and support you. You may want to:

- Talk to family or friends that have successfully quit.

- Talk to your family and coworkers about your intention to quit. Seek their support.

- Talk to your doctor about methods of quitting and quitting aids. Your pharmacist (or diabetes educator) can also be a great help, and is easy to access.

- Ask about quit smoking programs and support groups available in your community. See below.

- Ask for the number of your local toll-free quit line or on-line quit smoking service. See below.

- Ask if your health plan covers the cost of quit-smoking aids (for example, nicotine patches).

Support Groups and Phone Support

- Canadian Cancer Society

- American Cancer Society

- American Lung Association

- National Cancer Institute

- Addiction support organizations

These organizations can provide you with more detailed information to help you quit. They also have resources for you if you're thinking about quitting but aren't ready yet.

At these organizations, you can talk to someone in person to get advice and support. A variety of services are available depending on where you live including:

- toll-free telephone counseling

- web-based message boards

- handouts and booklets

- support groups

2. Set a Quit Date

It's natural to keep putting off quitting, this is a very hard but important change. You might find it easier, if you set a quit date. Then you have a goal to work towards. Don't set the goal too far away or it becomes unreachable. Consider setting a quit date within the next month. Try to choose a time without a lot of stressful events planned. You need to be prepared mentally and physically for quitting.

It's easy to give excuses for not quitting. Write your quit date on your calendar – and stick to it.

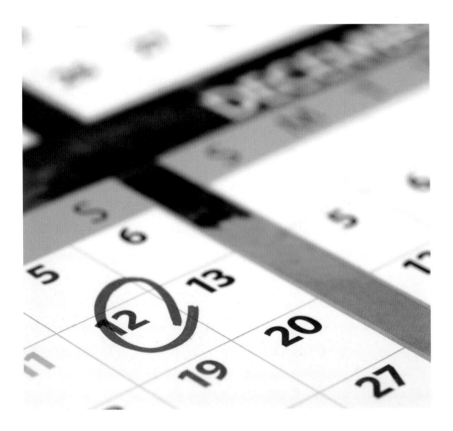

Imagine yourself as a non-smoker
If you can imagine it – you can do it!

3. Choose "Cold Turkey" or Reduce Slowly

Sometimes people quit cold turkey with great success after a major life event such as a heart attack or stroke. Please don't wait that long to make your change.

Cold turkey

This means when you reach your quit date, you quit totally that day without any quit-smoking aids. While most people who quit do so "cold turkey" this often involves numerous attempts to quit. Research shows that people who use quit smoking aids or toll-free quit phone lines are able to quit with fewer attempts. If you tried to quit cold turkey in the past, and then returned to smoking, next time consider using some of the tools available to you.

Cut back slowly

This means you cut back on smoking gradually over several weeks until you reach your quit date. Some people find it helpful to smoke the cigarettes that they feel are the hardest to give up (say first thing in the morning, or after a meal). Instead, wean off smoking at other times of the day. Then gradually cut back on the harder times. Each cigarette you don't smoke puts you closer to your goal of becoming a non-smoker.

Using nicotine gum to help cut back

Are you trying to cut back but not quite ready to quit yet? Perhaps you are cutting out smoking in your home, during work hours, when driving in your car, or when non-smokers are present. Good for you! Chewing on a piece of nicotine gum (see page 271) can help you with your cravings during these times. The good news is that research shows that when you stop smoking in your home, you are significantly more likely to quit. You are on your way to becoming a non-smoker.

4. Consider Quit-Smoking Aids

A variety of quit-smoking aids and medications are available. Research shows these help many people quit.

If you tried to quit with one method and it didn't help, consider trying it again, or trying something else. Find out about quit-smoking aids from your doctor or pharmacist or contact an organization, see page 268.

Nicotine replacement products

Smoking is more than a habit, it's an addiction. Nicotine replacement products can help you wean off the nicotine in cigarettes. They provide nicotine, but do not give you the carbon monoxide and toxins that comes from burning tobacco leaves and inhaling the smoke of cigarettes. These replacement products include nicotine gum and lozenges, the patch, or inhaler and in the U.S., nicotine nasal spray. Nicotine substitutes help decrease the physical symptoms of withdrawal so you can deal with not having a cigarette in your hand.

Deciding which one to use is up to you. Some people don't like the taste of the gum or lozenges, so prefer the patch. Some get some throat irritation with the inhaler or nasal irritation with the nasal spray. With advice from your doctor, you may want to use a combination of products.

Nicotine gum or lozenges

The gum and lozenges are sugar-free and contain nicotine. Follow the directions on the package. If you have an urge to smoke, take a piece of gum or a lozenge. Follow the recommended amount listed on the package (the gum comes in two different strengths). Some people will only use the gum or lozenges for a short period of time, while others may use them over 4–6 months.

Talk to your doctor or pharmacist

You can buy all these over-the-counter (except the inhaler needs a doctor's prescription in the US). Talk to your doctor or pharmacist for information about how to use these products. They can tell you how much to use and for how long. This is important if you have other health problems or are pregnant or breastfeeding. You need to use the products in the correct way so that you don't get too much nicotine.

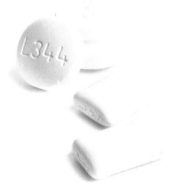

Nicotine lozenges and gum

Nicotine patch

If you smoke more than ten cigarettes a day or if you have a strong craving for a cigarette as soon as you get up in the morning, doctors recommend the patch. You attach the nicotine patch to your skin. The patch releases nicotine into your blood. You wear a patch for 16 or 24 hours, and then replace it with a new patch the next day. You start off with a stronger patch and decrease to a lower dose. Over 6–12 weeks, you can decrease the nicotine levels with patches containing less nicotine. The patch is easy to use.

Some people find that nicotine patches plus an occasional nicotine gum or lozenge works well together. Perhaps because the patch provides a steady supply of nicotine and the gum or lozenge provides a boost for an extra craving.

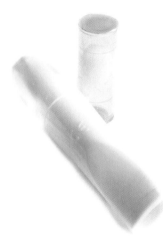

Nicotine oral inhaler

Nicotine oral inhaler

This is a small tube that looks like a cigarette. When you inhale you get a smaller dose of nicotine than if smoking a cigarette. You might use 6–12 cartridges each day and then you would slowly decrease the daily amount, and quit when you are down to 1–2 a day. The inhaler should not be used for more than six months.

Nicotine nasal spray

It comes in a small container that you spray into each nostril. You might use the spray 8–40 times a day. Use it for the length of time specified on the package. This may not be a good choice for you if you have hay fever or a sinus infection.

Menthol cigarettes, flavored cigars and other flavored smoking products are bad for you:

Menthol cigarettes may seem to be more "soothing" but they are just as hazardous as regular cigarettes.

Some people are tricked into thinking that online products such as electronic cigarettes (e-cigarettes) are safe – beware, they have nicotine just like cigarettes and should be avoided. In Canada they are not approved for sale. There is no such thing as a safe cigarette.

Medications that help you quit

There are several prescription pills to help you quit smoking. These don't contain nicotine but have other substances that reduce withdrawal symptoms and the urge to smoke. You can take some of these pills along with a nicotine product. Discuss this with your doctor or pharmacist as some of these pills have side-effects.

Hypnosis, acupuncture and laser therapy

Some people say these treatments helped them stop smoking, although it is difficult to prove why they work. Perhaps part of the reason these treatments work is that these approaches may be combined with nicotine replacement products such as the patch. Also, they often include counseling, support and education about quitting smoking, and help you to learn to relax. Studies do show you are more likely to benefit if you have numerous treatments with a skilled health worker.

Hypnosis: Only a medical doctor or psychiatrist is qualified to do this. It involves putting a person into a "hypnotic trance." In this relaxed state, the hypnotist will teach you behavior skills for coping with withdrawal and the urge to smoke. Treatment is typically for three months or longer. Not everyone can be hypnotized.

Acupuncture is a type of traditional Chinese medicine. It involves the insertion of very fine needles into specific points of the body (called acupuncture points). The aim of acupuncture is to help the body achieve its natural balance. There is some research that shows this approach may help smokers cut back or quit smoking.

Laser therapy uses fine beams of pulsating light. These beams shine on specific spots on the body (often the acupuncture points). This may help release endorphins which help to relax you.

New Research

A vaccine is being studied that would encourage your body to make antibodies to prevent nicotine from entering the brain. In early trials, the vaccine is being given in combination with other drugs. It is showing some promise in helping to reduce nicotine withdrawal. However, there are some side effects and support is still needed to break the repetitious habits of smoking.

If you choose one of these techniques, make sure the practitioner is reputable. Ask your pharmacist, doctor or local quit-smoking organization.

5. Time to Quit

Your quit date has arrived. It's time to put all your cigarettes, matches, lighters and ashtrays in the garbage. Take some deep breaths.

Take it one cigarette less at a time, and one day at a time.

This is the first day of your new life as a non-smoker. It will be challenging – but this is something you have wanted to do for a long time. It will be worth it! Remember, quit-smoking aids and the toll-free quit phone lines are there for you. It is helpful to know that generally the first one to three days of not smoking are the hardest. It gets a little easier as the weeks, months and years go by.

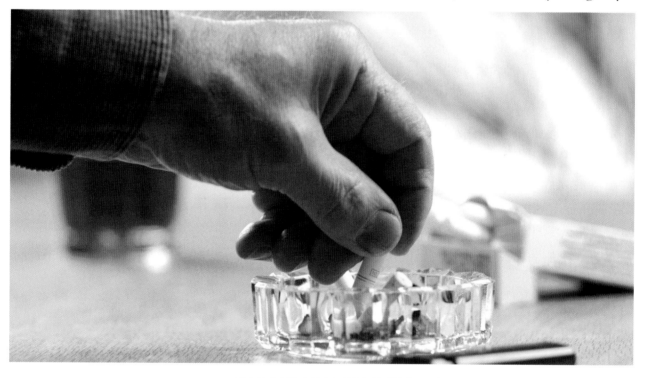

Tips for family and friends of someone who has just quit smoking:

- Quite likely the person who has just quit will be grouchy… they are fighting a very difficult addiction withdrawal. Quitting smoking isn't easy and isn't fun for them. Please be sensitive to their moods. Let them vent. Give them space but be a wall of support for them. Be understanding. It will pass. They will get easier to live with and they will be smoke free and so will you.

- If you are a smoker, don't smoke in their company.

- If they slip or relapse, don't make them feel guilty. Be supportive. This is a long process and they will need you to be there for them every step of the way.

6. Control Cravings

Each craving for a cigarette comes in a wave. It is the strongest at the beginning, then will get less, and will tend to last a couple of minutes. Get through each craving one at a time. Cravings will taper off over time.

Change your smoking routines

- Reduce your time spent in your favorite smoking places. For example, if you have your usual "smoking chair" in your home, sit on a different chair to begin with. If you are at home most of the day, go to a non-smoking location such as a library or mall. Go for regular short walks.

- If you smoked in front of the TV, then limit your TV watching at first. Maybe tune into the radio or music instead of smoking. You will quickly save enough money to buy yourself a portable MP3 music player and stock it with all your favorite songs. Each time you want to smoke, put on your earphones and focus on a special piece of music.

- During the first critical days and weeks after you quit, avoid smokers who want you to smoke with them. Reduce activities that you associate with other smokers. For example, homes of friends or family who smoke, bars, bingo halls and smoker coffee breaks. Look for non-smoking facilities.

- Is smoking a cigarette part of your getting–ready-for-bed routine? If so, before you quit it's a good idea to think about a different bedtime routine. For more ideas about sleep, see pages 362–363.

Fill the void left by no cigarettes

If you were a one pack-a-day smoker you put a cigarette in your mouth more than 400 times a day. Each time you think of reaching for a cigarette, take several long deep breaths. Put into action the three **D**'s of Dealing with cravings: take a **D**eep breath, **D**rink water and **D**istract yourself. The next page has some suggestions to distract yourself and keep your hands busy.

Three D's of Dealing with cravings:

Deep breath

Drink water

Distract yourself

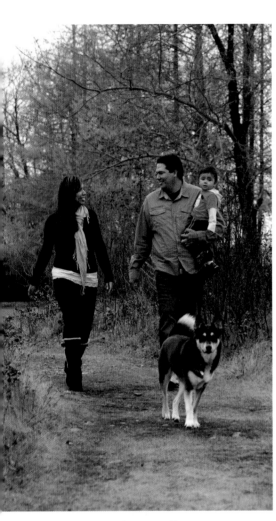

Go for a walk.

Distract yourself

- Get up and walk around for a few minutes.

- Do a few stretches.

- Chew a stick of sugarless gum.

- Do your nails.

- Some people find it helpful to take a small sniff of lavender oil, peppermint oil, or black pepper oil. These have a strong scent and can help break the association with smoking.

- Drink a cup of peppermint or strong flavoured herbal tea.

- Suck on a sugar-free peppermint, small wintergreen mint, or cinnamon stick.

- Play a hand of solitaire (with cards or on the computer).

Keep your hands busy

- Roll a pencil or coin in your hands.

- Play with a rubber band.

- Count the beads on a necklace. Prayer beads work well.

- Twiddle a key holder with an interesting ornament.

- Doodle.

- Massage your fingers and hands, or your feet, with a moisturizer or, massage someone else's.

- Do a puzzle, or some needlework or knit.

- Read or write down how you are feeling in a journal.

- Wash dishes or clean your home. This is a great chance to wash walls, curtains and furniture to get rid of the smoky stale smells and stains.

- Squeeze a stress ball (a soft spongy ball) or some play dough.

- If you are musical, strum on a guitar or play the piano. If you aren't musical, try playing a ukulele, it's one of the easiest instruments in the world to play and you can find free lessons on the internet!

- If you have a cell phone, text a friend and tell them you're texting them instead of smoking.

Review your reasons for quitting.

7. Prevent Weight Gain

A small or moderate weight gain is less of a health concern than a lifetime of smoking. However, if you exercise and eat right when you quit smoking, you can avoid weight gain or gain very little weight. Exercise increases your metabolism, offsetting the effect of nicotine withdrawal. Here are some tips to lessen or prevent weight gain after quitting smoking.

Before you quit smoking

Talk to a dietitian about healthy meal choices. This way you can make a plan of what foods you should have (and shouldn't have) in your home, when you quit. It is also good to have regular follow-up to monitor and manage weight. If you don't have access to a dietitian, contact an addictions counsellor, diabetes nurse or toll-free smokers' help line.

No weight gain alternatives to smoking

Instead of an after-meal cigarette

- Eat regular meals. Follow the meal plans in this book and in my first book, *Diabetes Meals for Good Health*.

- Slow down your eating. Drink water, both with your meal and at the end of your meal. Put your knife and fork down between bites.

- If you want a dessert, choose a fruit, mini pudding, or one of the light dessert recipes in this book.

- Try to resist going for a second helping. As soon as you finish your meal, get up from the table and do something else. This keeps you busy and distracted. (Try something different than you did when you were a smoker.)

- A small candy such as a Tic Tac, cinnamon heart or sugar-free candy after a meal can also help. Even one with sugar will have a lot less calories than going for seconds.

- After a meal, brush your teeth, rinse out your mouth, or chew on a small piece of mint or parsley, rather than smoke. This helps break the smoking craving.

- Go for a walk, around your home or outside. Even a short walk removes you from that familiar place where you used to smoke, and also gets your lungs invigorated. It helps you deal with the anguish and tension you will be feeling because of withdrawal from nicotine.

Take one step at a time

Eating healthy foods, keeping active and quitting smoking are all helpful. Making change is a process. You might decide to first try to get more active. When you have achieved this go on to making another change.

Nicotine withdrawal can affect metabolism. However, it's more likely that people who quit smoking tend to substitute food (especially sweets) for cigarettes.

Exercise is one of the best ways to control cravings and prevent weight gain.

277

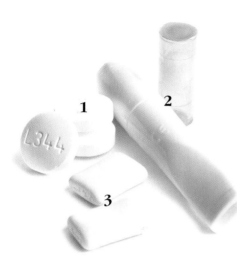

When you have a craving, try one of these:

1. a nicotine lozenge

2. a puff from a nicotine oral inhaler

3. a piece of nicotine gum

Instead of evening smoking

- **Plan small portioned snacks.** Before you quit smoking, stock your house with lots of low-calorie snacks and snacks that fit in the small and medium snack categories (try light popcorn, fruit, vegetable juice or crackers). See pages 196–200, and for additional ideas for snack choices see my book *Diabetes Meals for Good Health*. Cook up a large pot of vegetable soup. A bowl of this comfort food is an excellent replacement for a cigarette. Some people find if they add extra chili or other herbs and spices to their foods, it can intensify the flavor and help deal with cravings. Perhaps try a spicy vegetable soup!

- **Keep food out of sight – out of mind.** Don't have tempting foods sitting around. Chips, donuts and chocolate bars are not a good replacement to cigarettes. Better yet, don't have these tempting foods in the house at all.

- **Delay your snack.** When you are craving a snack, try to wait a pre-determined time, say 5 minutes. Go brush your teeth and have a drink of water. Progressively increase the length of time before each snack, and you may find you can eventually omit it altogether.

- **Try to distract yourself with a non-food related activity.** Go for a walk. Do a hobby, go outside, wash the dishes, or sweep the floor. Your home will never be so clean!

Instead of smoking at social events or "smoke breaks"

- In the first few weeks after you quit smoking, avoid these social events if possible. You may find that as you cut back on smoking you may also cut back on social drinking, which would also be a positive change.

- Go for a short walk instead of a coffee break at work. Also, see pages 78–79 for tips to manage overeating in the workplace. Have a drink of water or a diet beverage. A piece of fresh fruit is always a good choice.

Instead of smoking when drinking coffee

- Drink your coffee out of a different type of mug, or in a different location in your home or workplace.

- Change your drink. Cut back on drinking coffee and replace some of your coffee with tea, water, or a diet beverage.

8. Tips for Other Changes

Irritability or anxiety

Irritability is common when people quit smoking. Warn those around you! Going for a walk perks up your happy hormones and helps you burn off steam. Instead of yelling or getting mad at someone close to you, talk on the phone or text a supportive friend, family member, or even a stranger on a smoker's support phone line. Try deep breathing or easy meditation (see pages 363–364). Also see other stress management tips on page 351–364.

Sore throat or coughs

You may experience this for the first few days. Your lungs are cleaning out the tar leftover from smoking. It's good to get this out of your body by coughing. Drinking lots of water or herbal tea can help speed this up. If your throat is sore, sip on water or suck on a sugar-free cough drop. Usually this problem goes away in a week or two.

Difficulty falling asleep

You may find you are more nervous and restless at night as you go through your initial withdrawal. Earlier in the evening, do something that will help tire you out so you sleep better – try a short walk or just 5–10 minutes on your exercise bike or treadmill. Cutting back on caffeine at night might help; try switching to water, decaffeinated coffee or tea, herbal tea or other caffeine-free diet beverages. Take a short bath or shower to help yourself relax.

Dizziness

This usually only lasts for a few days and is because your body is getting more oxygen than it's used to. Sit down and have a drink of water. Get some fresh air. The dizzy feelings should pass.

Headaches

The stress of quitting smoking and the nicotine withdrawal can cause headaches. Lie down in a quiet dark room and rest. Do relaxation exercises. Treat a headache with your usual over-the-counter medication.

Constipation

Nicotine stimulates bowel movements. So some people have difficulty going to the bathroom after they quit smoking. Eating lots of vegetables and fruits can give you the needed boost of fiber. And, drinking water and exercise also helps.

Consider going to see a doctor or a mental health worker if your feelings of anxiety worsen, and you think you may be depressed (see pages 365–366).

Are you using the 24-hour nicotine patch?

As a smoker, did you sleep through the night without getting up to smoke? If so, then the nicotine released from the patch during the night might be keeping you awake or making you restless. Try removing the patch before going to sleep for the night.

For more sleeping tips: *See pages 362–363.*

9. Manage Slips

Most people make mistakes, that's part of being human.

Slip-ups could be minor – an occasional cigarette here or there. Or this might involve a day or two where you go back to smoking. The important thing is to get right back to your non-smoking pattern as soon as you can.

Remind yourself of your goal.

Revisit your reasons for quitting.

Re-enlist help. Smoker help lines are there at any stage — even months down the road. Call them again.

If you lose your footing, don't be hard on yourself – keep focused on sticking to your quit plan. Ask yourself, "What triggered this?" "How can I prevent it next time?" Learn from your mistake. Call the toll-free smokers help-line, or reconnect with a support group if needed (see page 268).

Keep your list of reasons to quit handy and visible. Look at it regularly.

Mistakes can also mean a full blown return to smoking. This doesn't mean you won't be able to quit smoking. For most people there will be several tries before you become a permanent non-smoker. When you are ready, get back to your non-smoking routine, but don't wait too long. Good luck!

10. Enjoy Being a Non-Smoker

Once you're a non-smoker, you have achieved an incredible milestone in your life. You have reversed something that quite likely you began in your teenage or early adult years. You will now begin to reap the benefits of being a non-smoker. Enjoy deep breaths, fresh air and better health!

Reward yourself
Use a jar to deposit daily or weekly cigarette money and watch your savings grow. Consider rewarding yourself along the way, or save your money for something larger. Whatever you decide, reward yourself in some way. You have earned it!

Consider a visit to a dental hygienist for a teeth cleaning. She'll remove that tar build-up and you'll enjoy your whiter smile.

Celebrate your success
After a month, celebrate your anniversary of quitting smoking. Then look forward to celebrating your first year anniversary of being a non-smoker.

Congratulations!

4. Preventing Infections

Keeping your feet healthy   **282**

1. See a doctor right away for urgent foot problems   282
2. Maintain good blood sugar, blood pressure and blood cholesterol   283
3. Check your feet every day   284
4. Ask your doctor or nurse to check your feet   286
5. Wash, dry and moisturize your feet   287
6. Trim your toenails properly   288
7. Do not use heaters, razors and chemicals   289
8. Wear comfortable socks and shoes that fit well   290
9. Take care of small problems at home   294
10. Medical care of an ulcer   295

Good skin care   **296**

Ten tips for mouth care   **297**

Avoiding urinary tract infections (UTIs)   **301**

Treatment   301

7 things for women to think about to prevent a UTI   302

UTI prevention tips for men   305

Preventing a flu, cold or food poisoning   **306**

Keeping your Feet Healthy

1. See a doctor right away for urgent foot problems

Information on why you may be at risk for foot problems is on page 29-32.

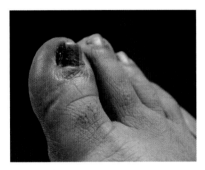

What are urgent foot problems?

- An ingrown toenail that is infected.

- Any cut or sore that doesn't heal within two days. Act sooner if it gets worse or there are any signs of infection.

- Any unusual pain, swelling, warmth, redness, coldness or cramping in your legs or feet.

- Pus draining from your foot or leg.

- Any part of your foot or leg turns dark blue or black. If you are a dark skinned person, watch for a darker color or change in color.

An infection can spread quickly, within one or two days. If you can't get an appointment with your doctor, go to a clinic or your hospital's Emergency Room.

Warning Signs of Infection:

- Redness or spreading (it can move from the toe up the foot or from the foot up the leg)

- Swelling

- Oozing pus

- Unusual pain (although there may be no pain)

- Fever, chills or fatigue

- Sudden unexplained increase in your blood sugar

2. Maintain good blood sugar, blood pressure and blood cholesterol

Follow steps 1–3 on pages 54–280.

- Step 1: Eat well
- Step 2: Become active
- Step 3: Become a non-smoker

Step 1: Eat well

The amounts and types of food you eat make a big difference to your blood sugar and circulation. If you need to lose weight, try cutting back gradually on portions and becoming more active. Weight loss will reduce the weight on the soles of your feet. It also improves blood sugar, blood pressure and blood cholesterol.

Step 2: Become active

In addition to the ideas for becoming more active outlined on pages 218–262, here are some specific tips to help improve circulation to your feet.

If you've been sitting for an hour, get up and walk around, peddle an exercise bike or do foot or leg exercises (see below).

- Wiggle your toes
- Starting from your ankles, move your feet in circles, up and down and side-to-side
- Ankle rotations (page 239)
- Chair exercises (pages 248–249)

Step 3: Become a non-smoker

Smoking significantly narrows blood vessels and decreases blood flow to the feet. It also reduces healing. As a smoker, having diabetes puts you at high risk for foot problems and amputations.

Other tips to increase circulation to your feet:

- *If your feet swell, raise your feet when you are sitting or lying down.*
- *Try not to sit with your legs or feet crossed as this reduces circulation and compresses nerves.*
- *Gently massage your feet if they are cold.*

3. Check your feet every day

You may have lost feeling in your feet, so you need to look and touch your feet with your hands daily. Then you'll notice infections and problems early.

To help remember, it's a good idea to check your feet at the same time every day (for example, after your bath or shower, or before going to bed). Then, checking your feet becomes a habit – a good habit!

If it's difficult for you to bend to look at the bottom of each foot, try one of these options:

- Extend your leg backwards with the top of your foot flat on the floor. Look back at the sole of your foot.

- Sit on a chair in front of a full length mirror. Put your foot on a stool and look in the mirror.

- Put a mirror on the floor or hold a mirror. You can buy special mirrors that are on the end of a long handle (like the type a dentist uses to look in your mouth, but larger). Hold this mirror to look at the bottom of your feet.

- Get help from a family member, friend or home care support person.

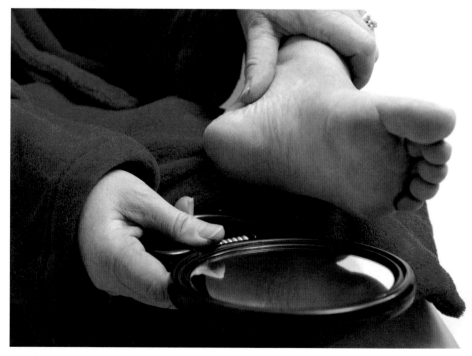

Is it difficult for you to see your feet?
Many people who are visually impaired do learn to check their own feet by carefully feeling them. However, you could still miss a problem area. It's best if you have someone help you.

Caution

You are looking for redness, blisters or sores, swelling, dryness or cracks, or a change in shape. Be aware of any change that wasn't there yesterday. Check the top and bottom of each foot and between your toes.

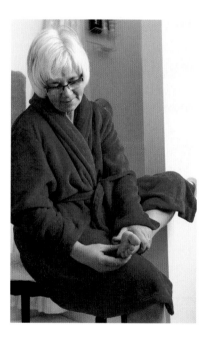

What to check for:

(1) Redness or color change
- bruising, or white or darkened or red areas
- red streaks
- skin that lightens for a few seconds after being pressed and released, which could mean decreased circulation

Look for redness or blisters.

(2) Swelling
This could be a sign of poor circulation or infection.

(3) Cold or hot spots
- A cold spot can mean an area is not getting enough circulation.
- A hot spot could mean an infection underneath your skin. This could turn into a blister or sore.
- Is one foot warmer or cooler than the other?

See pages 29–32 for more information on what these changes can look like.

(4) Sensation changes
You might feel "pins and needles," numbness or burning in your feet that can mean decreased nerve function. Your feet may feel like "blocks of wood."

(5) Cracks, bleeding, sores or ulcers, or blisters
- Dry skin can cause cracks in your skin (typically on your heel).
- Tight shoes, irritation or dry skin can cause a blister, cut or sore.
- Look in between your toes for cracks or cuts, or athlete's foot (flaky, red or white areas, itchy and cracking).
- Pus or bad odor could be a sign of an infection.

An ulcer *is an open wound (sore) with severe skin breakdown.*

(6) Changes to toenails
- Ingrown toenails will look red and bleeding at the edge of the nail. Tight shoes or bad nail trimming can cause this.
- Toenails that are thick, brittle and yellowish-green may have a fungus infection under the nails (it usually starts in the corner or end of the nail).
- If the whole toenail is discolored this may be due to poor circulation (lack of oxygen to the toe).

(7) Corns
A corn is a small, round hard spot on the top of your toe, or it could be a thickened but softer spot between your toes. Most corns occur because of friction from a tight, poorly fitting shoe.

(8) Calluses

A callus is thickened skin on the side or bottom of your foot. A callus is usually larger and flatter than a corn. Like corns, friction usually causes calluses. Pressure on the bottom of your foot can also cause this. An infection can develop underneath a callus (or corn).

(9) Changes to the shape of your foot

Changes to your bones will happen more gradually. Examples are the formation of a bunion, or a change in the arch of your foot (typically a flattening). Arches allow your foot to absorb pressure as you walk, and when the arch is lost, pressure points develop on your foot. Hammertoes (toes that rise up at the knuckle) are a kind of foot change that might also happen.

(10) Loss of hair

Reduced or no hair growth on your feet or lower legs could be a sign of reduced oxygen flow and nerve damage.

4. Ask your doctor or nurse to check your feet

- He/she should check your feet once a year, or more often if you have foot problems.

- If you have concerns during the year, **take off your shoes and socks while waiting for your doctor or nurse.**

- Urgent Foot Checks: See your doctor or nurse right away about some concerns – see page 282.

What will my doctor or nurse check?
He will check for the same things that you look for such as cracks, sores, color changes and swelling, and how your feet look and feel. In addition, he may examine:

- Your nerve sensation on the top of your big toe or on the bottom of your feet, using either a monofilament or a tuning fork. These tests don't hurt at all.

- Your circulation, by measuring the pulses in your feet or legs.

- Your blood pressure in your legs or feet. If lower than the blood pressure in your arms, this indicates reduced blood flow to the legs or feet.

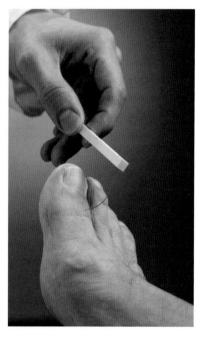

A check for nerve sensation using a monofilament.

5. Wash, dry and moisturize your feet

Gently wash your feet every day

- Wash your feet with mild soap every day with warm (not hot) water.

- If you are taking a bath, check with your elbow or wrist that the water isn't too hot before you get in. This is important because if you have nerve damage on your feet, you may not realize the water is too hot.

- After use, clean your tub with soap, and rinse well. To remove grime, use baking soda, then rinse well. Do not use bleach or harsh cleaners. If you leave behind traces of bleach, this will dry your feet further.

- If you have an open sore, check with your nurse or doctor about whether you should put your foot in water.

Dry your feet with care

- After your daily shower or bath, dry your feet, tops and bottoms and between the toes. This stops fungus and germs which need moisture to grow.

Moisturize your feet

- Put moisturizing lotion or cream (such as a hand moisturizer) on dry or cracked areas, and gently work it in. Avoid putting lotion between your toes, or on cuts or open sores. Common moisturizer brands are Nivea, Vaseline Intensive Care, Aveeno and lanolin-based creams. Vaseline is also an option. Strongly perfumed creams aren't a good idea, as they often have an alcohol base which dries the skin.

- Put the cream on every day, or twice a day, to get rid of or reduce dryness. If after several weeks the lotion has not helped, ask your doctor or nurse to recommend a different moisturizer.

- Try using a lotion at night after your bath or shower and after you have dried your feet. Then put on a pair of socks with a loose band; the moisturizer will continue to work as you sleep.

- Chlorine in swimming pools can dry your skin. Also public showers and swimming pools often are a source of athlete's foot (fungus). Wearing water shoes (aqua socks) at a pool can help protect your feet from germs. After swimming, thoroughly wash and dry your feet, then moisturize your feet and skin.

Problems with soaking

Soaking removes your natural oils and dries out your feet. Dry, scaly skin is more likely to get cracks and sores. Don't soak your feet, or limit soaking in a basin or bath to no more than 10 minutes.

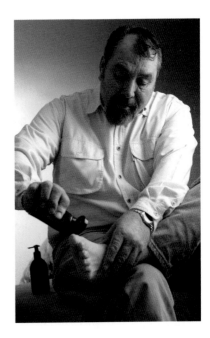

6. Trim your toenails properly

Carefully cut or file your toenails straight across.

- Use nail clippers or nail files rather than scissors, as you may be more likely to cut your toe with scissors.

- Cut or file your toenails straight across, and slightly rounded to the shape of your toes. Gently file any sharp edges. This will help avoid ingrown toenails. Properly fitting shoes also helps prevent ingrown toenails (see pages 291–292).

- Do not cut your nails too short (cut even with the ends of your toes).

- It's easier to cut your toenails after washing or a bath, as your nails are softer. If you have thick toenails this is especially helpful.

- You should cut your toenails at least every 4–6 weeks.

Get help with nail cutting if you need it.

- Please get help from a foot care nurse or podiatrist (foot doctor) for regular toenail trimming if:
  – You have lost feeling in your feet
  – You can't see or reach your feet.
  – Your nails are thick and difficult to cut.
  – Your hands are shaky.
  – You have ingrown toenails.

- Many senior centers employ nurses who know how to cut toenails. It is worth the cost to save your feet.

Ask your doctor or diabetes educator to recommend a foot care nurse with special training in diabetes foot care.

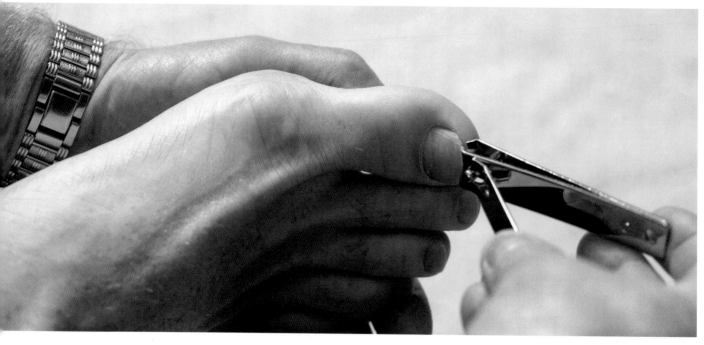

7. Do not use heaters, razors and chemicals

If you lack feeling in your feet, you can't tell if something is too hot.

- Avoid using heating pads and electric blankets as they might overheat.

- Don't put your feet close to a fireplace or radiator.

Never use sharp razors, knives, corn plasters or wart removal chemicals on your feet to remove calluses, corns or warts.

- Some people are tempted to use a metal grater on their feet, or to shave or cut off calluses, corns or warts using a razor or knife. This can be dangerous. One little slip and you can cut yourself and get an open sore. Also, sometimes there can actually be a sore or infection underneath a hard callus making cutting or filing very risky.

- Corn plasters can rip your skin. Wart removal products can cause open sores that might get infected.

- See your doctor, foot care nurse or podiatrist about how to treat calluses, corns or warts that won't go away. See page 294 about home treatment for minor problems.

Nail polish
If you have discolored toenails you may be tempted to hide them under dark nail polish. However, if you leave on nail polish for many days, this could hide a bigger problem, such as an infection. If you polish your toenails with dark nail polish, remove it after a day or two. Wash your toes with soapy water to remove all traces of the nail polish remover.

Hair removal on lower legs and feet
Both getting older and having diabetes can reduce hair on your legs. However, if you do still grow hair and want to remove it, avoid the use of hair removal chemicals. These can be harsh on your skin. Waxing isn't recommended as your skin can be torn when you or some else rips the wax off. Also hot wax can burn your skin. If shaving your legs with a razor, moisten and lather your skin with soap or shaving cream, and be extra careful. Don't shave if you have any blisters or boils on your skin, because you could break the skin and cause an infection.

If using a hot water bottle, check the water with your wrist to make sure it isn't too hot, and wear socks to protect your feet. Never fill a hot water bottle with boiling water or put it directly next to your skin.

8. Wear comfortable socks and shoes that fit well

Socks

Most injuries to the feet happen in your house – protect your feet by wearing shoes and socks in the house and outside.

Unless your doctor recommends it, avoid wearing:

- *support hose for varicose veins, or*
- *compression stockings (these control swelling in legs and feet).*

Clean and comfortable

- Clean socks worn inside your shoes, help protect your feet from rubbing. This is especially important when walking.
- Pantyhose can be worn but avoid elasticized knee highs.
- If you have swelling in your legs, you may need socks that are wide at the top (or have a loose band) so that your circulation is not restricted.

Cotton, wool or cotton-acrylic blends

- Cotton or wool socks are good as they have natural fibers and absorb moisture.
- A good quality athletic sock, often a blend of cotton and acrylic, is good for walking or sports.

White socks

- If you have a bleeding hangnail or sore, the blood will show on a white sock. This will alert you to take care of it.

Limit lumps and bumps

- Get rid of old or mended socks.
- Wear the correct size socks. If the socks are too small, they will press seams into your foot. If they're too large, the socks will bunch up.
- If your skin is thin and fragile, buy socks with no seams to avoid rubbing, or wear the socks inside out so the seams are on the outside.

Padded on the bottom of the socks

- This helps cushion the soles of your feet.

Dry and warm

- If your feet sweat a lot, change into a dry pair of socks during the day.
- Wear warm socks to bed (and during the day) if your feet get cold.
- In the winter, wear warm socks in your boots.

Shoes

- Look in your shoes, feel inside, and quickly shake them out before you put them on. You want to make sure there are no cracks, rough seams, pebbles or grit inside that could hurt your feet.

- Closed-toe shoes protect your feet better than open-toed shoes or sandals.

- Don't go barefoot, even when walking around the house. Think about it – where do you most often stub your toe or step on something sharp? For most people, the answer is "at home." When you have diabetes, a stubbed toe can lead to an infection. At home, wear either a pair of hard-toed slippers or "house shoes."

- On hot days, avoid barefoot on cement by a pool, or on a deck. You may not feel the heat on the soles of your feet and you could get a burn.

- At the beach, wear rubber-soled shoes. These protect your feet from hot sand, sharp shells, and sunburn. Also put on sunscreen as needed. Check frequently that sand doesn't rub against your feet and between your toes.

- In cold weather, wear warm dry socks and waterproof boots to prevent frostbite.

- If you have very few changes to the shape of your foot, a good quality athletic or walking shoe is ideal. If you have changes to the shape of your foot, you may need a specialty or prescription shoe.

At the shoe store – making sure your shoes fit well

- Shop for shoes in the afternoon or evening. This is when your feet are generally the most swollen, so you'll choose shoes that aren't too tight.

- Try on both shoes, and stand up and walk around. Shoes should be comfortable the first time you try them on. They shouldn't rub or pinch. There should be enough room at the toe.

- Wear new shoes for less than two hours at first. Check your feet afterwards to make sure there are no red areas where the shoes are rubbing.

- When you try on shoes at the shoe store it is sometimes hard to feel if your foot or toes are being squished into the shoe. One good solution is to stand on the removable insoles and see if your feet fit inside. Some shoes don't have a removable insole so it's a good idea to bring along an outline of your foot (see sidebar).

It's best if you have more than one pair of shoes, so you don't wear the same pair every day.

Leave on a light at night if you get up to go to the bathroom.

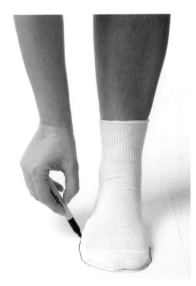

You may want to measure your feet before you go to the shoe store.

At the end of the day, stand on a piece of paper and draw around your foot. Take this piece of paper with you to the shoe store. Place the shoe over the outline to see if the shoe fits.

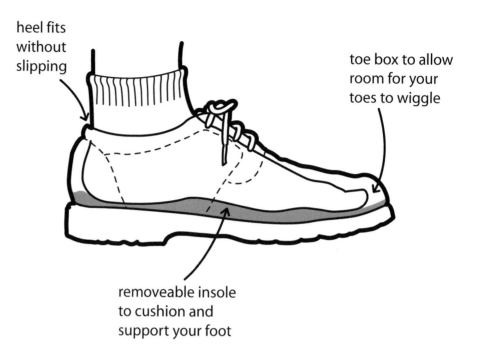

heel fits without slipping

toe box to allow room for your toes to wiggle

removeable insole to cushion and support your foot

- Shoes shouldn't be too tight. Allow room for your toes with a deep and wide toe box. Your longest toe should be a finger-width away from the end of the shoe. You will need the shoes to be wide enough to fit bunions or angular bones.

- Leather or canvas upper material is breathable and is a good choice.

- An insole helps cushion the bottom of your feet and absorb the jolts of walking.

- Choose shoes with removable insoles, as you can replace them when they wear out. You can also remove the insoles that came with your shoe, and insert a more cushioned insole or an orthotic. Remember to make sure there is still wiggle room for your toes.

- Avoid heels higher than 2 inches (5 cm). High heels increase the pressure on the ball of your foot and your toes.

- Avoid shoes with bare seams or bulges on the inside which may rub your feet.

- Shoes with laces, Velcro or buckles help hold your foot in place in the shoe.

Orthotics or specialty shoes

Orthotics

Made from foam or hard plastic, orthotics are devices that you insert into your shoes to support your feet. You can buy orthotics over-the-counter. There are also custom-made ones, which are more expensive but specially designed for your feet problems. Properly sized orthotics help manage pain in your feet, and support a fallen arch, bunion or curled toes. It can also help relieve skin irritation, an ulcer or callus.

Modified shoes

Sometimes a specialty shoe shop can modify your existing shoes to relieve a pressure point. This is usually less expensive than buying custom shoes. For example, they could cut open your shoe at a pressure point and attach Velcro straps.

Custom shoes

If you have a foot that is particularly difficult to fit, you may need a custom shoe ordered. A specialist will then make the shoe specifically for you. This shoe specialist may be called a pedorthist.

You may need to see a foot doctor (podiatrist or chiropodist) or go to a specialty shoe store if you need orthotics, shoe modifications, or custom shoes. Ask your doctor for a referral if your health plan covers this.

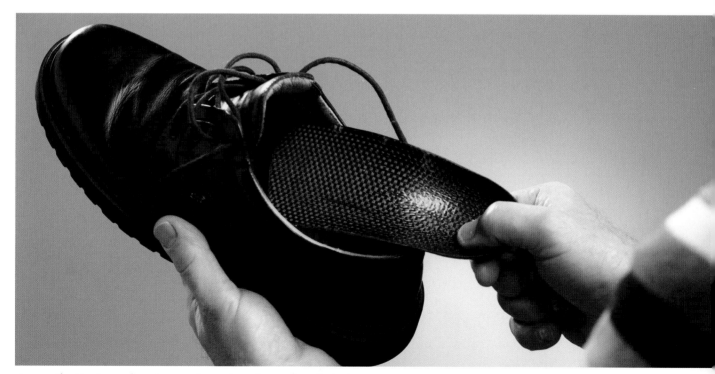

An orthotic is only as good as the shoe that it is in.

If your skin is particularly fragile, a bandage could rip your skin when removed. In this case, hold the dressing in place by wrapping it with gauze or attaching the bandage or tape to the gauze, but not your skin, or use paper tape which is less sticky (sold in drug stores).

Keep your cut or blister clean and dry.

9. Take care of small problems at home

Corns or Calluses

- Most important is to remove the source of the pressure that is causing the corn or callus in the first place. This may require you to change shoes, or alter or put an insole or orthotic in your shoe (see page 290–293).

- To soften a callus, apply a moisturizer first (but not between your toes). If needed, *gently* rub the callus with a moistened pumice stone. Do this once or twice a week.

- Talk to your doctor or diabetes nurse about corns or calluses that won't go away or are getting worse.

Cracks in the skin of your feet

- Wash your feet and gently dry them.

- Then put on a moisturizer every day, and twice a day if needed.

- If the cracks are deep – see your doctor or nurse. They may recommend an antiseptic and that you avoid walking on the injured foot.

Small cut or sore

- Wash with mild soap in warm water. Avoid rubbing alcohol, salt, vinegar, iodine or other ointments or antiseptics unless recommended by your doctor. These harsh antiseptics are drying and can slow the healing of a cut. Soap and water is the best treatment.

- Cover with a dry sterile dressing or bandage.

- Wash and cover twice daily. Each time, look to see if it's healing or if there are signs of infection (see page 282).

Moist, white or crinkly skin between or under your toes

- After washing, dry between toes gently with a towel or clean tissue.

Blister

- Don't burst the blister. Wash it with soap and water, pat it dry gently, and cover with a sterile dressing.

- If it bursts on its own, gently squeeze out the fluid, then wash, dry, and cover.

10. Medical care of an ulcer

Steps your doctor or foot care nurse may take to treat an ulcer (an open wound):

- **Take weight off the ulcer.** This may be as simple as wearing a different pair of shoes, or using insoles or orthotics in your shoes. If the ulcer or infection is on the bottom of your foot, your doctor may ask you to use a pair of crutches or temporarily use a wheelchair. With more serious ulcers, the doctor may have you rest in bed or put a cast on your foot to remove all pressure on the ulcer.

- Give you an **antibiotic**, *if* the ulcer is infected. Take the full dose prescribed, even if the sore looks healed.

- **Clean the ulcer** to examine what's underneath and to allow it to heal from the inside out.

- Apply **sterile dressings, medicated ointments, antiseptics or tissue healing products.**

- **Pain medication**, if needed.

- **Insulin or diabetes pills.** If your blood sugar is up, it is very difficult to get rid of an infection because the germs keep growing on the extra sugar. If you are taking insulin or diabetes pills, the doctor may increase your dosage. If you aren't on insulin you may temporarily need some.

- **Heart or blood pressure medications** may be changed to improve blood flow to the ulcer.

- You may need **surgery** to improve blood flow. Your doctor may refer you to a vascular surgeon or foot doctor.

Once healed, another infection or ulcer can be prevented by:

- Ongoing diabetes management to improve blood sugar.

- Daily foot checks and proper foot care.

- New shoes, insoles or orthotics, if the ulcer was due to your shoes being too tight or worn out.

- If necessary, surgery to correct the shape of your foot.

- Surgery on the blood vessels which go to your feet, to increase the blood flow and healing.

Some ulcers take time to heal

Any treatment will depend on your particular foot problem. Ulcers may take a long time to heal, sometimes six months, a year or more. Closely follow your doctor's advice to ensure complete treatment and healing.

Nutrition for healing:

Good nutrition and certain nutrients in particular help improve immunity and aid healing of infections. Include protein at every meal (see page 57), drink lots of water and eat foods rich in vitamin C, vitamin A and zinc, (see pages 132–133). If you have an infection, your doctor might also recommend you limit alcohol and take a vitamin and mineral supplement.

You can prevent or treat these concerns just like foot problems, with good blood sugar control, regular washing and skin care. Some skin problems are rare and hard to diagnose. If you have a skin problem that doesn't improve, talk to your doctor, or see a dermatologist (a doctor specialized in skin care). She may prescribe medications or treatment.

What kind of soap should I use?

Strongly perfumed soaps or deodorant soap can be drying to your skin. Some people find that soap with added oils (such as Dove) is less drying to your skin.

Corticosteriod creams:

In some cases, your doctor may recommend a corticosteroid cream or pill. Talk to your doctor about long-term use of these as they can increase your blood sugar.

Good Skin Care

1. **Keep your skin clean** with a daily shower or bath.

2. **Limit baths to ten minutes.** Don't use bath salts in your bath as they can make your skin dry. Check the bath water with your elbow to make sure it isn't too hot.

3. **Dry your skin well.** Prevent fungus and yeast infections by avoiding excess moisture on your skin. After bathing, dry your skin well, especially in moist areas where skin touches skin. For example, the groin, in the armpits, under breasts or at your waist, and your feet. Some people find it helpful to dust these areas with corn starch using a powder puff. For women, if the rash is under the breasts, wear a clean supportive bra to hold up your breasts. Warm temperatures or exercise causes skin-fold areas to get damp, so as needed, wipe and dry.

4. **Apply moisturizers to dry skin,** such as heels, elbows or hands.

5. **Use a humidifier in your home** in the winter if your house is dry.

6. **Your doctor may recommend skin ointments** depending on the cause of your specific condition such as fungus or bacteria.

7. **Drink lots of water.**

8. **Avoid excess sun exposure (tanning).** Some sun exposure (for example, 15–30 minutes a day while walking) helps your body make vitamin D and can be healthy for your skin. However, too much sun, or tanning at the hottest time of the day (10 am–2 pm) is unhealthy.

9. **Wear rubber gloves** when using harsh cleaning agents, solvents, bleach or hot water.

10. **Treat cuts right away.** As with foot infections, clean minor cuts right away. See your doctor if a skin problem isn't healing on its own.

Ten Tips for Mouth Care

1. The ABCs

Take steps to achieve a good **A**IC (good blood sugar), good **B**lood pressure and blood **C**holesterol. These things together help your blood vessels and nerves be healthier and reduce your risk for infection. When your sugar is high, bacterial and yeast infections in your mouth cannot heal.

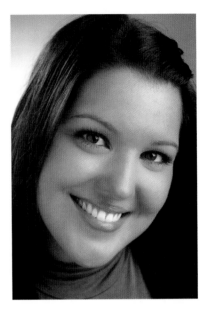

2. If you smoke, quit.

If you've struggled with smoking in the past, please give it another try. See pages 263–280 to learn more about quitting smoking. It can take several tries before you manage to stop smoking for good. Each time you quit, your chance of success goes up.

If you smoke, you are more at risk for cancer on your lips, sides of your tongue or floor of your mouth. Look in your mouth once a week to make sure there are no lumps, bumps, red spots or sores. Report any changes to your doctor.

3. Walk and do other exercise daily

This helps improve blood sugar and keeps the blood vessels and nerves in your mouth healthy.

4. Eat well

Eat less sugar and sweet foods, and drink less soft drinks and juice. Eating smaller portions helps reduce your blood sugar. Good nutrition helps infections heal.

Certain foods are especially important for your gums and teeth:

- Milk and milk products have calcium, vitamin D and phosphorus. These nutrients build strong teeth and a strong jaw bone to support your teeth. They reduce the acid in your mouth that comes from other foods.
- Vitamin C found in fruits and vegetables is important for healing gums.

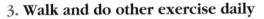

Fruits and vegetables have another important role. As you chew these foods, the roughness of the food fiber acts a little like a toothbrush to break up particles of food between your teeth. These foods also stimulate glands in your mouth to make more saliva. This helps to wash away bits of food, helping to clean your teeth.

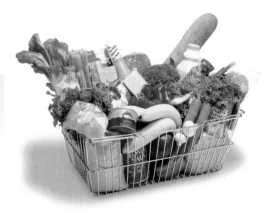

For more information about roles of vitamins and minerals in healing see pages 295 and 132–133.

Fluoride

Water with added fluoride is important for hardening tooth enamel and healthy teeth.

Sugar-free candies or sugar-free gum

For a product to be sugar-free and safe for your teeth, it should have no dextrose, sucrose, maltose, fructose or any word ending in "ose." These are all forms of sugar.

5. Drink water

After brushing and flossing, rinse your mouth well with water. Also, rinse your mouth or brush your teeth after eating these sticky, sweet or acidic foods:

- candies, toffees or fruit roll-ups
- any food that can get stuck in your back teeth (molars) like potato chips or stuck between your teeth like strands of meat or chicken
- fresh and dried fruits, fruit and vegetable juices, tomato sauces, ketchup and vinegar are acidic
- carbonated soft drinks (regular and diet) and sports drinks are highly acidic

At the end of a meal or snack, a small piece of cheese, a small glass of milk or a piece of sugarless gum made with xylitol can help reduce acid in your mouth. However, this is NOT a substitute for rinsing your mouth or brushing your teeth.

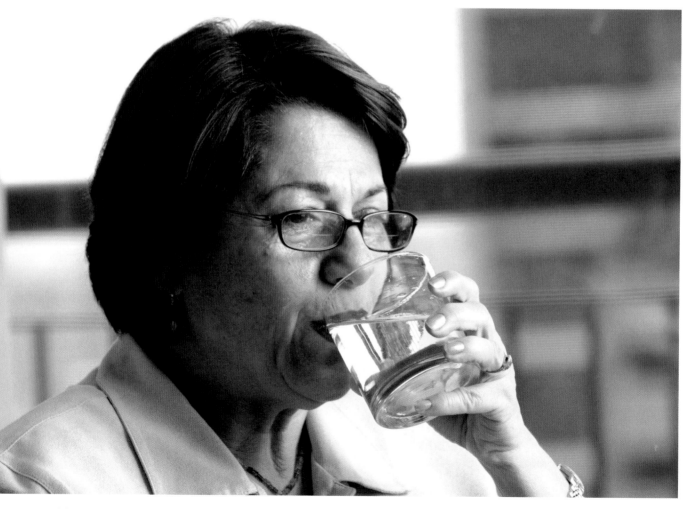

6. Brush

- Brush two to three times each day.
- Use a toothbrush marked "extra soft" or "soft."
- Buy a new toothbrush at least 3–4 times a year.
- Brush gently for about two minutes each time.
- Put your toothbrush bristles where your gums and teeth meet (gum line). Gently massage or vibrate and bring the bristles away from your gums. Brushing gently and properly is important – if you brush too hard, or up and down, this can actually damage your gums.
- Brush the inside, outside and chewing surfaces of your teeth. Make sure you brush all your teeth, including your back teeth. Don't forget to brush your tongue.
- The most important time to brush is before going to bed.

7. Floss

- Floss at least once a day.
- Floss cleans between the teeth where your toothbrush bristles don't reach, and helps remove plaque (see page 44).
- The best time to floss is at night before you brush.
- Use a piece of floss that is approximately 18 inches (45 cm) long.
- Wrap the floss around your middle fingers. Use a sawing motion, and gently press the floss between your teeth. Curve the floss around one tooth at a time and move the floss up and down making sure to get under the gums.
- If you find using floss is awkward, you may find it easier to use disposable floss-picks.

8. Care for your dentures.

- Rinse your mouth and dentures after every meal.
- If you wear a partial denture, remember to brush and floss your natural teeth!
- Always take your dentures out at night or sometime during the day for 4–6 hours. Now that you've taken out your dentures do the following:
  1) Brush them with a denture brush and liquid soap or dish detergent, then rinse with cool water. Toothpaste is too abrasive.
  2) Soak them in a commercial cleaner or in a solution of 1 teaspoon (5 mL) of vinegar and 1 cup (250 mL) of water. Rinse them well with water before you put them back in your mouth.
- If your dentures don't fit properly or cause sores, talk to your denturist or dentist.

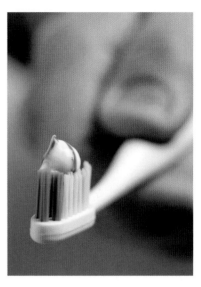

Use a soft toothbrush and a pea-size drop of toothpaste (with fluoride). After use, keep your toothbrush standing up and not touching another toothbrush. Don't share toothbrushes!

If your dentures have metal parts, ask your dentist or denturist what solution you should soak them in.

Is the cost of dental care a hardship for you? Find out if there is a dental hygiene training school nearby, or perhaps a public dental clinic where care may be more affordable.

9. **See your dental hygienist every 6 months,** even if you think your mouth is healthy. She will examine your mouth and clean your teeth. Sometimes x-rays may be recommended to look for problems that otherwise can't be seen. This helps the dentist know whether you have gum disease, tooth decay, or another mouth problem.

If you do not have gum disease:
Your dental hygienist will clean your teeth to remove plaque by scraping and polishing your teeth (see page 44 for description of plaque). If you have decayed teeth, fluoride may also be applied to your teeth.

If you have gum disease:
Your dental hygienist or dentist will help treat this infection by doing deep cleaning around your gums. For some people, this cleaning may be uncomfortable enough that an anaesthetic may be used to numb your gums. Your dentist may recommend that you have a professional cleaning more often than every six months.

Low blood sugar risk if you are on insulin

With your meter, check your blood sugar before your appointment. Tell your dentist or dental hygienist if you have had low blood sugar at the dentist office before. Then, they can watch for signs that you might be low, and help you treat it right away. You might also get low blood sugar if you take a Pancreas "Insulin Booster" pill (see page 318).

High blood sugar when at the dentist office

At the dentist's office you may be asked how well your blood sugar is controlled. In some cases they may ask for blood sugar reports from your doctor. Take your blood sugar at your dentist office, prior to having gum treatment or a tooth pulled. If your blood sugar is too high, your dentist or dental hygienist may rebook your appointment for a day when your blood sugar is better. Having dental treatments when your blood sugar is high may increase your risk of getting an infection.

**If you have
a gum infection**

Your doctor may temporarily increase your insulin (or start you on insulin) to reduce your blood sugar. He may need to change your diabetes pills. Make sure to take all the antibiotics prescribed for you when you have an infection.

10. **See your dentist or doctor for the following problems.**
    - Your gums are swollen and red, and bleed regularly.
    - Your gums or teeth hurt.
    - Your gums are pulling away from your teeth.
    - When you press your gums, puss comes out.
    - White patches on your gums or tongue – this could mean you have "thrush" which is a type of fungus infection.
    - You have loose teeth.
    - You develop sores on your gums from dentures.
    - You have bad breath, regardless of what you eat.

Avoiding Urinary Tract Infections (UTIs)

This section will explain the treatment of a UTI.

If you've already had a UTI, the prevention steps mentioned here can help reduce your risk of getting another one.

Treatment

Go to the doctor

An untreated infection can worsen blood sugar and become a serious health problem. Go see your doctor if you have symptoms of a UTI that won't go away. For women, this includes symptoms of a vaginal infection. Your doctor may determine your problem based on your symptoms. In some cases, he may order urine or blood tests. Women may have either a bacterial or yeast infection, so may also need a pelvic exam to determine this. Men may need a rectal exam so the doctor can feel the size of the prostate.

Take medication to treat the infection

For a UTI, your doctor will usually prescribe an antibiotic. (Unfortunately, needed antibiotics kill off "good bacteria" as well as "bad bacteria." Antibiotic use can actually lead to a vaginal yeast infection.) If you have a yeast infection, your doctor will suggest an over-the-counter or prescription medication. While taking the medicine, if you avoid having sex, this helps you heal and keeps your partner from getting the infection.

If your symptoms don't clear up after you finish the medication, go back to see your doctor. You may need a different medication, or additional tests.

Improve your blood sugar

Usually, the reason for the infection is that your blood sugar was high. Although medication treats the UTI, the benefit may only be temporary. If your blood sugar remains high, the infection can return once you finish the medication. To better control your blood sugar, you may need a change in your diabetes medication, or a temporary addition of insulin. You may also need to improve your diet and exercise. Eating healthy foods in the right amounts and being active are important. Doing this improves your blood sugar as well as your ability to fight infection.

Review the *Diabetes Complications* section on pages 46–48 to learn the symptoms of a UTI and why you might risk getting this infection.

Here's a quick review of how you could get a UTI:

- high blood sugar
- extra sugar spills into your urine
- germs feed on sugar in the urine
- infection develops
- blood sugars get even higher

Take your medicine according to your doctor or pharmacist's instructions.

If it's an over-the-counter drug, follow the package instructions. Continue taking the medicine for the amount of time recommended, even if the symptoms begin to go away.

Seven things for women to think about to prevent a UTI

1. **Maintain good blood sugar control.**

2. **Drink lots of water** – so that your urine color is pale (try six to eight 8-ounce/250 mL glasses a day).

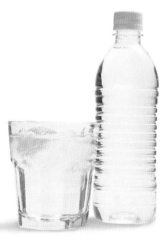

While drinking water is healthy – avoid excessive consumption.

3. **Pee regularly.** Don't wait until your bladder feels full. Try peeing at least every two hours during the day. Try to fully empty your bladder each time. This, combined with drinking water, helps flush germs out of your bladder. Also, pee after intercourse.

4. **Wipe front-to-back.** After you go to the toilet, wipe yourself front-to-back. This will help reduce the spread of bacteria from your back end. Wash your hands afterwards. If experiencing diarrhea or incontinence, take extra care to keep clean.

5. **Healthy sex means a healthy you.** Everything that touches your vagina should be clean so that you don't introduce germs. For example, this includes your hands, a diaphragm or a vibrator. If you have a partner, consider both showering before sex. If your partner is uncircumcised, ask him to wash under his foreskin where germs can hide. Be sure to pee after sexual activity – peeing will flush out your urethra. If you have vaginal dryness, this can cause itchiness and friction – consider using a sterile lubricant (see page 397), that you can buy at any pharmacy.

Using a diaphragm or a spermicide may increase your risk of a UTI. If you use these and are having recurrent UTIs, you may want to consider another birth control method (talk to your doctor; also see page 391).

Condoms protect you from germs that cause UTIs.

If your partner hasn't washed before having sex, consider using a condom. They also protect against sexually transmitted diseases and unwanted pregnancy and are a good idea for anyone who isn't in a long-term relationship.

6. **Keep dry, clean and perfume free.** Keep your genital area dry and clean. If you have heavy upper legs, make sure all skin folds are dry. You may find it helpful to dust areas that get moist. You can apply corn starch or talcum powder using a powder puff. Shower daily, then dry well. If you prefer to bathe, keep it short, avoid bubble baths, and ideally follow with a shower or rinse. Be gentle – extra washing, rubbing and the overuse of soap can lead to irritation and itchiness.

- If you are itchy, try not to scratch your genital area; it needs a chance to heal. Applying a cold clean cloth may help reduce itchiness.

- If you have heavy periods, gently wipe the area with a damp tissue or damp clean cloth or commercial un-perfumed wipes, then dry with a tissue. Change your sanitary pads or inserts regularly. If you use a menstrual cup – make sure the cup and your hands are clean prior to inserting the cup.

- If you have incontinence, change your pads regularly and keep the area as clean and dry as possible.

- Wear clothes that breathe! Don't wear nylons or tight pants for extended periods. These don't allow air to get to your genital area. Loose clothing is a better choice. Wear cotton, or cotton-lined underwear. It may be helpful to double rinse your underwear to remove all soap. Avoid using fabric softeners.

- Avoid vaginal deodorants, scented towelettes and "feminine douches" – these kill off the healthy bacteria in your vagina.

Anemia can contribute to vaginal itch

Ask your doctor to check your iron levels to make sure your body isn't low (this can be caused by heavy periods).

Have you recently changed soap, detergent or toilet paper brands?

Perfumes can sometimes cause itching, and worsen infections. Avoid wearing perfumes or using products such as toilet paper, soaps and lubricants that are perfumed. Change to another brand to see if there's improvement, and buy brands without perfume.

There is not enough research as to whether other cranberry products (such as whole cranberries or dried cranberries), or other foods such as yogurt or blueberries, help UTIs. At this time, none of these are recommended for preventing recurrent UTIs.

Interaction with medications

If you are taking an antibiotic, or a blood thinner such as warfarin, cranberry in large amounts may affect your medication. Talk to your doctor or other health professional.

7. **Cranberry juice or cranberry pills may help prevent recurrent UTIs.** A compound in the cranberry helps reduce the growth of bacteria in your bladder. *Cranberry is not effective in treating an existing UTI.*

> ## Caution
>
> **Regular cranberry juice cocktail** is sweetened and is not recommended as treatment. 1–2 cups (250–500 mL) daily of this sweetened juice can significantly increase your blood sugar and calorie intake.

Based on present research, estimates of how much cranberry juice or pills would be needed to have a benefit are listed below. If you get recurrent UTI's, you might want to try one of the following amounts daily for 1–6 months, to see if you can ward off another infection:

1. Drink ¼–⅓ cup (60–75 mL) of pure cranberry juice (with no sugar or water added). Buy this at most health food stores. It is an excellent choice – but it is sour! You can sweeten it with a low-calorie sweetener if you'd like. It has only 20 calories per ¼ cup (60 mL) so is a low-calorie choice.

2. Drink 1–2 cups (250–500 mL) of low-calorie cranberry juice (sweetened with sucralose). Cranberries will be the first ingredient, and there should be no added sugar. This has about 40 calories per cup (250 mL).

3. Take 400–800 mg cranberry pills twice a day. Choose ones made from powdered whole cranberries, not an extract. Cranberry pills have few calories so will not affect your blood sugar or weight.

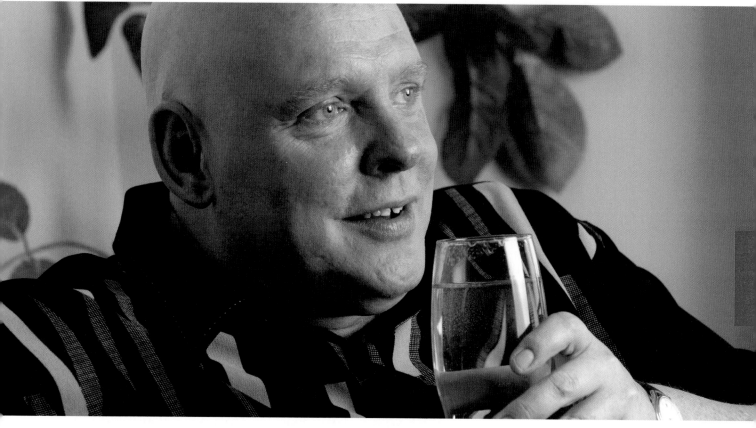

UTI prevention tips for men

1. **Maintain good blood sugar control.**

2. **Drink lots of water** – so that your urine color is pale (try six to eight 8-ounce/250 mL glasses a day).

3. **Pee regularly.** Don't wait until your bladder feels full. Try peeing at least every two hours during the day. Try to fully empty your bladder each time. This, combined with drinking water, helps flush germs out of your bladder.

   Pee after sex or masturbation to flush out bacteria from the urethra.

4. **Empty your bladder fully.** If you find it hard to fully empty your bladder, try sitting down when you pee, rather than standing. If you press gently on your bladder, (located in the middle, below your stomach) this may help. If these steps don't help, talk to your doctor about other options.

5. **Shower daily.** A daily shower or bath is important to keep your genitals and rectum clean. If diarrhea or incontinence is a problem, take extra care to keep clean.

6. **Consider cranberry juice or pills.** *Possible* benefits are listed on page 304.

Try unsweetened herbal teas as an alternative to water.

Preventing a Flu, Cold or Food Poisoning

Your immunity or resistance to infection is low when your blood sugar is high. This makes you more susceptible to flu, colds or food poisoning. Also, if you get sick, you risk becoming sicker than a person without diabetes. The flu, a cold or food poisoning, like all other infections, will make your blood sugar go up or be hard to manage.

Preventing a flu or cold

1. **Flu vaccine.** The flu shot is your number one weapon against the flu virus. All people with diabetes should get seasonal or other flu shots. Your second weapon is to boost your immune system through healthy habits. If you feel worn down, have high blood sugar, and don't look after yourself, you are more susceptible to getting a flu or cold.

2. **Wash your hands** frequently, especially if you have touched surfaces that other people have touched. Always wash your hands before eating.

If you do get sick, see pages 138–142 for information on managing.

Pneumonia vaccine

High blood sugar means your body has less ability to fight infection. If you get pneumonia, your lung infection can get worse. People with diabetes should therefore get the vaccine to prevent pneumonia (called pneumococcal vaccine). You are only given this vaccine once in your lifetime, usually after the age of 65.

To remove the germs from your hands, wash your hands for 15 seconds with soap and water. Give a good wash between your fingers, palms and tops, then rinse well.

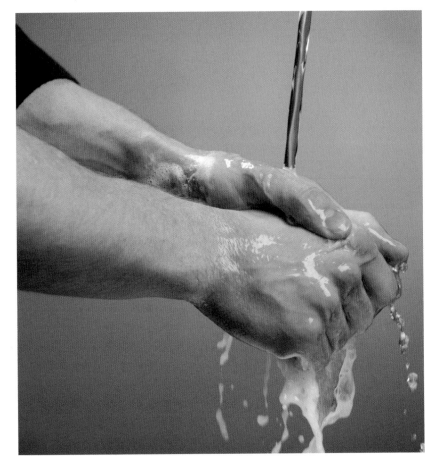

3. **Limit eating in restaurants and coffee shops.** Avoid places where lots of people handle your dishes and foods.

4. **Keep blood sugar in good control.** This helps your immunity.

5. **Exercising every day** also boosts your immunity. Exercise helps white blood cells – the special cells that fight infection – flow throughout your body.

6. **Drink lots of water,** about 6–8 cups (1.5–2 L). This helps flush germs out of your body. This also helps prevent dehydration, which can happen if your blood sugar is high. When you're dehydrated, tiny cracks can form inside your nose, and viruses have an easy way of getting in your body.

7. **Eating a healthy diet helps keep your immune system strong.** For example, choose foods rich in vitamin C and A and antioxidants (like oranges, sweet peppers and broccoli). Vitamin D may also have a role in a healthy immune system. Good dietary sources are milk, fish and margarine. Sunlight is our best source! In northern locations, we get less sunlight in the winter, when the flu or a cold tends to hit. Taking a vitamin D supplement, at least during the winter, (and especially if you have darker skin) is a good idea. See page 130.

For a list of food sources of vitamins and antioxidants see pages 120 and 132–133.

8. **Try to get a good night's sleep.** This reduces stress hormones and improves your immune system. Also see page 362–363.

9. **Limit or avoid alcohol and smoking.** These make you more susceptible to the flu. Also, when you are smoking or drinking, you will recover more slowly.

Food poisoning can be from something you ate earlier that day or even from the day before. It is the germs in food (and the toxins from the germs) that can upset your stomach and make you sick. Foods that are improperly prepared, cooked or stored can cause food poisoning. Food poisoning can occur anywhere. Contaminated restaurant food, food from your home, or the home of a family member or friend.

When you have diarrhea and vomiting, it's important to rest and drink lots of fluids. See pages 138–142. If you had a high fever, or your symptoms last more than 24 hours, it is important to see your doctor.

Your immune system may not be as strong as it used to be, so be extra careful handling your food.

Stomach upset can also be caused by a chemical on a fresh food or an ingredient in a processed food that you don't tolerate well.

Preventing food poisoning

Many times when you think you have a touch of flu or indigestion, you might actually have mild food poisoning. Severe food poisoning causes vomiting, diarrhea and fever.

Ten rules to prevent food poisoning

1. **Wash your hands with soap,** especially after touching raw foods or touching your mouth or nose, or after going to the toilet.

2. **Keep your kitchen clean and dry,** especially counter tops, dishes and utensils. Use clean dish cloths and allow them to dry between uses.

3. **Thaw frozen food properly;** in the fridge is safest.

4. **Do not cross-contaminate.** Don't let raw meat or raw eggs touch cooked food. Never place cooked food on an unwashed counter, plate or cutting board.

5. **Cook meat properly,** for example, no pink showing in hamburger meat or chicken.

6. **Keep hot foods very hot.** Germs grow when you leave foods at a warm temperature. Refrigerate or freeze hot food as quickly as possible.

7. **Keep cold food cold** at refrigerator temperature. Do not leave food sitting out on the counter.

8. **Use up leftovers quickly,** within 2 or 4 days, depending on the food.

9. **Do not eat raw eggs,** unpasteurized milk or unpasteurized cheese.

10. **Throw out bad foods.** That means – if it smells "off," doesn't look good, or you don't know how old it is or how long it has sat on the counter unrefrigerated. If in doubt—throw it out!

Gastroparesis or kidney disease

You may get sicker if you have gastroparesis (see page 51) and get food poisoning. This is because your stomach digestion is slowed by the diabetes, and the food and germs sit in your gut for longer. Kidney disease can also make you sicker as the kidneys can't clear toxins as easily.

5. Taking Medications and Tests

Appointments with health care providers **310**

 Appointments at diagnosis 310

 Appointments down the road 314

Pills and insulin **315**

 Diabetes managed without medications 315

 Medications can help you manage 315

 The right medications for you 316

 Common diabetes pills 316

 Insulin 323

Low blood sugar **331**

 Who can get low blood sugar? 331

 What causes low blood sugar? 332

 Symptoms of low blood sugar 333

 Four steps to treating low blood sugar 334

 Preventing low blood sugar 336

 Low blood sugar safety guidelines 338

Regular laboratory tests **339**

 Blood sugar tests and other tests 340

 Important diabetes tests (a record sheet) 343

Testing your own blood sugar **345**

 What is a meter and how to use it 345

 Do I need to test my blood sugar at home? 345

 Blood sugar goals 346

 How often should I test? 347

 Benefits of testing 348

 Challenges of testing 349

 Blood pressure testing 350

5

Appointments with Health Care Providers

When you are acutely ill or in the hospital, the doctors and nurses are the most important health care providers. When you feel well and live with diabetes, the most important health care provider is you. Others will help you, but only you can make lifestyle changes, take your medication and seek advice from your doctor and health workers. At diagnosis, you will need to see your doctor, and ideally a dietitian, diabetes nurse, pharmacist, and an optometrist. If you are not used to medical visits this will feel like a lot of appointments – but this is the time to learn about your diabetes. You may also want to do some reading on your own about diabetes. After you've had diabetes for a while, you may develop some early diabetes complications. Then you may need to see other health specialists so that you can stay as well as possible.

Appointments at diagnosis

Your doctor

Your doctor may want to see you regularly until your blood sugar is under control. Most people with type 2 diabetes continue seeing their usual doctor and don't see a diabetes specialist doctor. However, if your diabetes is difficult to manage, your doctor may suggest you see a diabetes specialist, sometimes called an endocrinologist.

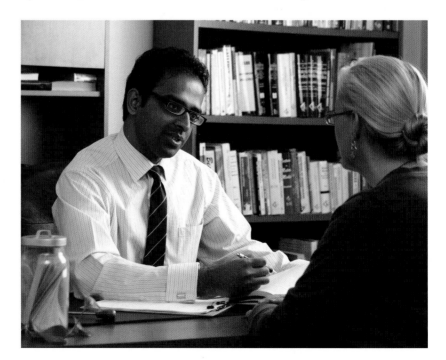

Question and Answer with Karen Graham: about your doctor visit

Kevin: When I go to see my doctor, he is so busy. He doesn't seem to have enough time for me. I really like my doctor but I feel so rushed. How do I get him to answer my questions?

Karen's Answer: Feeling rushed at your doctor's visit is true for many people. I suggest you make a short Doctor List (see below) or write down your questions. Give the list to your doctor at the start of your appointment. Keep a copy for yourself. Your list will help your doctor ask the right questions to help solve your medical condition. It will also help you stay on topic.

Doctor list:

1. Key problem why you want to see your doctor.
2. How long have you been having symptoms?
3. What do you feel is contributing to your symptoms?
4. What you have done to feel better?

Here is an example:

1. Key problem: I feel tired all the time. Sometimes I can't even get out of bed.
2. How long: About three months, worse in the last two weeks.
3. Possible contributors: Lots of family visiting and busy working. I haven't been eating right and I'm not walking regularly.
4. Steps taken: Trying to get back in my routine, but still feeling tired.

A good doctor will understand this information. He (or She) will recognize that your recent poor diet, lack of exercise and disrupted sleep routine may contribute to high blood sugar.

Your doctor may ask if you are testing your blood sugar. He may order some blood tests. Your doctor will want to know why you feel you can't get out of bed. He may suggest some changes to your diet and exercise that you could make as a first step.

Your doctor has an important role in your health. He can guide you to lifestyle changes. Your doctor can recommend tests and medications, assess, diagnose and treat illness, and refer you for additional care as needed. Take the time to write down what your doctor recommends and look after yourself in a healthy way.

Sometimes your diabetes questions may not all be answered. A nurse or dietitian at a community or hospital diabetes center may be able to help. They often offer group teaching, and individual appointments that are for 15–60 minutes. They will have additional time to listen to you and answer your questions. They can identify when you need to go back to see your doctor for further assessment, lab tests or care.

Dietitian and nurse

Ask your doctor to refer you to a diabetes education center or clinic. Here you will be able to see a dietitian and/or a nurse. They will teach you about diabetes and what you need to do to improve your blood sugars.

Desiree's Story

I knew diabetes was a serious diagnosis. I was scared, just over 30, and knew I had to learn all I could. I went to the diabetes clinic and attended classes offered by our health region. They taught me how to eat a healthy diet and what my blood sugar should be. I knew I had to lose weight. I got a puppy, and began walking him every day. Now I work out five days a week, and curl once a week in the winter. Two and a half years later, I'm 35 lbs (16 kg) lighter, and there is no sign of diabetes. My last average blood sugar test (A1C) was normal (5.8). I am so proud of myself. I also am trying to teach my son, who is 15, to eat properly, so he never has to deal with this disease. I hope all others will take it this seriously, listen to their doctor, nurse and dietitian, to get it under control. It's worth it.

Pharmacist

Your pharmacist can help you learn about diabetes medications or blood sugar testing.

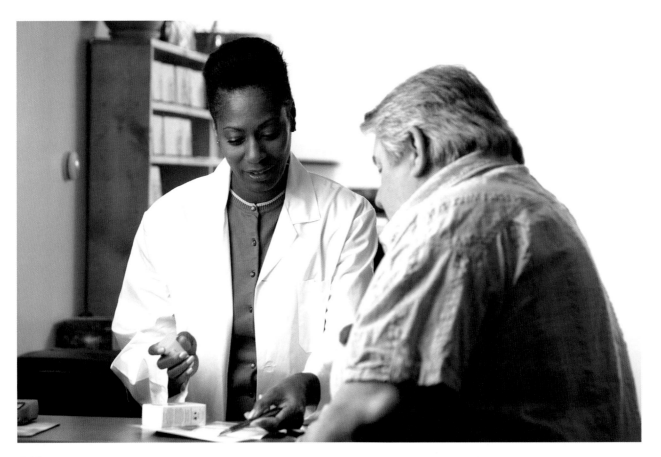

Optometrist

Make an appointment to see an optometrist for a diabetes eye check. This is called a dilated eye exam, see page 342. If your eyes are healthy, he will probably suggest you come back for another check-up in one or two years. If you get pregnant, you should also have your eyes checked during the first three months of pregnancy. Follow up with regular check-ups. Eye problems need to be found *early*.

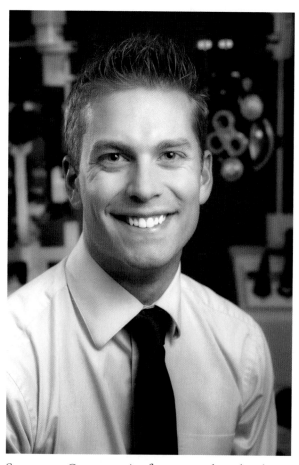

See your Optometrist for a regular check-up.

Optometrist or optician?

An optician can fit you for glasses, but is not qualified to do a diabetes eye check or to check your eyes for cataracts or glaucoma. See your optometrist or ophthalmologist for this.

Ophthalmologist?

An ophthalmologist is a medical doctor who has special training as an eye specialist. An ophthalmologist will do laser eye surgery or other types of eye surgeries. You might also see an ophthalmologist for your regular diabetes eye check.

Ruth's Story

About two months ago I had problems with my distance vision being blurry. I went to see my optometrist. He asked me if my blood sugar was running high, or going up and down. I said "yes" – I hadn't been eating properly. The optometrist did an exam and found a change in my prescription, but he said he didn't want to give me a new prescription. Not until my blood sugar stabilized. He said that while I might see better for a little while with today's new prescription, that if my blood sugar improved then days or weeks later I might just end up going back to my old lenses. He suggested that I go back and see my doctor for a checkup and a review of my medications, and then come back and see him again in one month if my vision hadn't improved. He also said that it was good that I had come in to see him as sometimes blurry vision can have more serious causes, such as macular edema, which may require treatment by an ophthalmologist. I learnt something new that day about how diabetes can affect my sight. I also had an incentive to go back to my doctor, *and* my dietitian. With changes and improvement in my blood sugar, sure enough the blurriness went away, and I didn't need to get new glasses.

Appointments down the road

Dentist or denturist

See a dentist within the first six months of your diagnosis (sooner if you have concerns), because diabetes can affect your gums and teeth. A dental hygienist should clean your teeth at each visit. Regular visits are a good idea.

Shoe specialist/podiatrist/diabetes foot doctor

- At some point, you may need to buy special shoes to protect your feet. Going to a store that specializes in diabetic foot wear is a good idea, especially if your feet are difficult to fit in standard shoes. A pedorthist is specialized in fitting you for custom shoes or shoe inserts.

- If your toenails are difficult for you to cut, you may need to hire a foot care nurse to trim your toenails. If your nurse notices significant problems, she may refer you to a podiatrist.

- A podiatrist is a doctor who provides foot care and does some surgery. For more serious foot problems, such as an infection that won't heal, you may need a specialist. This is a doctor who specializes in vascular surgery (surgery of your blood vessels) or more extensive diabetes foot surgery.

Other specialists

As needed, you may be referred to:

- An ophthalmologist, who is a medical doctor who can do cataract surgery or laser eye surgery for diabetes retinopathy.

- A mental health worker if you are feeling depressed or require emotional support.

- A sports medicine clinic or physiotherapist to help you develop an individualized exercise program, especially if you have challenges such as arthritis.

- An obstetrician if you are pregnant.

- A urologist, gynecologist or sex therapist if you have problems with your bladder or with sex.

- A neurologist or pain clinic, if you have pain related to diabetes nerve damage.

- A gastroenterologist for stomach or bowel problems.

- A dermatologist if you have diabetes skin problems.

- A cardiologist for further heart assessment.

- A nephrologist (a kidney doctor) as well as a renal dietitian (dietitian specializing in kidneys) if your kidneys are not working properly.

Pills and Insulin

Diabetes managed without medications

You may wish to avoid the side-effects and bother of taking medications. If you can manage your blood sugar through diet and exercise changes, this is a healthy option. It is usually easier to manage without medicine when you have had diabetes for a short period of time of perhaps less than five years.

When the doctor makes your diabetes diagnosis, your blood sugar may be high. If so, you may require pills or insulin right away. However in some cases, the doctor will decrease or stop the prescription once you are able to lose some weight and do more daily exercise.

Medications can help you manage

As the years go by, unfortunately your pancreas will make less insulin. Also your insulin can become less effective. Even though you may do all the "right things," such as eat well and exercise daily, you may still need diabetes pills or insulin at some point. If you need pills or insulin, take them. Keeping blood sugar in good control and preventing complications is what is most important.

I often hear comments such as "I am not taking any medication (or I am only on pills), so my diabetes is not as bad as so-and-so's because she or he is on insulin." The medications don't tell you how you're doing. Your blood sugar and A1C level tells you how "good" or "bad" your diabetes might be. A1C is a lab test that measures your average blood sugar over a three month period (see pages 340 and 343–344). If you are not on medications but your A1C is high, you are more at risk for complications than someone who takes insulin whose A1C is good. In years past, doctors prescribed insulin as "the last step" when a person's health was already bad. In those cases, blood sugar had been high for many years – it was too late to help. Today, doctors start prescribing pills and insulin earlier. The result is better blood sugar control and less diabetes complications.

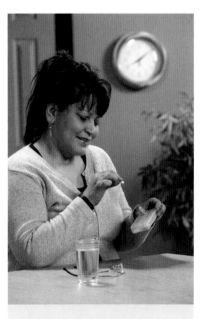

Take your pills as prescribed by your doctor.

Pills work best when you take them at the right times, regularly. Yet, it's so easy to forget whether or not you have taken your pills! You may find it helpful to use a pill container, or some pharmacies will organize your different pills into blister packs.

The right medications for you

Pills and insulin work in different ways. Your doctor may prescribe one or several pills, with or without insulin. He will decide on the right dosage for you, often starting at a lower amount, and gradually increasing it. Tell your doctor if you have any side effects. He may have to change your medication or dosage. There are many possible combinations of pills and/or insulin and it can take some time to find what works for you.

Common diabetes pills

We can group diabetes pills into the four main parts of the body that they help.

 Liver "Sugar Blockers" reduce the release of sugar from your liver.

 Pancreas "Insulin Boosters" help your pancreas make more insulin.

 Intestine "Sugar Blockers" slow the absorption of carbohydrate into your blood.

 Intestine "Insulin Boosters" stimulate your intestinal hormones that, in turn, help your pancreas make more insulin.

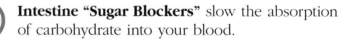 **Cell "Insulin Helpers"** help insulin move sugar out of your blood and into your cells.

Pages 317–322 lists some of the most common drug names in each group. It also lists how they work, and common (but not all) benefits and side-effects.

The doctor may prescribe you a pill that is not listed here. Please ask your pharmacist which group it fits into, and specific side effects for that pill. Some pills combine two types of pills together, for example, a Liver "Sugar Blocker" with a Pancreas "Insulin Booster." One pill can interact with another pill. For example, diabetes pills might interact with your heart medicine, so talk to your pharmacist about side effects that apply to you.

If you are trying to get pregnant (or are pregnant or breastfeeding), ask your doctor what medications are safe for you to take.

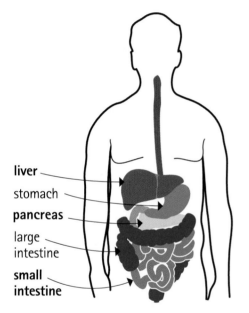

liver
stomach
pancreas
large
intestine
**small
intestine**

The common brand name of the drug (or insulin) is in capital letters. A "no-name" or cheaper version of the same drug is sometimes available. Ask your doctor or pharmacist about this.

Liver "Sugar Blockers"

Your doctor may call these "biguanides."

Reduce the release of sugar from your liver

This is often one of the first types of diabetes pills prescribed.

- metformin (Glucophage)
- metformin long-acting (Glumetza)

> ### How metformin works
> Your body stores extra sugar in your liver. When you have diabetes, sugar leaks out of your liver. This pill helps stop or reduce this leakage.

When to take it

Metformin works best if taken several times a day with meals. In some cases, with each meal and the bedtime snack. Improvement begins to show after 4–6 weeks. Take the long–acting version once daily with food in the evening.

Benefits

- It helps bring down a high fasting blood sugar (morning blood sugar before eating).
- If you are overweight, this is a good choice as it doesn't cause unwanted weight gain.
- It doesn't cause low blood sugar.
- It may help improve cholesterol level.

Most common side effects

- *Stomach upset and diarrhea, especially during the first month of use.*
- *If after a month or two, your stomach is still upset, tell your doctor. He may want to prescribe a different type of medication.*
- *Pregnancy risk: If you are a pre-menopausal woman, be aware that this pill could make you more fertile. If you need birth control, see page 391. If you are already pregnant, doctors don't recommend this pill.*

Not recommended if:

- *you have liver disease, advanced kidney disease or heart failure, or*
- *you are alcoholic or a binge drinker.*

Drugwatch.com is a website with information on drug side effects.

Pancreas "Insulin Boosters"

Your doctor may call these "insulin secretagogues."

Help your pancreas make more insulin

- glyburide or glibenclamide (Diabeta)
- gliclazide (Diamicron)
- glimepiride (Amaryl)

These kinds are sulfa free:

- repaglinide (GlucoNorm or Prandin)
- nateglinide (Starlix)

How they work
These stimulate your pancreas to make more insulin.

When to take it

- Take glyburide half an hour before breakfast and your evening meal.
- Gliclazide and glimepiride are "one a day" versions of this drug. You take them just before or with the first meal of the day.
- Take repaglinide and nateglinide with each meal.

Benefits

- If your blood sugar is high two hours after eating, these pills can help.

Most common side effects

- *Low blood sugar, especially with glyburide (and even more likely if you are elderly).*

- *Weight gain, especially with glyburide: To prevent this, be careful with what you are eating and keep active when you start on this pill. Also, have your dose decreased if you have a lot of low blood sugars, as these result in you needing to eat.*

- *Take with caution if you have liver or kidney disease.*

- *Less effective over time. After about 5–15 years, these pills can become less effective.*

Intestine "Sugar Blockers"

Your doctor may call these "alpha-glucosidase inhibitors."

Slow carbohydrate absorption from the intestines.

- acarbose (Glucobay, Prandase or Precose)
- colesevelam hydrochloride (WelChol or Lodalis)
- miglitol (Glycet) in the USA, but not yet available in Canada

---

How they work

Acarbose (or miglitol) slow absorption of carbohydrate from the stomach and intestines. These will reduce blood sugar spikes after a meal or a large snack. Then your pancreas won't be so overworked.

Colesevelam hydrochloride also slows the absorption of carbohydrate. Plus, it also removes cholesterol from the gut which can help lower the blood level of unhealthy LDL cholesterol.

When to take it

- Take acarbose (or miglitol) with your first bite of food at each meal that contains carbohydrate.
- Take WelChol once or twice a day with food.

Benefits

- Acarbose helps decrease blood sugar two hours after you have eaten.
- Do not cause weight gain or low blood sugar when taken on their own.
- WelChol also helps decrease LDL cholesterol.

Most common side effects

- ***Acarbose and miglitol*** *can cause stomach upset.*

- ***Colesevatam hydrochloride*** *can cause constipation or stomach upset. Doctors do not recommend this if you have an intestinal blockage, high triglycerides or a history of pancreatitis.*

- *Your doctor may not prescribe these if you have liver disease or intestinal disease.*

Intestine "Insulin Boosters"

Your doctor may call these "incretin therapies."

Help increase intestinal hormones that help lower blood sugar.

Pills:

- Sitagliptin (Januvia) and saxagliptin (Onglyza)
- Linagliptin (Tragenta/Tradjenta)

Injection:

- Liraglutide (Victoza) and exanatide (Byetta/Bydureon) are given by injection. Although given by injection, they are not insulin. Pramlintide (Symlin), another injectable drug with a similar action, is available in the U.S.

How they work

These help release intestinal hormones (called incretins) that help your pancreas make more insulin. This then lowers blood sugar after eating. The pills increase the release of your body's intestinal hormones. The drug that is injected has a similar action to the intestinal hormones.

Some of them also have other actions. For example, they may slow down the emptying of your stomach so sugar goes into your bloodstream more slowly, or they may help decrease your appetite. They also work a little like the Liver "Sugar Blockers." Unlike the Pancreas "Insulin Boosters," intestinal hormones are only secreted or produced in response to food. So these medications won't cause low blood sugar.

When to take it

- Take Januvia, Onglyza or Tragenta once a day with or without food.
- Victoza is a once daily injection. Byetta is a twice-daily injection taken before meals, and Symlin is injected with meals.

Benefits

- Helps decrease blood sugar two hours after you have eaten.
- Do not cause weight gain or low blood sugar *when taken on their own.*

Most common side effects

Januvia's side effects are usually minimal. The most commonly reported side effect is breathing problems.

Victoza and the other injectables may upset your stomach a bit.

Victoza is not recommended if you have chronic kidney disease. Talk to your doctor.

These medications work best in the early stages of diabetes, rather than for people who have had diabetes for many years.

Cell "Insulin Helpers"

Your doctor may call these "TZDs," "glitazones" or "insulin sensitizers."

How they work
These help sugar move out of your blood into your body cells. They do this by improving how your insulin works when it gets to your cells (especially your muscle and fat cells). These drugs improve insulin sensitivity.

Help insulin work better at the cell level
- pioglitazone (Actos)
- rosiglitazone (Avandia)

When to take it
Take pioglitazone once daily with or without food, usually in the morning. Take rosiglitazone once or twice a day, at breakfast and/or supper. It may take up to six weeks before you see a benefit to your blood sugar, and up to three months before you see the full benefit.

Benefits
- Reduces your blood sugar two hours after you eat a meal.
- Does not cause low blood sugar when taken on its own.

Caution
Avandia is now being prescribed less often due to concerns it may increase heart problems. Both the Canadian and American governments are taking steps to limit how it is prescribed.

Most common side effects

- *Fluid retention: If you are at risk for fluid on your heart or lungs, this is not a good choice of pills. Rosiglitazone, when used with insulin, increases this risk.*

- *Rosiglitazone compared to pioglitazone may have a greater risk for heart failure, stroke and heart attack. Heart failure is more likely if you are also taking insulin. Further study is being called for to assess the risks and benefits of these drugs.*

- *Weight gain.*

- *Muscle weakness, fatigue and headaches.*

- *For women, especially older women, it may increase your risk of breaking a bone.*

- *Pregnancy risk: If you are a pre-menopausal woman with irregular periods, this kind of pill could make you more fertile.*

Other common pills your doctor may prescribe for you

Pills to reduce your risk for blood clots

Doctors recommend low dose aspirin for adults with heart disease.

If aspirin gives you stomach problems, a doctor can prescribe another pill instead.

Cholesterol pills

If you are at risk for heart problems, your doctor may prescribe a cholesterol-lowering pill from a group of drugs called statins. Statins help lower the LDL (lousy) cholesterol. These have names that end in "statin" such as atorvastatin (Lipitor), rosuvastatin (Crestor), simvistatin (Zocor) and pravastatin (Pravachol). These drugs have great benefit for people who have had a heart attack. Although most people do okay when they take statins, if you experience any unusual bone or muscle pain after starting on this pill, report it to your doctor right away.

For information on LDL and HDL cholesterol and triglycerides, see pages 339–341.

TriCor is a fibrate – another type of cholesterol medication prescribed for some people with diabetes. These are not as effective as statins, but can lower triglycerides (blood fats) while boosting the HDL (healthy) cholesterol.

Blood pressure pills

For diabetes, the two types of blood pressure pills most recommended are "ACE inhibitors" and "ARBs." ACE inhibitors have names that end in "pril" such as captopril, enalapril, fosinopril, lisinopril, or framipril. ARBs have names that end in "sartan" such as candesartan, losartan, irbesartan or valsartan. These two groups lower blood pressure as well as protect your kidneys.

Pregnancy warning:

During pregnancy or breastfeeding, it is a good idea to stop taking statins, ACE inhibitors and ARBs. Your doctor can prescribe alternatives.

Sometimes, to manage your blood pressure your doctor may give you several types of blood pressure pills, including ones that are neither ACE nor ARBs. For example, the doctor might also prescribe water-losing pills (diuretics).

Weight loss pills

Orlistat (Xenical) is a kind of weight loss drug. It has some weight loss benefit but can cause significant diarrhea and urgency.

Talk to your doctor or pharmacist about any medication you are taking. Ask about side effects, how much to take and when to take it.

Insulin

An early start helps

High blood sugar over many years can permanently damage the insulin-making cells in your pancreas. Therefore, insulin has the greatest benefit when you start using it early – when blood sugar first starts to go up. Insulin can bring down blood sugar and protect these cells from damage. You may need insulin at the time of diagnosis if your blood sugar is very high, or after you've had diabetes for many years and you can't control your blood sugar with pills any longer.

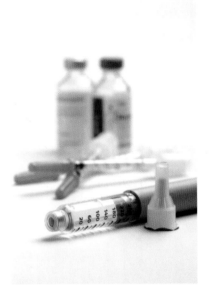

Becoming comfortable with insulin

Dealing with needles everyday is a difficult thought. Talk to your doctor or diabetes educator about how you feel. You can overcome difficult things when you learn more and have support. See the story on this below.

After starting on insulin, many say that it was not as bad as they thought it would be! They often feel so much better because their blood sugar improves. Some wish they had started sooner. They find the new microfine needles are really not so painful. This doesn't mean they want to be on insulin! No one wants something like this, but it does mean it is possible.

Bev's story about starting insulin and the benefit of seeking support:

When my doctor told me I had to take insulin, I was terrified. The nurse at the diabetes center taught me about using the needle. She showed me how to stick it in an orange. She was really supportive. At home, I just kept reading all the literature and kept going over everything that the nurse had said. I even went so far as to stab an orange a couple of times. And I thought, OK, I can do this, I can do this. That night at 10 o'clock I gave myself the very first real shot. And I was just sweating, so shaky, but I did it! But then, as I was pulling the needle out, I stabbed myself in my finger. My finger was bleeding and I was scared. I didn't know what to do, so I phoned the nurse at the toll-free health line. She was just wonderful. She calmed me down and told me everything was okay. She said I'd done a great job, and to wash my hands really well. That helped a lot. The next day I phoned the nurse back at the diabetes center. She was great, too! I told her about phoning the other nurse and feeling like an idiot. She didn't laugh about it or anything. I think if someone had started laughing I would have broken down again. She said, "Things like that happen. It was a sensible thing to do, to phone the health line nurse, because you would have worried all night about it." When I think back on it, I feel so silly. At the time though, I felt so worked up about it. I laugh about it today, but at the time, I was a "novice" so to speak. Today, I don't have the same fear of putting the needle in. It took me longer than some people to feel really comfortable with it but that was four years ago. Now I give myself two shots a day. I work really closely with my doctor, the diabetes nurse and dietitian to keep my A1C at a good level.

Your doctor will help

Your doctor will prescribe the type of insulin he feels is best for you. He will also tell you how much to take. He will start with a lower dose. He or your diabetes education team will review your blood sugar records. They will advise you to gradually increase the amount of insulin you take until your blood sugar improves.

Once your blood sugar is well controlled, he may tell you to take the same amount every day. In this case it is important to eat similar sized meals at regular times and to have a regular exercise routine.

If you have a lifestyle that is less predictable from day-to-day, your doctor might recommend a type of insulin that you can adjust. You'll be able to adjust your insulin from one meal to the next and from day to day. To learn how to adjust your insulin, you will need individualized teaching from your doctor or diabetes educator.

Side effects of taking insulin

Insulin does not have as many side effects as diabetes pills. It is a normal part of your body. The most significant unwanted effects that insulin causes are low blood sugar and weight gain.

Low blood sugar

If your blood sugar is usually close to the normal level, you are more at risk of it going low. Also, some older adults could have a serious low blood sugar. See pages 331–338 for information on low blood sugar.

Weight gain

You may gain more weight when starting insulin compared to diabetes pills. Here are tips to prevent or reduce unwanted weight gain:

- Reduce your blood sugar gradually during the first weeks or months after you start taking insulin. This can be done if insulin is increased gradually.

- Cut back on your food portions and salt.

- Keep active.

If your blood sugar does not improve, talk to your doctor about different options. That includes trying a different type of insulin or combining the insulin with a diabetes pill(s). You may also need to make some further lifestyle changes.

Why does insulin cause weight gain?

Insulin removes the extra sugar in your blood. Some of this sugar turns into body fat. Some weight gain may also be due to holding some extra water, as insulin tends to hold sodium in your body.

Using a syringe or insulin pen?

Talk to your doctor, pharmacist or diabetes educator as to what is the best option for you. Your choice depends on various factors such as how many shots you are willing to take, your budget (syringes can sometimes be cheaper) and how easy you find the insulin syringe to use compared to the insulin pen.

Learning to inject your insulin

Ask your pharmacist, doctor or nurse to show you how and where to inject with either your syringe or pen. Having someone show you is the best way to learn.

Storing your insulin

Keep the vial you are using at room temperature. This is okay for up to a month. Keep extra supplies in your refrigerator. If flying, always carry your insulin in your carry-on bag.

Different types of insulin

The names of insulins describe whether they work in your body for a long time or a short time: long, intermediate, short and rapid. Background insulin (basal) describes long and intermediate insulin. Mealtime insulin (bolus) is the term for short and rapid insulin.

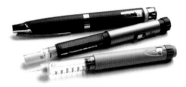

What is an insulin pen?
An insulin pen looks like a regular pen but it is a bit wider around. The pen has a small container of insulin inside at the top end and a needle at the other end.

Safely disposing of lancets and needles

Put them in a hard plastic food or bleach container, or buy a "sharps container" from a drugstore. When full, put on the lid and tape it shut. Ask at your drugstore where you can safely dispose of this full container.

The charts on the next four pages show how the main types of insulin work in your body. The information is approximate. Brand name drugs vary slightly in their actions. Also, absorption of the insulin can vary between people. Your reaction can depend on your dosage and where you inject it. Ask your pharmacist or nurse for a booklet or further information on the insulin you are prescribed.

---

1) Background insulin (long and intermediate)
These give you a fairly even amount of insulin over a 12–24 hour period. This helps to manage the sugar that is in your blood at all times. This includes the sugar that your liver releases into your blood at night.

2) Mealtime insulin (short and rapid)
These act quickly and then the effect wears off. They have a "peak" action, which is a period of strongest effect. These kinds of insulin mimic how blood sugar goes up after you eat. They give you a spurt of insulin over a ½–4 hour period. This helps to bring down the blood sugar rise after a meal.

BACKGROUND INSULIN: Long

detemir (Levemir)
glargine (Lantus)

Starts working in: 1½ hours

Very little peak: a slow steady release

Lasts for: up to 24 hours

When you take it: Usually once a day (at night), but occasionally a second shot can also be taken in the morning.

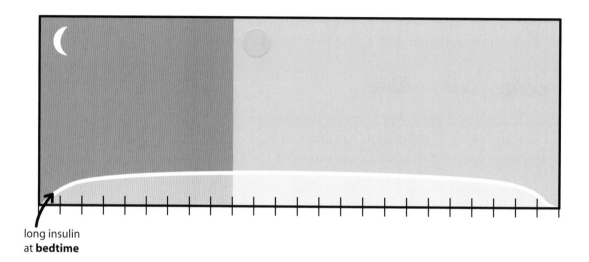

long insulin
at **bedtime**

This chart shows an evening injection of long insulin (over 24 hours).

If you are pregnant:

Long insulin is still being studied for safety during pregnancy. However, your doctor may recommend that you continue with, or switch to, long insulin so you can get the best blood sugar levels, as this is so important when you are pregnant.

Advantages:

• If your blood sugar isn't consistently high, a dose of this insulin in the evening may be all you need.

• Compared to intermediate insulin (see next page) it has a lower risk of causing low blood sugar in the middle of the night. It also causes less weight gain than intermediate.

Disadvantages include low blood sugar and weight gain, although less so than other insulins.

• Don't mix this in the same syringe or pen with another type of insulin. It needs to be taken as a separate shot.

• Typically it is more expensive than intermediate and is not covered by all drug plans.

326

BACKGROUND INSULIN: Intermediate

NPH (Humulin N or Novolin N)

Starts working in: 1–3 hours

Peaks in: 5–8 hours

Lasts for: up to 18 hours

When you take it: Usually two injections a day (morning and evening).

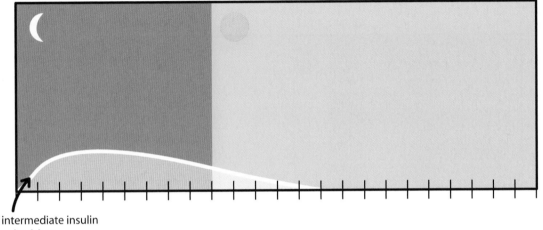

intermediate insulin
at **bedtime**

This chart shows an evening injection of intermediate insulin.

Advantages:

- It is less expensive than long insulin.
- Like long insulin, some people with just moderately high blood sugar may do well with just one or two shots of this insulin.

Disadvantages include low blood sugar and weight gain.

- An evening dose may cause low blood sugar in the middle of the night. Some people need to take a snack at night to prevent this low, yet they don't want to eat a snack because of the extra calories and weight gain.

- If you are only taking an evening shot, it doesn't cover your dinner meal. You may need extra insulin or diabetes pills.

MEALTIME INSULIN: *Short*

regular (Humulin R or Novolin ge Toronto/Novolin R)

Starts working in: ½ hour

Peaks in: 2–3 hours

Lasts for: 6–7 hours

When you take it: About half an hour before you eat. Sometimes you take it with just one or two meals (depending on your blood sugar). In other cases, people take this with every meal, as shown in the example below.

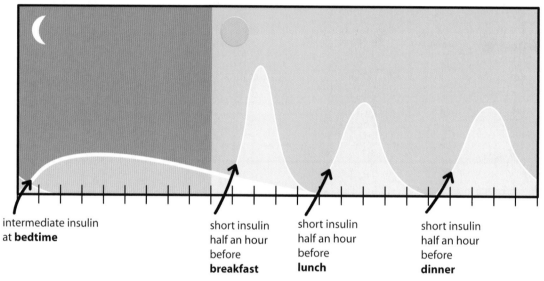

Intermediate and Short Insulins

intermediate insulin
at **bedtime**

short insulin
half an hour
before
breakfast

short insulin
half an hour
before
lunch

short insulin
half an hour
before
dinner

An example showing one shot of short insulin with each meal, taken with one shot of an intermediate at bedtime. The peaks of short insulin show how long the insulin is in your system. It is very similar to how blood sugar rises after meals and snacks.

Advantages:

This can be a good choice of insulin, if you:

- choose meals that have a lot of fiber, fat or protein and include low glycemic index foods, or

- digest foods slowly due to diabetes nerve damage to your stomach (gastroparesis), or

- like to have snacks between meals, as it lasts longer than rapid, so will cover for a meal and a snack.

Disadvantages include low blood sugar and weight gain.

MEALTIME INSULIN: *Rapid*

aspart (NovoRapid)
glulisine (Apidra)
lispro (Humalog)

Starts working in: 10–15 minutes

Peaks in: 1–2 hours

Lasts for: 3–5 hours

When you take it: Just before, or even after, a meal. You can take an extra shot to lower high blood sugar or to allow for extra eating. As with short insulin, sometimes you can take it with just one or two meals or with every meal, as shown below.

Please talk to a dietitian for advice about counting carbohydrates and see pages 85–93 and 150. Then you can learn to match the amount of rapid insulin with the carbohydrates that you eat at each meal.

Long and Rapid Insulins

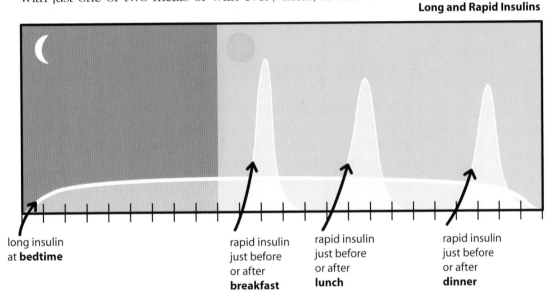

long insulin
at **bedtime**

rapid insulin
just before
or after
breakfast

rapid insulin
just before
or after
lunch

rapid insulin
just before
or after
dinner

An example that shows one shot of rapid insulin with each meal, taken with one shot of a long insulin at bedtime. These peaks of rapid insulin show how long the insulin is in your system. This is very similar to how blood sugar rises after meals.

Advantages:

- If your schedule changes from day to day, this insulin gives you flexibility. You can adjust the insulin amount you take to match the food you eat at each meal. You can adjust the time you take the insulin, so when you eat can vary. If you don't snack between meals, this insulin is a good choice.

- This insulin works well if you're ill and unsure of how much or when you will eat.

- You can get fewer lows and less weight gain with rapid insulin. This insulin is in and out of your body fairly quickly, and you can reduce the temptation to snack.

Disadvantages include low blood sugar and weight gain.

- This insulin gives you the flexibility to take more insulin when you want to eat more. If you do this frequently, you may eat too many calories and gain weight.

Premixed insulin

These contain a fixed amount of two types of insulin, either short and intermediate or rapid and intermediate. The bigger percentage is the intermediate insulin. Examples of brand names are NovoMix 30 (30% rapid and 70% intermediate), Humulin 30/70 (30% short and 70% intermediate) or HumalogMix 75/25 (75% intermediate and 25% rapid).

Premixed insulin works well if your diet and exercise are similar from day-to-day. You can take premixed insulin once a day (in the morning) and sometimes in the evening. You don't have to make daily adjustments to your insulin or draw out of two bottles. In a pen, it means one shot instead of two.

Insulin patterns

There are many different patterns for taking insulin and diabetes pills. Your doctor and diabetes education team will work this out for you. They will teach you how to adjust your own insulin if needed. Here are three examples of insulin patterns:

One injection

Background insulin (long or intermediate), at bed time: If you experience any low blood sugar in the middle of the night then long insulin is a good choice. This one bedtime shot often reduces fasting blood sugar. Your doctor will gradually increase the amount of insulin you take until your fasting blood sugar improves. Your blood sugar during the day will improve as you now start the day at a good level. Your exercise and healthy diet will have more of an impact. Any diabetes pills you are taking can also work better.

Two injections

Add in another shot of background insulin in the morning. Once your fasting blood sugar improves, then your doctor will need to look at your day time blood sugar. If this remains high, you may need more insulin added in during the day. This could be another injection of long or intermediate insulin.

Two to four injections

Add in some mealtime insulin (short or rapid) during the day, with some or all of your meals. A premixed insulin may be an option.

Your doctor may leave you on some or all of your diabetes pills when he starts you on insulin.

Sometimes it can take a month or two before you see your blood sugar coming down. Your body needs time to adjust and reset itself.

Insulin cannot work alone. It works best when you eat well and are active.

330

Low Blood Sugar

Low blood sugar is when your level is under 4.0 mmol/L (70 mg/dL). You feel dizzy and weak and you need to take sugar.

Who can get low blood sugar?

If you take insulin or certain diabetes pills you can get low blood sugar. The insulin or diabetes pills build up in your blood. This can cause your blood sugar to lower. If your blood sugar is usually close to normal, you are more likely to sometimes have low blood sugar.

Insulin: Long insulin (for example, detemir or glargine) is the least likely to cause a low. The other types of insulin all have a peak action time when the insulin is the strongest. This is the time when a low is most likely to happen.

Diabetes pills: The diabetes pills that can cause a low are mostly from the Pancreas "Insulin Boosters" group on page 318. Glyburide (Diabeta) is the diabetes pill that is most likely to cause low blood sugar. Gliclazide, glimepiride, repaglinide and nateglinide can also cause a low. If you take another kind of diabetes pill, you'll only have low blood sugar in unusual circumstances such as a lot of exercise.

False low blood sugar

I am not on insulin or diabetes pills but I feel like my blood sugar is getting low. Why is this?

You may have had a large swing in your blood sugar level. For example, if your blood sugar was high and then in a short period of time dropped down into the normal range, that shift can cause you to feel "low." This is not low blood sugar, but you may feel some of the same symptoms.

If you have a blood glucose meter you can check your blood sugar. This will tell you if you are low.

To help the symptoms go away, do not treat it with sugar if you are already in or above the normal range. Instead, sit down and rest for 5–10 minutes. Have a drink of water. Some people feel better after chewing sugar-free gum, or sucking on a small sugar-free candy.

Low blood sugar terms

The name for low blood sugar is hypoglycemia. You can also call it a low or a reaction.

It takes time to adjust to normal blood sugar

When your blood sugar has been high for awhile, it can take a month or two before you get used to normal blood sugar. Eventually, these low blood sugar feelings will go away.

What causes low blood sugar?

Illness

When you are ill, your blood sugar usually goes up, but sometimes it can go low. A low is more likely if you are vomiting and have diarrhea.

1) **Eating less carbohydrate than usual.**

2) **Doing more exercise than usual.**

3) **Taking too much medication.**

- You accidentally took too much insulin or an extra diabetes pill.

- Herbs or other drugs could contribute to a low.

- Your dose of insulin or diabetes pills is too strong for you. This could be because you have lost some weight or have kidney disease.

4) **Drinking alcohol without taking precautions.**

Examples of lows:

"My meeting went on longer than planned and my lunch was delayed an hour."
"It was such a nice evening that I walked longer than usual."
"I get more lows when I'm busy gardening, especially if I forget to cut back on my insulin."
"My wife and I had sex when we went to bed, and later at night I woke up with a low."
"I was visiting with friends and we had a few too many drinks."
"I was shopping at the mall and lost track of the time."
"I didn't remember if I had taken my insulin so I took another shot. I think I must have taken it twice."

Certain medications hide signs of low blood sugar. For example, a blood pressure pill called propranolol, a beta-blocker, does this. If you have hypoglycemic unawareness, ask your pharmacist if any of your other medications have an effect on blood sugar.

Hypoglycemia unawareness

This means you will not have any symptoms of low blood sugar until you are under 3 mmol/L (55 mg/dL), or not at all. If you don't know you are low, you don't know to treat it quickly, so this can be dangerous.

Cause of unawareness:

You may have a tolerance to low blood sugar if you have had frequent lows for numerous years. Also, if you have diabetes nerve damage, this can affect the release of certain hormones. These hormones often stimulate sweating, trembling and other symptoms of low blood sugar.

What can be done about it?

Regular blood sugar testing is very important. Your doctor may suggest that for a period of time you aim for a blood sugar that is a bit higher than the usual goal, to decrease your risk of having a low.

Symptoms of low blood sugar

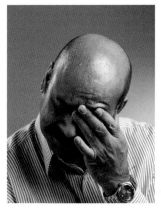

Sweating, dizzy, light headed,
or a headache.

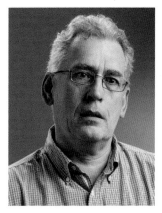

Looking pale or tingling around
lips that look a little blue.

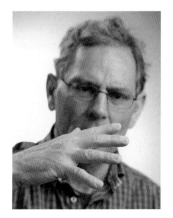

Hands or legs are shaky
(or unsteady on your feet).

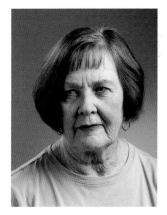

Suddenly confused or irritated
(you may be acting as if you are drunk).

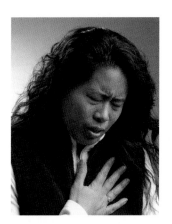

Weakness and heart
palpitations.

Other symptoms could
include extreme hunger,
tiredness, nausea, feeling
anxious, blurred vision
or difficulty speaking.

Four steps to treating low blood sugar

STEP 1. Test your blood sugar.

If you are under 4.0 mmol/L (70 mg/dL) go to Step 2. If your hands are shaking badly or your symptoms are severe, go straight to Step 2.

STEP 2. Eat or drink sugar.

Take 15 grams of sugar to raise your blood sugar quickly. See photographs of easy choices on the next page. Pure sugars that aren't mixed with fat or protein work best. For example, sugar works best on its own and not in a chocolate bar. Glucose tablets are the fastest.

If your blood sugar is under 3.0 mmol/L (55 mg/dL), take 20 grams of carbohydrate.

If you take acarbose (Prandase, Glucobay or Precose) or miglitol (Glycet), glucose tablets are the recommended treatment. These drugs can slow the absorption of other sugars. If you don't have glucose tablets, take honey or 1 cup (250 mL)skim milk.

STEP 3. Rest and wait fifteen minutes.

Try not to panic. Sit or lie down. Give the sugar time to work. If after fifteen minutes you still have symptoms of low blood sugar, then retest. If your blood sugar is still low, repeat STEP 2 and 3 until blood sugar improves. Call a friend or seek medical help if your blood sugar doesn't come up.

STEP 4. If you won't be eating a meal for an hour or more, have a snack.

This is so your blood sugar won't drop again. Your snack should include some protein or fat as well as carbohydrate. For example, eat a few crackers with cheese, peanut butter or ten almonds.

Do not try and treat low blood sugar with:

- *sugar-free soft drink*
- *sugar-free candy*
- *low-calorie sweetener*

These foods will not correct a low blood sugar.

15/15 rule

This means take 15 grams of sugar and wait 15 minutes.

If a person passes out call 911 or an ambulance

It is unusual for a person with type 2 diabetes to pass out with low blood sugar. However, you are more at risk if you:

- are elderly and in poor health
- drink excess alcohol
- have had significant change to your medication, or to your exercise or what you eat

---

*To treat low blood sugar, choose **one** of these 15 g carbohydrate choices:*

1. ¾ cup (175 mL) unsweetened juice or regular soft drink (this equals mini juice box or ½ can of 12-ounce/355 mL soft drink)

2. 20 gram fruit roll up

3. 3 sugar packages (1 teaspoon/5 mL each) stirred into a glass of water, or 5 sugar cubes (3 g each)

4. 6 Life Savers

5. 6 jelly beans

6. **3–5 glucose tablets (15 gram total); sold in pharmacies *BEST CHOICE***

7. 1 tablespoon (15 mL) honey

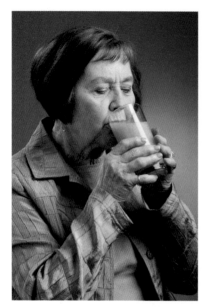

She is drinking too much juice to treat her low. This will cause her sugar to shoot up too high.

If you don't want to snack in the evening, ask your doctor for advice. Ask: "Can I change the kind or amount of insulin or pills I take? Can I adjust the time that I take them?"

Over-treating lows

When you have a low you may feel panicky and ravenously hungry. As a result, you may eat a lot more than the recommended tablespoon (15 mL) of sugar. Perhaps you drank a large glass of juice, then ate several pieces of toast with honey. The result is a roller coaster ride. You start out with the low but you end up with a high blood sugar. One suggestion that works for some people is not to treat with food, but to only use glucose tablets. They go in your system the fastest, so you feel better sooner.

Preventing low blood sugar

Each time your blood sugar goes low, your brain and organs are short of sugar. The lower your sugar, the more serious it is.

Eat meals and snacks at regular times

- Have a small snack if your meal will be delayed.
- If your meal is higher in fiber and has a lower glycemic index, you may need to delay taking rapid insulin.
- If you are taking rapid insulin, your meal time can be more flexible. Check your blood sugar before taking your rapid insulin. Take the right amount of insulin to match the type and amount of carbohydrates you'll eat.
- If you forget to eat snacks, you might be better off with rapid insulin as compared to short insulin.

Include snacks as needed to prevent a low at night

Many find it helpful to eat a snack at night that includes a slowly absorbed carbohydrate with a protein and/or fat. For example, one or two whole grain crackers with a small piece of cheese. The sugar then releases into your bloodstream gradually during the night. The snack portion size you choose will depend on blood sugar readings and your evening activity.

Adjust for alcohol

If you drink alcohol, have only one or two drinks. Eat extra food, or mix your drink with juice or a soft drink. You may need to decrease or omit your insulin or diabetes medication.

Adjust for exercise

- If you have taken your pills or insulin and then you do more exercise than expected, you may need to eat extra food. For example, eat an extra slice of bread or one piece of fruit or ¾ cup (175 mL) of yogurt for each half hour of moderate exercise. High intensity exercise requires more food. For planned exercise, you can reduce your insulin or pills, or adjust the time you take them. If you are trying to lose weight, this is a better choice.

- Don't exercise at the time that your insulin "peaks."

- Don't exercise soon after injecting into a muscle that you will be using to exercise. For example, if you will be walking, that might be your leg. An exercising muscle absorbs insulin quickly.

Adjust for sick days

- When you are ill your blood sugar usually goes up, but sometimes it can go low, especially if you are vomiting or have diarrhea. It is important to test your blood sugar at least every 4 hours when ill.

Adjust insulin or diabetes pills as needed

- Work with your doctor or diabetes educator to learn how to safely adjust your insulin. To reduce lows, they may suggest you adjust the times when you take medication.

- As you lose weight, you generally need less insulin or fewer diabetes pills.

Test your blood sugar

If low blood sugar is a problem for you, regular blood sugar testing is important. For example:

- *Test your blood sugar before and after exercise and during, if your exercise is intense. Blood sugar can drop up to 24 hours after an extended exercise session.*

- *Test before going to bed.*

- *Test when drinking alcohol.*

- *Test when you are ill.*

When to talk to your doctor or diabetes educator:

- If you regularly have more than two lows a day or 3–4 lows a week, especially lows that drop under 3 mmol (55 mg/dL).

- If your blood sugar low causes you to lose consciousness, even for just a short time.

Record your lows and other blood sugars and take this to your appointment.

337

Low blood sugar safety guidelines

Always have some kind of sugar with you

Consider putting it in your pocket or purse, in your car (tucked under the visor or in the glove compartment), and by your bed. Always have sugar with you when you are walking or doing other exercise.

Wear a diabetes identification bracelet or necklace

Carry a card in your wallet that says you have diabetes and lists your medications. Ask your diabetes educator to give you information about a diabetes bracelet. You can also ask your diabetes educator for a wallet card.

Tell others you could have a low and how to treat it

Talk to your family, friends, work associates or a walking partner.

Take precautions with drinking alcohol

Alcohol can cause seriously low blood sugar. This is a particular concern when you live alone. If you have been drinking heavily and took your insulin, someone needs to check you every 2–4 hours throughout the night to make sure your blood sugar doesn't drop dangerously low.

Driving safety

- Check your blood sugar before you drive to make sure it is not too low or too high. Do additional tests as recommended by your doctor or diabetes educator.

- If you have low blood sugar, pull over, stop the car and treat yourself immediately. Before driving, test to ensure your blood sugar is 5 mmol (90 mg/dL) or more. Eat a small protein/carbohydrate snack if a meal is more than an hour away. Check your blood sugar one hour later.

- Talk to your doctor about whether it is safe for you to drive if: 1) you have had a severe low where you lost consciousness even for a just a short time, or 2) you have hypoglycemia unawareness.

- Don't drink alcohol before or during driving. This also applies to marijuana and other street drugs, as well as prescription or over-the-counter medications that cause drowsiness.

You may appear drunk when you are low

If you wear a diabetes necklace or bracelet, people passing by are more likely to help you.

If you live alone

If you are elderly or in poor health, low blood sugar can cause you to feel disoriented. In addition to these precautions, you might want to consider wearing a "life line." (This is a device that you wear around your neck or keep by your bedside when you sleep. You can press it in an emergency to get help.) Talk to your doctor or diabetes educator about a possible change to your medication. There may be a better choice of medication that is less likely to cause you to go low.

Be safe!

Check your blood sugar.

Regular Laboratory Tests

Why are laboratory (lab) tests important?

You may not feel any difference when blood sugar, blood pressure or cholesterol is high – yet damage is happening. Blood tests and exams will tell you and your doctor how healthy you are. The tests also explain what medications you need and how your lifestyle changes help improve your wellbeing.

Which lab tests are important for you?

Pages 340–342 describe the lab tests that are important for you as a person with diabetes. The chart on pages 343–344 lists these tests and how often you should have these tests done. It also shows what healthy levels for each test are. The name for those healthy levels is the target. If you live in Canada, use the chart on page 343. Information for Americans is on page 344. If you'd like to photocopy the chart, go ahead. Put your name at the top and fill in any lab information that you have. When you see your doctor or diabetes educator, ask them to help you fill in the blanks from their records. This chart is a reminder to you of the important tests to have done on a regular basis. Your doctor is busy. It is often up to you to request lab work be done.

Tip: *Consider asking your doctor for a lab requisition for 3–6 months down the road. Then you can get your lab work done two weeks prior to your next doctor visit. When you see your doctor, he will have your lab information.*

Individual targets and frequency of tests

Your doctor may set slightly different targets for you than what is on the chart, especially if you are older. Also, you may need to take some tests more or less often.

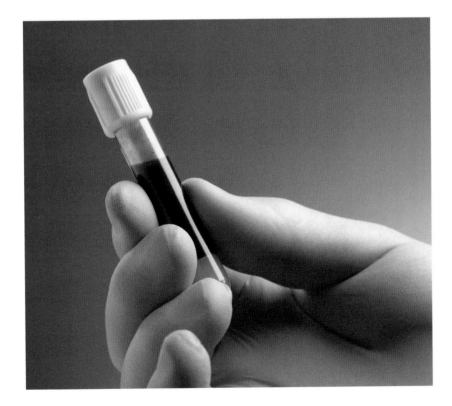

Blood sugar tests

A1C ("A-one-C")

This is a very important test for you as a person with diabetes. The higher your A1C, the higher your risk for complications. It is an average of all your blood sugar ups and downs over about a three month period of time. This test will give you the "big picture" of how you are doing and supplements your home blood sugar testing results. If your A1C is above normal, your doctor may want you to have it taken every three months. In between, try and make changes to improve it. When your A1C level is good, he may suggest taking it just once or twice a year.

At home A1C tests

At this time, results from these kits can't be guaranteed to be as accurate as one done at a lab. If you are seeing your doctor at least every 3–6 months, there is really no need for additional home testing. Your doctor can order the A1C for you.

Fasting blood sugar

This is a test done in the morning before eating; either at home or at the lab.

Random blood sugar

This test can happen at any time of the day. At home, write down the time.

Blood pressure

Good blood pressure helps protect your blood vessels, eyes and kidneys from diabetes complications. The doctor should check this at every appointment. You may also be able to get it checked at a local pharmacy, your diabetes education center or at a drop-in seniors' center. Testing at home is another option (see page 350).

Weight

Extra body weight makes extra work for your heart and body organs including your pancreas. When you weigh more, your pancreas needs to make more insulin. Keeping track of your weight is therefore an important tool to monitor your health. A small weight loss and even preventing weight gain are successes. In addition, a few times a year, you may want to measure your waist. Putting weight on around the waist is the most dangerous to your health.

Cholesterol panel

LDL cholesterol ("Lousy" cholesterol)

This cholesterol builds up and clogs your blood vessels.

HDL cholesterol ("Healthy" cholesterol)

This cholesterol helps clear unwanted deposits from the insides of your blood vessels. You want more of this one.

Triglycerides

This is a type of blood fat that clogs your blood vessels. It goes up when your blood sugar is high or you are drinking alcohol regularly. Excess sugar or alcohol in your blood turns into triglycerides.

Kidney tests

Albumin Creatinine Ratio (ACR)

The ACR is a urine test that measures the amount of albumin (a type of protein). Albumin usually stays in your blood, but when kidney damage begins, it leaks into your urine (see pages 33–37). Another name for this is microalbuminuria (meaning, micro or small – albumin – in your urine). The ACR is a really important test because it can pick up kidney problems early. It can also indicate if you are at risk for a heart attack. This will alert you and your doctor to take steps to protect your kidneys and heart, including improving blood sugar and blood pressure. You may need some new medication. Your doctor may also do further blood or urine tests to measure the health of your kidneys. For example, estimated Glomerular Filtration Rate (eGFR) measures the rate that fluid flows through your kidney filters.

Foot exam

It is very important to check your feet daily. See your doctor right away for urgent foot problems. In addition, there are certain things that your doctor (or diabetes nurse) can pick up when they check your feet. A monofilament or tuning fork can determine how much nerve sensation you have on the bottom of each foot (see page 286). If you have damaged nerves, you are more at risk for foot problems. (Read pages 29–32 and 282–295.) When the doctor measures your pulses, he is getting an idea of how much blood flow you have going to your lower leg, feet and toes.

Your ABC's:

A1C, Blood Pressure and Cholesterol tests are three important tests for you as a person with diabetes. Together they measure the health of your blood vessels.

If you have had a recent kidney or bladder infection, you may have extra protein in your urine. This returns to normal after the infection is gone.

To gently remind a busy doctor or nurse to check your feet, you might want to remove your shoes and socks before he or she comes into the examining room. You will be all ready for a quick 5-minute foot exam!

Dilated eye exam

For information on diabetes eye problems see page 38–41.

When an optometrist (or ophthalmologist) looks into the back of your eye, he actually can see inside your blood vessels. The only other way to see inside blood vessels is for a doctor to do surgery. Your eyes are like a window into the health of all blood vessels in your body. If your eye blood vessels seem damaged, there is also likely damage in your kidneys and other parts of your body. On a routine eye check, an optometrist is sometimes the first one to realize you may have diabetes. He would advise you to go right away to see a physician.

The reason for regular eye checks is to pick up eye problems early. This way, you have time to make changes to make it better. If you need any laser eye surgery, you can do this early to keep the problem from getting worse. Once your optometrist has seen you for your first diabetes visit, he will tell you how often you need to come back, usually once a year.

How does a dilated eye exam work?
It means the optometrist will put drops into your eyes to make your pupils go large. When they are large, he looks through your pupils and can completely see the back of your eye. After a dilated exam, your eyes can be blurry and sensitive to light for a few hours. Someone else should take you home. Wear a pair of sunglasses if you are outside or in bright lights, until your pupils go back to normal size.

Other tests

This section covers the most important diabetes-related tests. However, there are many other relevant tests that your doctor might order such as thyroid and complete blood count (CBC) tests, which measure the health of hormones and blood cells.

Important Diabetes Tests

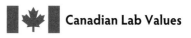 **Canadian Lab Values**

The Canadian Diabetes Association has updated their diabetes guidelines (Clinical Practice Guidelines) based on the latest evidence for treating diabetes. The chart below lists the tests used to assess diabetes and the usual targets. The targets that are right for you will depend on questions such as:

- How long have you had diabetes?
- Is your A1C high?
- Do you often have low blood sugars?
- Are you pregnant?
- Are you elderly and quite frail?
- Have you had a heart attack or other health problems?

For example, if your A1C is above the target of 7%, your doctor may recommend that you keep your random blood sugar level lower than the 5–10 mmol/L shown. However, if you are elderly and likely to get a low blood sugar, your doctor may instead recommend a higher target. Another example: if you have had heart problems, your doctor may recommend a lower target LDL cholesterol than shown.

Show this page to your doctor and ask, "What targets are right for me?"

Test & Target	Record result and date in the squares below.			
Usually tested at diagnosis and every 3 months				
BLOOD SUGAR TESTS, BLOOD PRESSURE AND WEIGHT				
A1C (average blood sugar over the past 3 months) Target: 7% or less				
Fasting Blood Sugar (in the morning before eating) Target: 4–7 mmol/L				
Random Blood Sugar (any time during the day) Target: 5–10 mmol/L if 2 hours after eating				
BLOOD PRESSURE　　　Target: 130/80				
WEIGHT　　　Your target: _____				
Usually tested at diagnosis and once a year, more often if abnormal.				
CHOLESTEROL TESTS				
EITHER LDL Cholesterol (8-hour fast) Target: 2 mmol/L or less				
OR apoB (no fast needed) Target: 0.8 g/L or less				
Non-HDL-C Target: 2.6 mmol/L or less				
KIDNEY TESTS				
Albumin Creatinine Ratio (ACR) urine test Target: less than 2 mg/mmol				
Estimated Glomerular Filtration Rate (eGFR) Target: more than 60 ml/minute				
FOOT EXAM				
Includes monofilament or vibration test, pulses and general foot exam. Do daily foot checks at home. Target: Sensation present and pulses felt				
DILATED EYE EXAM				
Eye drops will be given. Target: no retinopathy				

Source: *The Complete Diabetes Guide* (Robert Rose, 2013).

Important Diabetes Tests

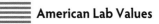 American Lab Values

The American Diabetes Association has updated their diabetes guidelines (Standards of Medical Care in Diabetes) based on the latest evidence for treating diabetes. The chart below lists the tests used to assess diabetes and the usual targets. The targets that are right for you will depend on questions such as:

- How long have you had diabetes?
- Is your A1C high?
- Do you often have low blood sugars?
- Are you pregnant?
- Are you elderly and quite frail?
- Have you had a heart attack or other health problems?

For example, if your A1C is above the target of 7%, your doctor may recommend that you keep your random blood sugar level lower than the 70–130 mg/dL shown. However, if you are elderly and likely to get a low blood sugar, your doctor may instead recommend a higher target. Another example: if you have had heart problems, your doctor may recommend a lower target LDL cholesterol than shown.

Show this page to your doctor and ask, "What targets are right for me?"

Test & Target	Record result and date in the squares below.			
Usually tested at diagnosis and every 3 months				
BLOOD SUGAR TESTS, BLOOD PRESSURE AND WEIGHT				
A1C (average blood sugar over the past 3 months) Target: less than 7%				
Fasting Blood Sugar (in the morning before eating) Target: 70–130 mg/dL				
Random Blood Sugar (any time during the day) Target: less than 180 mg/dL if 2 hours after eating				
BLOOD PRESSURE Target: less than 140/80				
WEIGHT Your target: _____				
Usually tested at diagnosis and once a year, more often if abnormal.				
CHOLESTEROL PANEL				
LDL Cholesterol (L for "Lousy") Target: less than 100 mg/dL				
HDL Cholesterol (H for "Healthy") Target: more than 40 mg/dL (men) more than 50 mg/dL (women)				
Triglycerides (blood fat; goes up when blood sugar is high) Target: less than 150 mg/dL				
KIDNEY TESTS				
Albumin Creatinine Ratio (ACR) urine test Target: 30 mcg/mg or less				
Estimated Glomerular Filtration Rate (eGFR) Target: more than 60 ml/minute				
FOOT EXAM				
Includes monofilament or vibration test, pulses and general foot exam. Do daily foot checks at home. Target: Sensation present and pulses felt				
DILATED EYE EXAM				
Eye drops will be given. Target: no retinopathy				

Source: *The Complete Diabetes Guide* (Robert Rose, 2013).

Testing Your Own Blood Sugar

You can test your own levels of blood sugar using a blood glucose meter (monitor) designed for home use. Along with A1C results, regular blood glucose monitoring can provide you and your doctor with valuable information. These results can show you what time of the day your blood sugar is high and low. You'll also learn what's working with your lifestyle choices and medications, and what's not working.

What is a meter and how to use it

Blood glucose meters are compact and easy to carry. While they are quite easy to use, some instruction is always helpful at first (see side bar). Every meter works a little differently but they have some common features. Basically, you prick the side of your finger with a lancing device, and then put a drop of blood on a test strip that is inserted in a small machine (glucose meter). This meter measures the amount of sugar in the drop of blood.

Do I need to test my blood sugar at home?

This is something that you should talk to your doctor about. If she wants you to test your blood sugar, ask her how often you should test. If you are on insulin or the pills that are Pancreas "Insulin Boosters" (that can cause you to have a low blood sugar), you will likely be told to test your blood sugar for safety reasons. Otherwise, testing may be optional for you.

Testing your blood is only a tool. On its own, it does not improve your blood sugar. It only tells you what your blood sugar is. To improve your numbers, you need to change medication, or adjust what you eat or your exercise. If you go to the expense and bother of testing your blood sugar, please do something with the results to make it worthwhile.

Learning to use your meter:

- *Ask the store or pharmacy where you buy it to show you how to use it.*

- *Seek assistance from a nurse working at a diabetes center.*

- *Read the instruction manual or call the manufacturer. Most companies have a toll-free phone number where you can get help from a customer support person.*

- *View step-by-step online instructions with visuals or videos. Find these on the company website or on youtube.com. Search the name of your meter.*

Your doctor may suggest blood sugar goals for you a bit higher or lower than these. See pages 343–344

Blood sugar goals

You've been testing your blood sugar and have written down the numbers. Use this guide to assess how you are doing.

Fasting blood sugar (FBG) or before meals:
under 7 mmol/L (130 mg/dL)

2 hours after eating:
under 10 mmol/L (180 mg/dL)

To avoid a low:
Always stay above 4 mmol/L (70mg/dL)

An occasional high due to a large meal is less of a concern than if your numbers are consistently above these goals. If the numbers are consistently high, is there something you can do to bring your levels down? Do you need to see your doctor about additional medication?

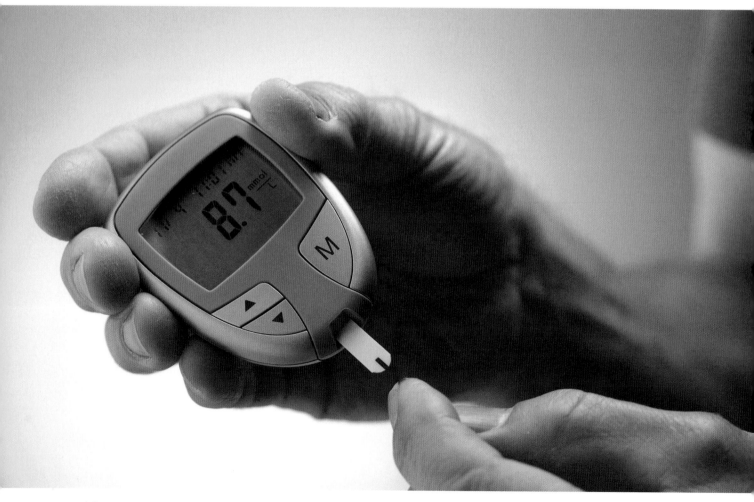

How often should I test?

Discuss this with your doctor or diabetes educator, as your testing plan is unique. Some people test a few times a week, while others test numerous times a day. More testing will give you a better picture. Here are some guidelines.

If you are not taking insulin or diabetes pills, these are possible testing times:

- Fasting – first thing in the morning before you have eaten.
- Two hours after eating a meal. Your blood sugar peaks at one hour and by two hours should be coming down.
- Before and after exercise – wait till you cool down.
- Any time you are not feeling well.

If you are on insulin or pills that are Pancreas "Insulin Boosters," here are some other times to test in addition to the above testing times.

- Before meals – this is critical if you are taking rapid insulin that you want to adjust.
- Before going to bed – to determine whether or not you need to take a snack or adjust your evening dose of insulin.
- Any time you think your blood sugar might be low or high.
- Before driving.
- After drinking alcohol.
- After prolonged exercise, check blood sugar to assess long-term effect over 12–24 hours.

Your doctor or diabetes educator may suggest you test more often when you:

- are ill
- are pregnant, or planning a pregnancy
- have started a new medication
- have an infection
- have been having a lot of low blood sugars.

Benefits of testing

You can't always know by "how you feel" whether or not your blood sugar is high or low. Testing gives you an answer. Then you know and you can do something about it.

Manage highs

If your blood sugar is high, you can go for a walk or get on an exercise bike for ten minutes. Another option is to cut out a snack or eat less at your next meal. If you measure your blood sugar before and 2 hours after eating, you can learn which types of meals tend to make your blood sugar stay high. If you take rapid insulin, you could take extra insulin to help bring down your high blood sugar.

Testing results tell you if you should increase your dose or change the timing or type of medication. For example, if you consistently have high blood sugar first thing in the morning (fasting), you may benefit from pills that are Liver "Sugar Blockers." These will help slow down the release of sugar from your liver in the early morning hours. If your blood sugar is good in the morning but consistently high after meals, you may benefit from another kind of pills or from insulin.

Manage lows

If you test and see your blood sugar is low, you can treat with sugar and prevent it from dropping lower. If you have hypoglycemic unawareness (see page 332), testing is essential. If you have had a low, testing can let you know when your blood sugar comes back up into a safe range.

It helps motivate you

Many people find that if they test their blood sugar regularly, it helps keeps them on track. For instance, if they find it is a bit high before supper, they'll cut back a bit on their portions. Also, because they discover that certain foods make their blood sugars too high, they will cut back on eating these to excess.

Helps you deal safely with changes such as:

- Eating or exercising more or less.
- Traveling, for example through time zones.
- Drinking alcohol.
- Illness, when blood sugar can go very high or low.

Write down your results

Although your meter may store a large number of results, it is often helpful to write them down. If you already record what you eat or your exercise, then put your blood sugar results in the same notebook. Now you can see trends and patterns. This helps you identify highs and lows, and problem areas needing correcting.

Challenges of testing

Expensive
The cost of doing one or several tests a day adds up.

Uncomfortable
Although the new lancet devices are quite small, testing can hurt if you have sensitive fingertips.

It takes learning and record keeping
You'll need to learn how to test your blood sugar, but you also have to learn what to do with the numbers. If you take your blood sugar at the same time every day and find similar results, then you are not learning anything new from the testing. If when you test, your sugar is high, but you don't change how you eat or exercise, then you need to ask yourself, "How is this helping me?" Testing and action need to go together.

It takes time
If you check your blood sugar three times a day that might take 15 minutes of your time (5 minutes each time). It might be more beneficial if you walked around for 5 minutes three times a day instead. That would total 15 extra minutes of exercise.

It can cause you to feel stressed
You might feel upset when you see high blood sugar numbers. If you don't do something positive about it, then worrying about it can actually make your blood sugar worse. You may be unsure what the numbers mean and this can cause anxiety. Stress hormones cause blood sugar to go up. In this way, testing could actually make your blood sugar worse. High blood sugar numbers make some people so upset that they turn to food and end up eating more!

You know yourself best as a person, and how you respond to stress and what motivates you. Ask yourself, "Will blood sugar testing help or hinder me?" If it hinders you, then rely instead on the A1C test, and just periodically test your blood sugar, and test to ensure safety.

Whether or not you are testing at home, it's important to have an overall picture of how you're doing. Have an A1C done every three months (or as recommended by your doctor) to check on your health.

Testing works best if it motivates you to make lifestyle changes.

Blood Pressure Testing

Advantages and disadvantages of blood pressure testing

These advantages and disadvantages are similar to blood glucose monitoring. Higher results can be worrisome and aren't valuable if you don't do something about it. If the blood pressure results motivate you to go for a walk, eat more fruits and vegetables, or cut back on your salt, then the testing helps you! If you keep a record of your results and take it in to your doctor this can help him know how to change your medication. Testing can also alert you if your blood pressure is dangerously high. If so, you need to seek immediate help.

What is a blood pressure machine and how do you use it?
Home blood pressure machines are compact and easy to use, although not as portable as the blood glucose meters. Make sure you have the right cuff size for your arm. Relax for five minutes in a quiet place. Avoid smoking or caffeinated drinks for 30 minutes beforehand. Now you are ready to take your blood pressure. Place the cuff on your bare upper arm, push a button and it will pump up by itself (it's run by batteries) and give you a reading. Get detailed instructions at a pharmacy, from a diabetes educator, a doctor, or online. Learn about how to test your blood pressure just as you might seek more information on glucose meters (see page 345).

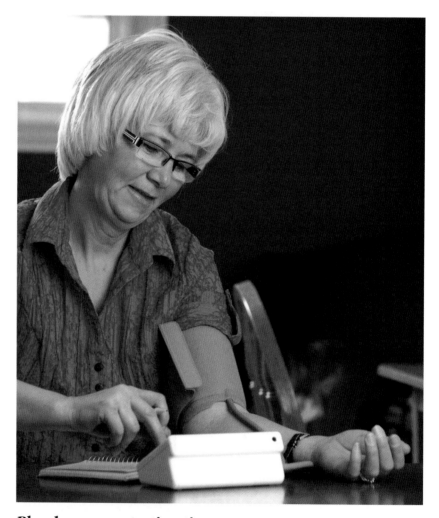

Blood pressure testing times
A good time to test is first thing in the morning before you have eaten and before going to bed.

6. Staying Upbeat

Coping with stress   **352**

    How much stress do you have?   352

    Stress and diabetes   353

    Tips to help manage stress   354

Coping with depression   **365**

    If you think you might be depressed, take this short test   365

    Depression and diabetes   366

    When to seek help?   366

6

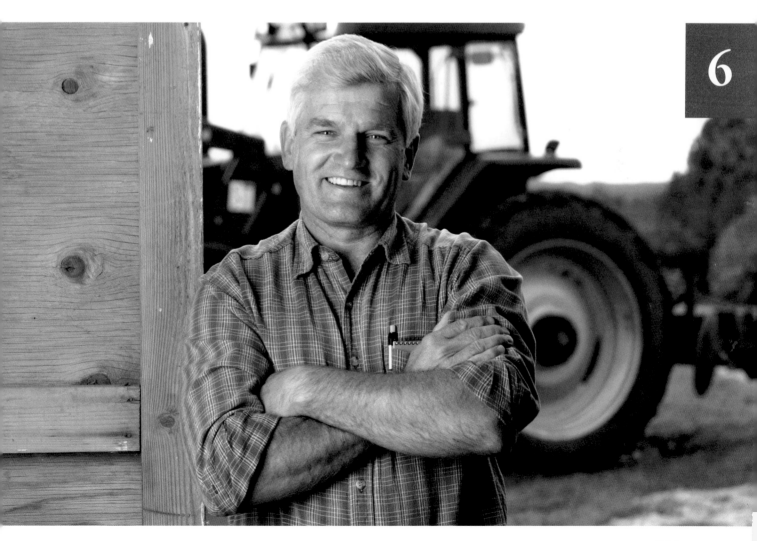

Coping with Stress

Stress is an inevitable and a normal part of everyone's life. We stress ourselves because of our own expectations, or others around us can also stress us. Stress is part of human relationships and the reality of paying bills, work, and looking after yourself and others. Even people with the picture perfect life have stress.

Stress helps you set expectations and goals for yourself.

A certain amount of stress is a good thing. It helps you get up in the morning. It motivates you and moves you to get things done. It helps you live up to your potential. Stress makes the world go round, and makes life challenging and always interesting.

Keep your mind healthy to keep your body healthy, too!

Stress is a bad thing when it overwhelms you, and you don't know how to handle it. Then it can have a serious impact on your diabetes, blood pressure and health. Please don't ignore stress. If you have too much stress, take steps to lower it.

How much stress do you have?

What number (out of ten) would you rate your level of stress now?
This is a question that I ask many of my clients at the diabetes clinic. I ask them to rate their own level of stress on a scale of one to ten. One would be very low stress and ten would be very high stress. Think about it for awhile for yourself. At different times of your life your level of stress changes.

Very low (0–1)
I have never met someone who told me they had no stress at all (zero out of ten), or even a stress level of 1/10. Can you think of anyone with a level of stress that is zero or one? I suspect that this might be next to impossible. Perhaps such a person would be so unmotivated and unbothered by life (or overmedicated) that they aren't contributing or caring about what is going on around them.

Low (2–4)
A small percentage of my clients have told me they have a level of stress of two, three or four. That would likely mean that in spite of their diabetes, they have a lot of support around them. It may also mean that they have a medium level of stress but they know how to manage it in a healthy way. With careful management and support, they reduce their stress to low levels.

Medium (5–7)

Typically on diagnosis of diabetes, clients tell me their stress level is five to seven. When diagnosed, you may have felt this way as well. It usually isn't just the diabetes causing stress. It's also the stage of life that is most common at the time of diagnosis. Lots of things can cause stress, no matter where you are in life. You may be a middle-aged bachelor or a mother of teenagers. You could be working at the peak of your career or be a grandparent. You may be dealing with an excessive work load or financial debt. Do you have multiple health conditions or suffer from chronic pain? Have you recently gone through a divorce, a loss of job or loss of a loved one? You may have family members or friends who weigh you down with their demands or complaints. Are you caring for an elderly parent or getting older yourself and frustrated with the unfair changes of aging? Although you can't make it go away, there are steps you can take to manage your stress.

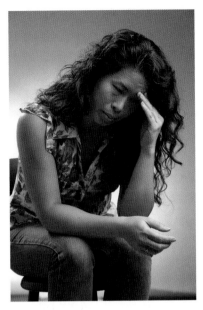

Feeling stressed

High (8–10)

Constantly high stress levels, because of your own life circumstances, can push you up to an 8, 9 or 10. Grieving the loss of a husband or wife, or dealing with the loss of a long-time job, creates change that can overwhelm you. Perhaps personality conflicts in your workplace or at home have escalated. Verbal, physical, or sexual abuse also creates high level stress. Your diabetes diagnosis or dealing with diabetes complications can then shoot your stress up to a 9 or 10. This stress then worsens your blood sugar. If you score yourself as having a ten, the highest stress level, you probably know the source of your stress. Your stress level can improve as you learn to cope with the diabetes or as crises resolve. Bringing your stress down from this dangerous level is critical. Please read the rest of this section for tips on managing stress

We can't always control the causes of stress, **so we need to change how we respond to stress.** *Pages 354–364 suggest steps to manage stress, and lessen your risk for diabetes complications. Not all these suggestions will work for you, but please read through them to find a stress buster that will work.*

Stress and diabetes

Changes in your body with medium-high stress

Your body makes stress hormones when stress levels are constantly high or escalate to a medium to high level. These hormones circulate in your blood and affect your body in different ways. For example, stress hormones increase your blood sugar and blood pressure, reduce immunity, increase inflammation inside your blood vessels, and cause over-stimulation of your nerves. You may feel unwell, have an upset stomach, be sleeping poorly, and be agitated and unhappy. Over time, high stress levels increase your risk for diabetes complications including a heart attack or stroke.

When stress becomes unmanageable

It is wise to seek help before stress leads to a serious health problem. If you don't handle stress in a healthy way, it can cause problems. Stress leads some people to addictions, including abusing food, alcohol, and drugs. Addictions may feel good in the short-term, but over the long-term, they can devastate you and your family. If you think you may need help, please ask for it.

Seek professional help if needed:

Talk to your doctor or diabetes team. You may need a referral to an addictions counselor, mental health worker, social worker, psychologist or psychiatrist (medical doctor specializing in mental health). You may require medication for awhile to help you cope or to help you sleep better. If you are experiencing abuse you may need shelter in a safe home.

Tips to help manage stress

Slow down a bit

Are you feeling down, sad, angry, on the edge?

I know how you feel. I experience that sometimes when things get a bit overwhelming and desperate. I get out of it by slowing down a bit. I try and get back to basics. I try and remind myself that I can only do what I can do, and no more. This may help you too.

Stress can motivate you, but it can also cause burn out. Think about how slowing down a bit would help. Once you've identified the main source of your stress, see if you can change it. For example, if it is your job, is there any option for change? Are you a perfectionist? Remind yourself that you may be the only one who feels something needs to be perfect. Staying in a bad situation that causes you to get sick is not worth the risk.

Take one day at time, one step at a time. Set small, reachable goals.

Ask your doctor, health worker or friend, "What do I need to do right away?" Make a plan for other changes that can happen a little later, when you are ready.

Think in healthy ways

Some ways of thinking are like diseases.

Do you have a lot of negative thoughts?

Negative thoughts build up, one on top of another, and are like poison. If you say, "I will never be able to control my diabetes" you feel discouraged – so you may eat more and do less. Try to replace this with a positive thought. For example, "I can start making one small change every few days to make my blood sugar better." Now you have changed your outlook. You work towards a positive mood and give yourself motivation to move forward. Focus on the positive changes you have made and good things in your life. This is what is most important.

Do you sometimes "over-think" things?

Was the situation really as serious as you thought it was? Could you solve that problem? Did your friend really think that bad thing about you that you imagine they did? We are not all good communicators. Sometimes our relationship problems stem from misunderstandings. We think we know how another person thinks and feels, or feels about us, but do we really? Words are often misunderstood, or silences taken in the wrong way. Sometimes our emotions bring us stress when that was not the intention of the other person. Don't save correspondence or reminders if it causes you stress or pain. Sometimes as hard as it is, the best way is to let the past alone. Old grudges and arguments are very difficult to give up, but if they are increasing your stress, ask yourself if you can relax them a bit so they don't burden you.

Thinking too much can complicate matters. The world is simpler than we sometimes imagine. Sometimes you get less overwhelmed if you don't over-think. Instead, step back once in a while and breathe. Things will get better.

Talk it out

Sometimes we're angry. Sometimes we laugh, and it's wonderful to laugh. Sometimes what we need most is to be alone, and be silent. Mostly we talk to express our emotions, because this is what helps us most. It's good to share our troubles and our pain. If we don't talk, all these troubles stay inside us. They build up and we start getting sick.

Thoughts are powerful

When you replace negative thoughts with positive thoughts, you start seeing good results. Tell yourself something positive – and give others compliments.

Journaling

Writing down how you are feeling can be beneficial (see pages 62–63) especially when you are trying to find out how your emotions affect your habits. It can also be a good way to vent your emotions (to yourself). However, this doesn't mean you need to keep these words. Sometimes it's best to erase or delete this because when we are upset we don't always see things clearly.

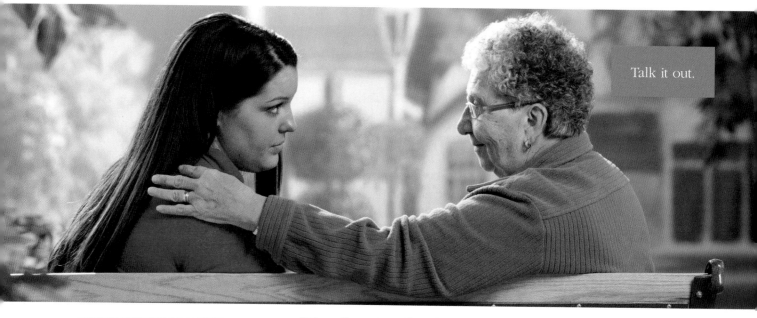

Talk it out.

It's okay to let it out sometimes

Don't pretend you're happy when you are not. Sometimes we cry, and crying is good too. We would not have tear ducts if we weren't meant to cry. It is an essential part of being human. It's a way to relieve tension that builds up inside us. It is a way to get out our feelings. The problem is when we can't stop crying, we may need to seek help.

For some of us, even screaming is good now and again! Not a scream at someone else or at ourselves, but just to get it out. Use a private place where no one else will hear and think we are strange. Perhaps this is one reason that roller coaster rides are popular. On a roller coaster, you can let out a great scream of terror and next thing you know it's a scream of joy. It's over and you feel like a kid again. It works to let out your emotions this way.

Keep learning

You may be blue because of a misunderstanding with someone. Being bored, idle or feeling drained also causes the blues. Try learning something new that involves you completely. Make good use of books, magazines, the radio or computers. Learn about diabetes and managing stress, so you don't feel helpless. Enjoy games, crafts, crossword puzzles, playing cards, gardening or travel to stay stimulated.

Do you find that sometimes you learn more from other people than on your own? Consider group learning or classes. Could you help and teach others, be a role model, work or be a volunteer? If you work with those in high need, this can help you put your own concerns in perspective. You will also know that others need you.

Finding someone to talk to in confidence can be difficult. You may be lucky and have a friend or family member with whom you can talk. It's a good idea to talk to a spiritual leader, a counselor, your doctor or a diabetes worker. Talking and having someone hear you are parts of your mental health.

Sadness is an integral part of life. It is fair to say that the good times are better when we've also gone through hard times.

Keep yourself busy. There is nothing worse than sitting around and worrying about your problems.

Have fun

Smiling makes you feel positive. Sometimes it's hard to smile, but it does work!

Keep in touch with things that make you happy – friends and family, pets, keepsakes, music, plants, sports, hobbies or television. Simple and familiar things and routines help us feel good. Get out of the house now and again for a social outing. Enjoy a cup of tea (or if it fits for you, an occasional beer or glass of wine) with friends or family. Laugh and have fun. Start planning a vacation now!

Laughter – a wonderful medicine

What could be funny about following a meal plan, exercising and taking pills or insulin? Well, nothing really! That's exactly why we need some humor and laughter to balance our lives.

Sometimes we need to think about our problems with more relaxed emotions. This can help us realize that some problems are not the big events they seem to be at the time. Laughter helps us accept our limitations, and still get on with taking care of ourselves the best we can.

Keep good things close to you. Focus on short moments of happiness. Tuck these moments away, folded like a napkin, and take it out when you need a good thought. Write down happy things. Bring out the photographs. Happy memories are the ones to keep.

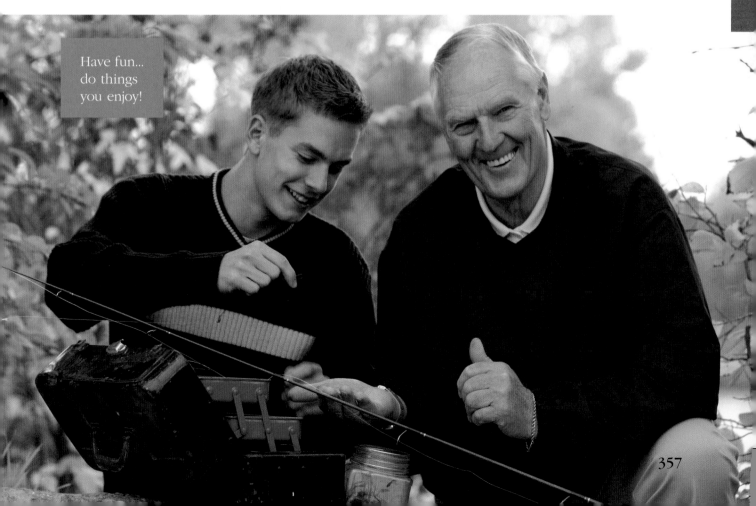

Have fun... do things you enjoy!

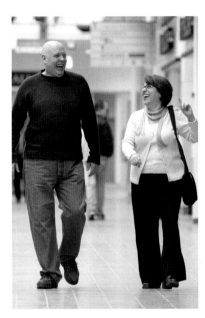

A good hearty laugh can also:

- lower blood pressure and protect your heart,

- improve your brain functioning,

- help you relax and feel good,

- help take away anger,

- and connect you to others.

Isn't it true?

For the most part, small everyday moments make up our lives – not great occasions or successes. Enjoy those moments.

Why laughter is good for our health

Laughter may help us live longer – longer and happier. Amazingly, laughter helps improve our resistance to disease and infection, and it encourages healing. When we laugh, we breathe deeper. Then the oxygen-enriched blood and "happy hormones" (endorphins) flow through our body.

When you think about all the bad things that could happen with diabetes – your stress can go up and so can your blood sugar and blood pressure. Humor and laughter can help you cope. This helps you overcome troubled times.

How to bring laughter into your life

Kids have a wonderful way of laughing and giggling, even in the face of adversity. We don't have to always be grown up. Sometimes we feel good when we act like kids again. Let's learn from the children in our lives, and play and laugh along. If you have grandkids or young kids around, it can be healing to play in the sand or make things out of clay or play dough. Remember the roller coaster as a good place to let out a scream? For some of us, a ride on one of the easier rides at a fair is fun.

Who helps you laugh? Spend more time with those people. Some of us laughed more when we were young – you may want to try to reconnect with your friends from when you were young. If you can't connect with old friends, do activities where you might meet new friends.

What makes you laugh? A favorite radio or TV show, a movie, a book or comic strip, an email joke, that old family story – go ahead and enjoy it. If it makes you laugh, it's good and you need it. Better yet, share it with someone else who has the same sense of humor as you – and the laughter will be even better. Laughter is contagious.

Believe in something

A belief in something gives us hope. Hope renews itself, like flowers in the spring after a long hard winter.

The most important thing is for you to believe in yourself. Be proud of who you are and where you have come from. Don't measure success by the position you are in life, but by the obstacles you overcame to get to where you are today. You may have had some big obstacles to overcome. Good for you.

Believing in things bigger than ourselves gives many people hope and comfort. Regular attendance at a place of worship is like scheduled stress reduction. It is a chance to relinquish your everyday worries to a higher power, if even for a short time. Studies show that spiritual belief in a greater being, and prayer, can be very important to good health and longevity. You become part of a network of support with others in your community and around the world. Prayer and meditation provide an opportunity for quiet reflection. When you sing hymns and chants you may feel a communion, but you also breathe deeply and relieve tension. Hearing these familiar sounds can calm you.

Love of nature is a form of spirituality whether or not you are religious. Many of us now live in large cities, where nature is out of our reach. Modern technology draws us further away from the outdoors as we spend more hours indoors in front of a screen. Yet, deep inside us all is a need to connect to nature. Perhaps this is one reason why gardening is so popular. Some cities have scenic nature trails and park areas, and we also have wonderful national, state and provincial parks that offer chances to hike. There is something very basic about feeling the soil in your hands, feeling the wind on your face and at night, gazing at the stars.

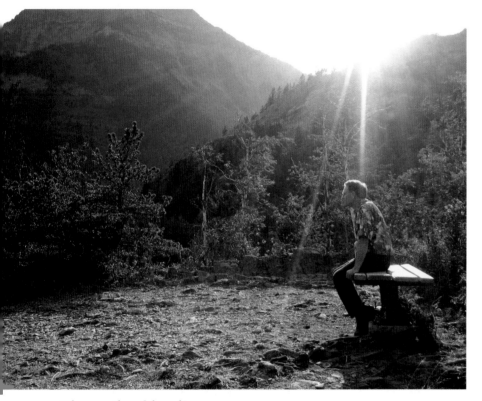

The path of healing

Nobody is perfect. Human nature is both good and bad – we do wonderful things *and* make mistakes. Making room for compassion, forgiveness and respect can give you and others hope. It is the struggle to overcome terribly hurtful things in your life. It is learning the path of healing. You can express this in privacy or in support groups and counseling, or time spent with your family and friends. Some find it is easier to travel this road called life when you help others. One of the greatest benefits of helping others and volunteering is that it can help you grow. There are many volunteer opportunities. Choose something that you will enjoy and that makes use of your special qualities. Look for your own path.

Reducing clutter in your home can help you lose weight – here's why:

- *Clutter causes stress and a feeling of failure, this can lead to overeating.*

- *If your fridge, freezer, counters and cupboards are cluttered with high-calorie food, you'll be tempted.*

- *When your dining area is clean and tidy, you'll enjoy eating at home more.*

See the vitamin charts on pages 132–133 for information on food sources of vitamins and minerals. Page 58 and 119 have information on omega-3 fats.

The "winter blues" are more common in people who live in northern latitudes or are shift workers. A lack of light may be part of what causes these blues. Spending a half an hour a day sitting near a specially designed fluorescent light that acts like day light helps some people. For more information, ask your doctor or your local mental health association.

Make your home your nest

Keep your home tidy, comfortable and safe. A vase of freshly picked flowers (or spring flowers from the grocer) can pick up your mood for days. Easy renovations can cheer you up – try different pillows on your couch or hang up a new picture. A fresh coat of paint on your walls can make quite a difference. Consider calming wall colors of pastel or paler colors (try a pale sage green or light sky blue) complemented with shades of white or ivory. Soothing scents in your home (such as cinnamon, orange or lavender) might help relax you.

Feed your brain good food

Your brain controls your mood and it needs nutrients to work properly. Adequate magnesium, B vitamins (especially niacin, vitamin B6 and folic acid) and omega-3 fats, help improve mood and reduce stress. Foods that have a type of protein called tryptophan also help boost your mood and help you sleep better. Milk is especially rich in tryptophan, and other good sources are yogurt, cheese, eggs, bananas and peanuts. To get the nutrients you need, eat a colorful variety of healthy foods in the right amounts for you. Eat regular meals and eat slowly – share meals with family and friends. Enjoy the occasional indulgence. If your weight causes you stress, think about getting rid of your scale. As long as you monitor your weight with your doctor, you don't need to weigh yourself every day.

Exercise and sunlight

Keep active at home or work. Walk away from stress. Walk, bike or do other exercise – even a large body can be fit and strong. When you exercise you pump out "happy hormones." These relax you and bring down your blood sugar and blood pressure, and reduce inflammation in your body.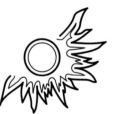

An extra bonus of walking outside is that you are getting light. Sunlight (even through a window) helps stimulate your senses and lift your spirits. The vitamin D that we get from sunlight outdoors may also help lift your mood.

Alice's story:

When I started walking, I could only walk for 5 minutes, and then I went to 10, then 15, then 20, then I was really happy with 30 minutes. And I found that it helped me in many ways. It didn't just help me physically but I feel it helped me emotionally also. You're just in a better frame of mind. Whatever comes up you seem to be able to handle it better. And as we age, we have children and grandchildren and there's always something going on. I found it helped me to be more positive, whatever came up. I'd say, "Well okay, it's not that bad, we'll look at the half full glass of water, forget the half empty."

Look your best

Enjoy a relaxing shower or short bath daily. Keep your nails and hair well groomed. Wandering around your home in your pajamas or sweat pants is comfortable, yet dressing up has a way of making you feel better about yourself.

Your smile is the most important thing you can wear.

"Look good" clothing tips:

- Clothes that are too oversized or too tight may not show you off at your best.

- Black or dark pants help balance your hips and waist and make your body seem longer. Also try standing and walking tall.

- Try wearing a solid covered t-shirt or tank top, and then layer with a lighter or brighter-colored shirt or jacket (solids, small prints or thin vertical lines work well). Choose V-necks and shorter hems on fitted tops (just to the bottom of your stomach).

- Complement your look with a nice watch, bracelet or belt.

Music

Music can improve the health of children and adults, including those with chronic diseases. To reduce stress, choose music that reminds you of positive and happy times. You can listen to music on an MP3 player while you are walking, or on a stereo while you are on your exercise bike or treadmill. Tap your feet (or dance) to your favorite rock, country, pop or gospel, or relax with your feet up to classical. Musicians can work out stress by beating on a drum, strumming a guitar, or playing the piano. If you don't consider yourself to be a great singer, but love to sing, then sing along at church, or at home in your shower. Singing and being sung to (even by poor singers) has ancient and comforting traditional roots.

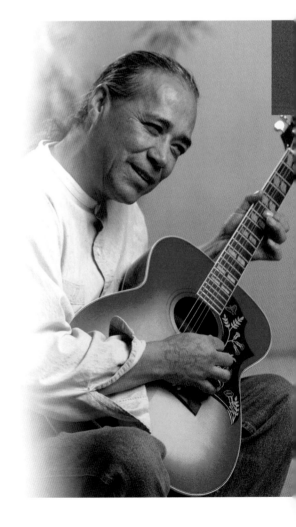

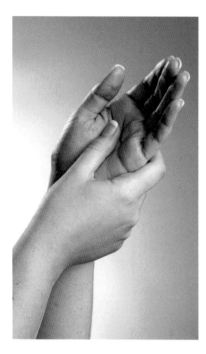

Touch

Appropriate and invited touch comes in many forms. Touch has the power to relax and improve health. Shaking hands, holding hands, hugs and kisses, cuddling, hand manicures, foot or back massages, a "wash and cut" at the hairdresser, brushing a child's hair, holding a baby or child, or dancing with a partner can all be good touches. Petting a dog or cat is a wonderful opportunity for touch. Pets need our attention as much as we need theirs.

On your own, have a relaxing bath or shower and feel the touch of the warm water. When you feel stressed, your circulation decreases and you can get cold hands. Massage and warm your hands by working in hand cream. Start at your wrist and work down to each individual finger. Perhaps, later you may want to massage or stimulate other parts of your body. It's good to let go of tensions. When sex is enjoyable, you release "happy hormones" – whether you are with a partner or flying solo.

Get 7-8 hours of sleep

Lack of sleep can make stress worse, as well as increase your weight and your blood sugar. You may do well on less or more, but if you feel stressed, it's good to try and get 7–8 hours of sleep. The following tips to help you sleep may not all be suitable for you, but if you are having trouble sleeping it's worthwhile to try a couple. Sometimes, making just one small change can make a difference.

Have a regular bedtime routine

- Try to go to bed and get up in the morning at a similar time.

- Have a "before bed" routine, for example, brush and floss your teeth, then have a shower or short bath.

- If you have a TV, computer or cell phone in your bedroom, turn them all off 15 minutes before bedtime. Your mind and eyes need a chance to settle down. If you want to read just before turning off the lights, settle for something light rather than something that will keep you awake. Try to save arguments with family members for other times so your body can relax.

Avoid or limit caffeine, nicotine and alcohol 3–4 hours before bedtime. Also limit fluids 1–2 hours before to reduce needing to get up at night.

If your bedmate snores…

If this disrupts your sleep, think about options to resolve the problem. Consider ear plugs or a fan that might provide white noise. Can you sleep in a different room? Can your partner change something that will reduce his or her snoring such as treating allergies or sleeping on his or her side? Snoring can be a symptom of sleep apnea. Talk to a doctor to learn more.

Exercise during the day or earlier in the evening will help tire you out so you sleep better at night. The exertion of sex helps some people nod right off to sleep.

Avoid or limit large bedtime snacks. If feeling hungry prevents you from falling asleep or wakes you up, you may need to have a small evening snack. A glass of milk or a small banana is a good choice as the tryptophan helps you sleep. Large, heavy snacks will disrupt your sleep.

Limit long daytime naps if possible.

A comfortable mattress helps. See page 244 (point 9.), for information about sleeping positions if you have a sore back.

Keep your room temperature about 65°F (18°C), if possible. If your feet are cold, wear warm loose socks.

A dark and quiet room makes a big difference.

If you are lying awake for more than half an hour, get up. You may want to read a book or watch some TV until you feel tired again. Then repeat your regular bedtime routine. You may want to try focused relaxation (see page 364) or listen to some calming music (such as wave sounds that lull you to sleep).

Other ways to relax

Are you feeling stressed? Try one of these easy ways to relax. The first one takes less than a minute, the second one a couple of minutes. The third ones take ten or fifteen minutes.

Deep breathing → Less than one minute

Deep breathe during the day whenever you are feeling stressed. Just stop and take a couple of deep breaths. It only takes a minute, but it gives you an immediate oxygen boost and helps relax you.

Short exercises → One to three minutes

Doing a few short exercises can relieve tension building up in your muscles. For example, try shoulder shrugs, ankle rotations or stretches (see page 239). If the tension is in your neck, drop your neck to your chest, hold for ten seconds, then slowly move it from side to side.

Talk to your doctor *if insomnia continues to be a big problem for you. Do you think you might have sleep apnea? You may benefit from seeing a counselor, going to a sleep clinic or taking a sleeping pill. Sometimes taking a sleeping pill for just a short time might help get you over a particularly stressful time.*

If you spend only 1% of your day focusing on relaxing, that's just ten minutes. Yet, it can make a significant improvement in your blood sugar and blood pressure.

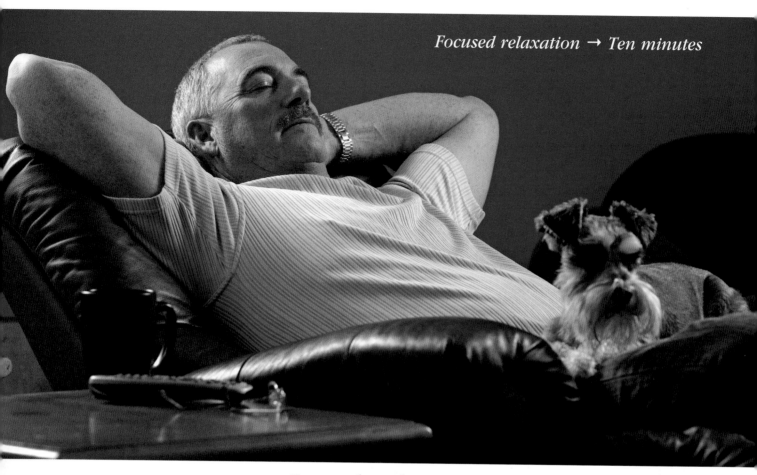

Focused relaxation → *Ten minutes*

For complete relaxation, find a quiet place with lights dimmed, then:

1. Sit in a comfortable chair or lie down.

2. Breathe deeply and slowly with your eyes closed.

3. Concentrate on slowly relaxing all the muscles in your arms and legs. Try to not think about anything else, just focus on your muscles relaxing.

4. Then focus on relaxing your stomach, bottom, back, face and neck. Keep relaxing until you feel no pressure on your muscles. You will feel like you have softly sunk into your chair or bed.

6. Continue breathing deeply. Each time that you breathe out, slowly say the word "calm" to yourself.

Yoga, Pilates and Tai-Chi → *Fifteen minutes or more*

These exercise routines all include relaxation components. They include slow controlled movements and poses that focus your attention away from outside distractions. They require different levels of fitness and flexibility. If you have never tried them, talk to an instructor at a local fitness club about whether it might be a good exercise for you. If so – consider giving it a try.

Coping with Depression

Depression is different than stress. Depression can be like a black cloud that hangs over your head. One day, for a reason, or sometimes for no reason, that black cloud drops down on you. You feel its pressure on you and it affects everything you want to do. It makes it difficult for you to get out of bed, to talk to family or friends and to do the work that you should be doing. It takes away joy, and it takes you away from people who love you. If you think you might be depressed, please talk to your doctor or a mental health professional. Also, consider taking the depression test below.

If you think you might be depressed, take this short test:*

Over the last two weeks, how often have you been bothered by any of the following problems? (Circle your answer then add up your circled answers.)	Not at all	Several days	More than half the days	Nearly every day
Little interest or pleasure in doing things.	0	1	2	3
Feeling down, depressed, or hopeless.	0	1	2	3
Trouble falling or staying asleep, or sleeping too much.	0	1	2	3
Feeling tired or having little energy.	0	1	2	3
Poor appetite or overeating.	0	1	2	3
Feeling bad about yourself – or that you are a failure or have let yourself or your family down.	0	1	2	3
Trouble concentrating on things, such as reading the newspaper or watching television.	0	1	2	3
Moving or speaking so slowly that other people could have noticed? Or the opposite – being so fidgety or restless that you have been moving around a lot more than usual.	0	1	2	3
Thoughts that you would be better off dead or of hurting yourself in some way.	0	1	2	3

0 + _____ + _____ + _____

Once you have your score, go to page 366 and read "When to seek help?"

Total score: _____

*These questions are from the PHQ-9 Patient Health Questionnaire. It was developed by Drs. Robert L. Spitzer, Janet B.W. Williams, Kurt Kroenke and colleagues, with an educational grant from Pfizer Inc. To access the original questionnaire which is designed for use by health professionals, go to www.pfizer.com. It includes ways to determine if depression is mild or severe.

Some, but not all, anti-depression medications can contribute to weight gain. This may increase your chance of developing diabetes or making your diabetes worse. Talk to you doctor about all your options.

Depression and diabetes

When you are depressed you feel lethargic and uninterested in making healthy choices. You may gain weight and this can contribute to diabetes. On the other hand, coping with diabetes is challenging, especially if you have developed some complications. This can contribute to depression. Treating the depression is an important first step. Once your depression improves, you feel better, and it can be easier for you to manage your diabetes.

When to seek help?

You *may* be depressed if you scored 5 or more on the test on page 365. Talk to your doctor or a mental health professional so he/she can assess you further. This is particularly important if your score was high or you have feelings of depression that don't go away. If your thoughts of hurting yourself or someone else are urgent, seek medical care or if needed, call an emergency help phone line.

If your doctor determines that you are depressed, ask your doctor whether you should see a counselor, and if so, who? Some people have success in managing their depression through exercise (see pages 217–262) and by making changes to help manage stress (see pages 354–364). A health counselor can support you in making some of these changes. Other people benefit from also taking anti-depressant pills. Your doctor may prescribe pills for a short time, or you may need them for life. Medications, if needed, can help lift a black cloud and let the sun shine in again.

7. Managing at Other Life Stages

Preschoolers to Teenagers   **368**

    Tips for parents or caregivers to establish
good exercise and eating habits in preschoolers   369

    Are you a teenager with type 2 diabetes?
Here are some things to think about   373

Pregnancy and Gestational Diabetes   **381**

    Problems that may occur   382

    Seven steps to having a healthy baby   383

        1. Keep active   383

        2. Gain a healthy weight   384

        3. Make wise nutrition and health choices   385

        4. Take insulin if needed   385

        5. Test your blood sugar   386

        6. See your doctor regularly   386

        7. Breastfeed to protect against future diabetes   387

    How many children do you want?   388

Sexuality and Diabetes   **392**

    Good solutions for sexual changes and diabetes   392

    Six approaches to sexual changes   394

        1) Boost your circulation and nerves   395

        2) Self-fulfillment   396

        3) Lubricants   397

        4) Build intimacy   398

        5) Medications and erection devices   401

        6) Bedroom alternatives   407

Preschoolers to Teenagers

Recommendations to prevent or reduce diabetes complications covered in this book also apply to kids and teenagers.

Healthy habits for preschoolers to help prevent type 2 diabetes is found on pages 369–372.

Teenagers who have already developed type 2 diabetes, please read pages 373–380.

Parents, or caregivers of a child or teenager with type 2 diabetes, please read through this section also.

Type 2 diabetes in children and teenagers was virtually unheard of thirty years ago. The risk of diabetes for today's youth is like a tsunami waiting to happen. Change needs to happen now to prevent this huge wave of life complications. Children and youth eat more, do less exercise and weigh more than ever before in history. Overweight youth will become overweight adults. As adults they will live a shorter life. They will suffer from diabetes, heart disease and cancer.

We can blame much of this problem directly on modern technology and an excess of sweet and fatty foods. Television, computers and internet, cars, vending machines, mega food stores and fast food restaurants cause health problems. Yet, in spite of this, we still have power to influence our children.

Genetics and the way we live, makes type 2 diabetes a family affair. Generally, if a parent(s) or caregivers are inactive and watch a lot of television, their children will have similar habits. If parents eat a lot of potato chips, soft drinks and rely on fast-food restaurant meals, this becomes normal for their children. Children take these habits with them into their adult lives. There are options for kids to be more active, and the earlier they learn how to shop for healthy groceries, cook meals and eat well – the better!

Make time to dine:

Eating together helps families talk and develop a support network for life. Studies show that children who eat dinner often with their families:

- *Are less likely to smoke, drink or use drugs.*
- *Earn higher grades at school.*
- *Eat healthier foods.*

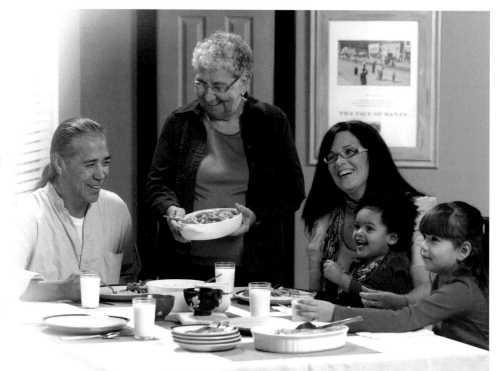

Tips for parents or caregivers to establish good exercise and eating habits in preschoolers

You have the power to make decisions about what your children eat and what exercise they do. You are the one doing the grocery shopping. You decide if you spend time and money on fast food or a home cooked meal. You are the one that can turn off the TV to reduce the impact of food advertising on your children. You know what is best for them. A two year old or four year old does not know, no matter how much they argue! The rules and guidelines you give them as toddlers and young children will carry them into their teenage and adult years. A variety of suggestions follow. To begin with, consider trying just one or two.

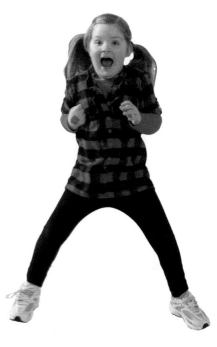

- **Keep kids active – limit screen time.** From an early age, it is wise to restrict use of electronic devices such as electronic games, computer and television. The more that screen time is restricted, the more opportunity there is for kids to play. Play includes structured time where you play with your child and unstructured time where the child plays on their own or with other children. Visit a playground regularly. Hang a swing in a backyard tree. Once outdoors, kids are moving and burning calories.

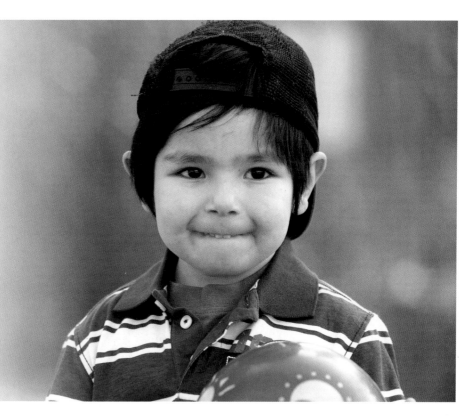

The Canadian Paediatric Society recommends limiting total screen time to less than 1–2 hours a day for the whole family. The American Academy of Pediatrics suggests no TV or screen time for children younger than two. For more information go to www.cps.ca or www.aap.org

At home and school, make water the #1 beverage choice.

Set a good example – eat healthy foods yourself!

Other resources:

There are many great books on infant and child care that you can borrow from a library or purchase at a bookstore or online. For example, borrow a recent edition of Dr. Spock's Baby and Child Care Book, or check out this website: www.ellynsatter.com

- **Limit juice, soft drinks and all other sweetened beverages.** Limit fruit juices to 4–6 ounces (125–175 mL) or less per day. Try to avoid giving young children soft drinks and sugared drinks. Also limit potato chips and high calorie "junk food." By limiting these drinks and foods, your child will come to the table hungry for their meal or snack, and will be less picky. They will also have a better appetite for meals if you encourage outdoor and active play time, summer and winter.

- **Offer water to drink throughout the day.**

- **Feed them regular meals and snacks.** Give them a routine they can count on. Help them learn to wait until the next meal or snack.

- **Provide healthy foods.** See pages 149–200 for meal and snack ideas. At snack time, offer nutritious foods, including whole wheat crackers and breads, fruits and vegetables (soft or thin partially cooked pieces, to avoid risk of choking), milk, cheese and yogurt, peanut butter, kidney beans or brown beans, hard boiled eggs, and slices of avocado. If you offer healthy foods, (instead of cookies and chips) kids will choose them.

- **Keep conversation light.** Turn off the TV when eating. Serve meals in a calm and casual way. Let everyone talk about their day. Try to avoid stressful topics.

- **Don't force feed.** Don't force, or even ask children to eat a food they don't want, nor to finish what's on their plate. You might think this is strange because our natural feeling as a parent is to encourage our child to eat. Too often this doesn't work because we all know kids can be pretty stubborn!

- **Encourage food manners.** It's natural for kids to have favorite foods and to dislike others. Everyone is different. Even if someone dislikes a food, it's best to avoid speaking rudely about it at the table. Consider setting a rule that they can't say "I hate that" or "yucky." In some cases, a child may dislike a new flavor, but more often kids say bad things about food to get attention at that moment. Over time if your child repeats that they hate a food without tasting it again, eventually they truly will. Instead, encourage and praise positive talk about foods.

- **Teach children to respect food.** Offer small portions of food, and let your toddler or child feed themselves. If your child does not want to eat some or all of the food, remove it from the table when the meal is over. Praise them for what they ate, and don't comment on the food not eaten. It's a good idea to not offer alternatives to what you are serving. If there is fussing, remove your child from the table and quickly give them a toy or activity. This takes the focus away from the food so your table does not become a food battleground. Your child won't starve because they've missed a food group or even if they miss a meal here and there. When you are on a routine of regular meals and snacks, the next food is always in just a few hours time (during the day). Be consistent. You will find your child will start enjoying their meals and leaving little on their plate.

- **Cook with children.** Children can learn cooking skills from as young as three or four years old. Show them the meal pictures in this book. Let them "help" you put together a meal. Start with really easy meals, such as Cold Cereal (Breakfast 1), Wrap (Lunch 2) or Hot Chicken Salad (Dinner 3). By the time they are teenagers, they should be able to prepare most of the meals found in this book. This will give them the knowledge and confidence to cook and try new recipes and healthy foods.

- **Allow for occasional treats.** Your shelves and refrigerator should hold mostly healthy food. Offer treats, in reasonable portions, occasionally. Kids love chocolates, cake, ice cream and candies as much as adults do. As long as they recognize that these are not everyday foods, they can go ahead and enjoy them!

- **Put children to bed at a regular time.** Sleep is important for appetite control. Inadequate sleep is associated with becoming overweight and getting diabetes. One of the biggest benefits of getting your children into a regular sleep pattern is that it gives you, the caregiver, a break. You need a break every night so you can be fresh to look after your kids the next morning. Keeping these rules consistent is important. If young children learn that bedtime is 7 or 8 o'clock, they adapt to this. If they are active earlier in the evening or day, this will tire them out. For the last half hour before bedtime, create a "healthy" routine that works for you. It's a good idea to get rid of distractions. Turn off all technology. Consider giving them a bath and brushing their teeth, and reading a bedtime story.

Use hand portions as a guide. See the Food Guide on pages 55–59. A toddler only needs portions that fit in their small hands on most days. At times they will have growth spurts and be hungry and will need more. As your child grows older, their hands get bigger, and so will their appetite.

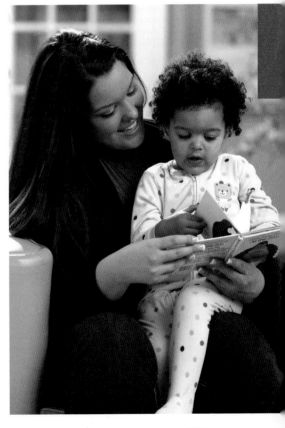

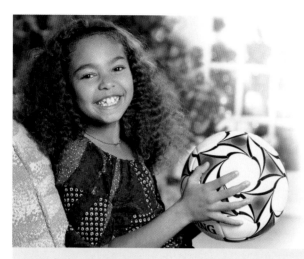

Gifts for Children

Keep them active and safe for outdoor play all year round

- balls of all kinds (soccer, basketball, volleyball, and football)
- baseball bat, mitt and ball
- bean bag tossing games
- Velcro ball catch games
- badminton rackets and birdies
- set of bowling pins and balls
- wiffle balls (plastic balls with holes in them) and plastic bats or plastic golf clubs
- frisbees in different styles and colors
- hoola hoops and jump ropes
- water wings, floating toys and life jackets
- set of flippers, mask and snorkel
- beach set of buckets with hand shovel and rake
- rollerblades or skateboards with safety pads
- bicycles, tricycles, wagons
- safety and fun gear for bicycles: helmets, handlebar tassels and bells, soft seats, baskets, and reflectors
- fishing tackle and poles (children sizes)
- butterfly net, water net, magnifying glass and bug containers
- child size shovels and rakes (help you in gardening)
- books on animals, birds, insects, weather and stars

Give active and healthy gifts for all family members

Gifts costing under $10
- Hand weights or resistance bands
- Tickets to skate, go the gym or swim at your local recreation centre or arena
- Water bottles
- Sunscreen
- Hand or foot lotion
- Socks
- Pill container
- Insulated lunch bag

Gifts costing under $25
- An exercise video
- A pedometer
- A music CD with a great beat to inspire one to do chair exercises or dance
- Car cleaning and polishing kit
- Neck and shoulder bean bag pillow (microwave to ease sore muscles)
- Sports bag, swim suit and special towel
- Clothing and gear for fishing or hiking
- A gardening gift basket, with a trowel, gardening gloves and vegetable seeds
- A gift basket of herbal tea, low-calorie drink mixes, and light hot chocolate
- A gift basket of low-sodium spice blends
- A diabetes cookbook or health book.

Gifts costing $50–$100
- A CPR lifesaving kit (contact your local heart organization)
- A mini-peddler; see page 229
- Nordic walking sticks; see page 225
- A good pair of walking shoes
- Nintendo Wii games
- A one month gym membership

Gifts costing over $100
- A recumbent bike which has a comfortable wide seat and back support.
- Regular exercise bike or street bike
- A treadmill

The best gift you can give your child or teenager is your time – listen and keep talking.

Are you a teenager with type 2 diabetes? Here are some things to think about:

Limit soft drinks, juices and other sweet beverages

Do you drink a lot of cola and eat a lot of chips at home? Do you have stores and coffee shops located near your home and school? Do vending machines tempt you to buy sweet drinks? If these vending machines and shops were far away, you might not think so much about drinking sweetened beverages. Did you know? – Both soft drinks and juice contribute to obesity. Many schools have replaced soft drinks with juice, but juice can also make you gain weight. Some juices even have more sugar than soft drinks (see pages 86–89). Many of the beverages in vending machines also contain caffeine. "Energy drinks" are particularly high in caffeine and sugar. It's okay to have sweet beverages now and then, but drinking them everyday is not good for your waistline. When you have diabetes, these drinks are really bad for your blood sugar. Think about drinking sweet beverages less often.

Encourage schools to say "no" to vending machines and "yes" to exercise

Some communities believe "out of sight, out of mind" is the way to go with tempting beverages and foods. They are taking vending machines out of schools. They are also making bylaws that restrict the building of new coffee shops and corner stores within a mile (2 km) of schools. Your parent(s) might also consider buying less junk food and more healthy foods. Do you think these changes might help reduce diabetes?

Some schools are also increasing the amount of physical activity that you get to do during the school day. When five minute exercise breaks occur half way through each class, this can total a half hour of exercise a day. Students learn better when their brains get a rush of oxygen.

Your school or local store make money when you buy soft drinks and junk food, but you still have a choice to drink more water and to spend your money instead on something that isn't bad for your health. You also have a choice to be more active. If you have concerns, talk to anyone who will listen – your parents, your student council, even your town or community council! Do you have parents, grandparents, or an aunt or uncle that wants to fight against diabetes? We need to keep talking about this and thinking of solutions. At home, start making healthy choices.

Teaspoons of sugar from 16 ounce (500 mL) servings:

- **Zero teaspoons:** water

- **7–9 teaspoons (35–45 mL):** sports drinks including Gatorade, Thirst Quencher or PowerAde

- **11–15 teaspoons (55–75 mL):** Energy drinks including Red Bull, Monster, Rockstar, Full Throttle and Amp; cola and cream soda; unsweetened orange juice or apple juice; sweetened milks; Slushees or Slurpees; or iced sweetened coffees

- **24 teaspoons (120 mL):** Gatorade Energy Drink

Sports drinks are sugared beverages that have salts (sodium and potassium) added to replace those lost when you are sweating hard. If you are not exercising, these are not good to drink as they just give you sugar and calories you don't need.

Energy drinks have even more sugar than sports drinks, plus they are also high in caffeine. Therefore they will raise your blood sugar more and are more fattening. Energy drinks can cause you to become dehydrated, see page 379.

Keep Active

Exercise and technology

Some studies recommend that youth get at least 90 minutes (1½ hours) of exercise a day. This is more exercise than the amount recommended for adults who wish to prevent chronic diseases.

Research shows that on average, youth spend 4–6 hours each day sitting in front of a TV. How much "screen time" do you have each day? Did you ever stop to think that the more time you spend in front of a screen (TV, computer, gaming, cell phone and texting), the less time you have in the day for moving around and being active? For good physical health, doctors recommend that you reduce your screen time to two hours or less. If this seems impossible, consider starting with just one or two of these steps below. You aren't going to change everything overnight, but start with a couple of small changes that will help your blood sugar and help you feel better.

- Consider cutting out one hour of television or being on the computer on most days?

Parents: Consider removing televisions and computers from bedrooms – your own and your teenagers. Explain to your children the negative impact that excess time spent in front of the television or computer screen has on anyone with diabetes.

- If you don't know what to do with this extra hour, try being active outdoors with friends, go for a bike ride, or help out around the house.

Parents: Are your kids bused to school? Are there safe options for your kids to walk to school or partway to school? What about safe ways for them to walk to friends and activities? When we are always driving our children, they forget to hop on a bike or walk to get to where they are going. They may come to expect to catch a ride everywhere. Are there older siblings that can assume the responsibility of walking with those that are younger? When kids walk to school together, there is safety in numbers.

The good news is that even small changes can make a big difference over time.

Try just one change every week. Check your blood sugar, and monitor what difference eating better and being more active can make to your sugar levels. You will feel proud when your A1C level and weight start coming down.

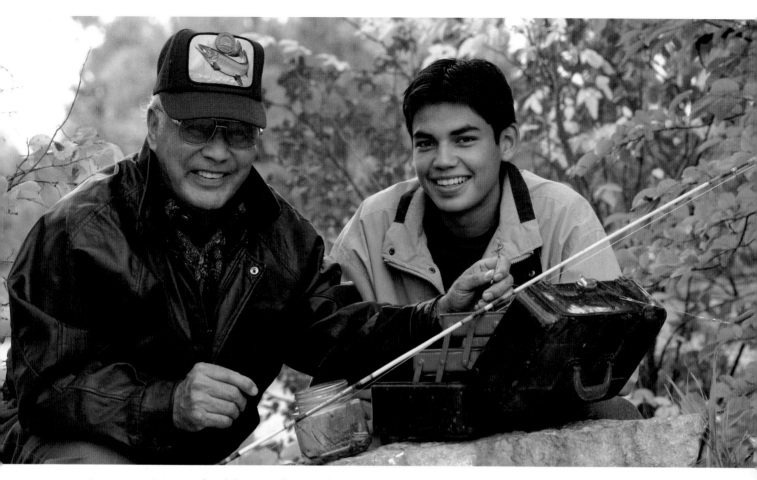

- Arrange visits with elders and grandparents. Some of them may have diabetes too. You can learn from them. Are you interested in helping out teachers or adults with after-school activities, or small jobs such as delivering papers, cutting lawn or babysitting? If you are an older teen do you have a part-time job? Keeping busy grows your mind and also keeps you away from sitting on the couch.

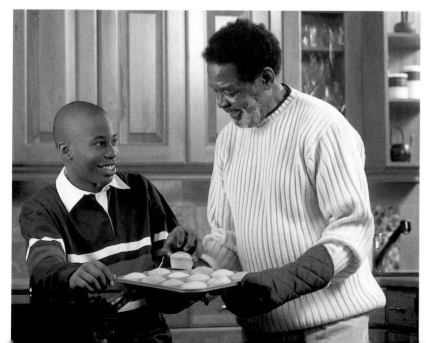

Does grandma, mom, dad or auntie like to cook? Help them cook some healthy meals. Try some of the recipes in this book. Learning to cook and eat well will help you grow strong and in control of your diabetes.

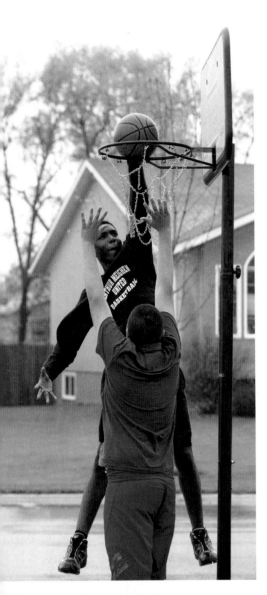

- After school, go for a walk with your parents or in a safe area with your friends or dog.

- Shoot some basketballs, or a soccer ball around an open field.

- Go for a bike ride with your brother, sister or friend.

- Go swimming, roller blading or skate boarding, and in the winter, skating, skiing or snow boarding.

- Some day you may want to do some team sports such as soccer, baseball or hockey.

- Ask an adult or older sibling to help prepare an area for street hockey (summer or winter) with movable nets. Stock up on hockey sticks and soft pucks or tennis balls.

Parents: If you live in a northern climate, a back yard hockey rink, even a small one, can provide great opportunity for your kids to get outside in the winter.

- Take your younger relative to a park to play outdoor games.

- Are there any recreational facilities in your communities such as arenas, swimming pools or bowling alleys?

- If you are musical, consider joining a local marching band or choir.

Parents: Try to go for a family walk or bike ride after dinner. On weekends, go for a hike on a nature trail, or throw a frisbee or football.

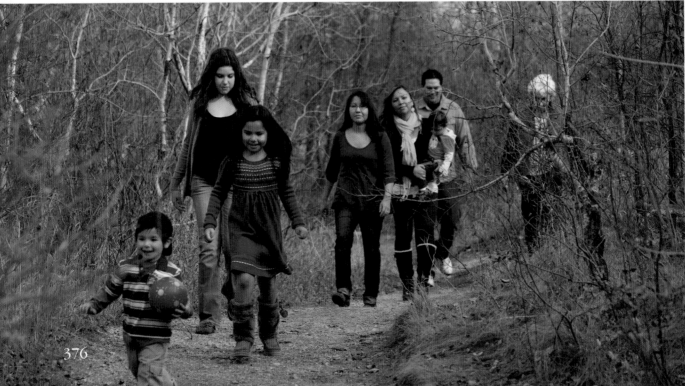

Parents: Be active and your kids will see you as a role model. Could you go biking, or even canoeing, with your kids? If you take a summer vacation, can you and the kids plan activities with exercise like kayaking, horseback riding, hiking or bike tours? Try to encourage your kids to develop interests and hobbies, and to get involved in physical activity. Take an interest in their school work so they stay in school. Studies show that if kids are more active, they will do better in school and are less likely to smoke and take drugs.

Parents: Will your children and teens protest changes? Yes, undoubtedly, unless you explain why he or she must exercise consistently. Emphasize how important healthy eating is for their bodies. Knowing why is important.

Active kids do better in school and are less likely to smoke and take drugs.

Medications and insulin

Insulin is often the medication recommended by doctors for young people with type 2 diabetes. When your blood sugar improves, your doctor may tell you that you can stop your insulin. Doctors also sometimes prescribe diabetes pills. When you start on insulin or pills, remember it is really important to also watch what you eat and to keep active or else the insulin or Pancreas "Insulin Booster" pills (page 318) can make you gain weight.

Pregnancy risks for girls with diabetes

Doctors usually don't recommend Metformin (a Liver "Sugar Blocker") for girls with diabetes who are sexually active. If someone on Metformin became pregnant, the pills could harm the growing fetus. In addition, pregnancy in a teenage girl with diabetes carries risks to the baby. See pages 381–382.

For more information on birth control see page 391.

All sexually active teenagers need to think about birth control and preventing a sexually transmitted infection (STI), but this is particularly important when you have diabetes. If you get an infection, this can increase your blood sugar. Girls with diabetes are also more likely to get a vaginal or urinary tract infection (see pages 46–47 and 301–304). If you get pregnant and your diabetes is not well controlled, you could put your fetus at risk for being born unhealthy. Using the pill and a condom is a whole lot easier than getting an STI for life or being pregnant and having a baby. If you don't feel you can talk to your parent(s) or caregiver about birth control or sexuality, please go see a school counselor or public health nurse. You can talk to them in private. You will also find some information on birth control on page 391.

If you are a teenager and pregnant, attend a diabetes program and prenatal classes to learn as much as you can about having a healthy pregnancy and delivery, and healthy baby. Also, read the Pregnancy and Gestational Diabetes section on pages 381–391. If you live in a northern community, healthy fresh food may be expensive. Eat local food such as wild berries and wild meats. Attend programs for pregnant women that support healthier food choices.

Low blood sugar - risks

Your blood sugar can go low (see pages 331–338) if you are taking insulin or a Pancreas "Insulin Booster" pill. Low blood sugar is especially dangerous if you are driving and/or drinking. Alcohol can cause a serious low blood sugar. Alcohol, marijuana and street drugs impair judgment and can mask low blood sugar.

When you have diabetes and are on medications, it is safest to not drink, but if you are going to drink, then talk to your parent or doctor about this. Your doctor will likely advise you to omit your insulin or pills prior to and during the drinking. Be safe, not sorry.

Parents: If you find your child drunk or high on drugs and you think they might have taken their insulin, you need to keep a close eye on them while they are sleeping. You may need to wake them every two hours to make sure their blood sugar isn't going seriously low. If needed, call a toll-free health phone line or Emergency department for advice.

Dehydration risk

No matter how old you are or how much medication you take, beware of mixing energy drinks with alcohol. High blood sugar plus drinking energy drinks (high in caffeine) in combination with alcohol can cause dehydration. This is more likely to happen if you are also exercising (or dancing). See page 138 for more on signs of dehydration.

> ## Caution
> **Low blood sugar and being drunk can look the same.**
> If your friends are also drinking, they won't realize you have low blood sugar and so can't help give you the sugar you need.
>
> Blood sugar can be low for up to 24 hours after you drink alcohol.
>
> For more information on alcohol, see pages 134–137.

> ## Caution
> ### Energy drinks
> Caffeine from all sources (such as herbs like yerba matte) is often not listed on energy drinks. Just one 16 ounce (500 mL) can of energy drink usually has 11–15 teaspoons (55–75 mL) of sugar plus as much caffeine as 5 cups (1.25 L) of coffee.

Seek out a qualified diabetes team (doctor, nurse and dietitian) to help you and your child or teenager look after their diabetes. It can be helpful if you can also connect with a social worker or mental health worker. They can help you (or caregiver) to work through the challenges of being a kid, plus having diabetes. Sometimes we all need someone to talk to, and lean on for help. An exercise specialist can give ideas for increasing exercise. If you live in a rural or northern location, ask your local nurse or doctor if you could access a diabetes children's team by computer (telehealth) or telephone.

Rules are like the guard rails along the edge of a bridge. They help guide you and keep you safe.

Don't let diabetes hold you back

Having diabetes isn't easy, but it helps to realize that all your friends have challenges too. If you make small gradual changes, it is easier to cope, and this will help you feel better day by day. The things that you need to do to be healthy are the same for all teenagers. A diabetes lifestyle will be a good friend for you as you get older. Set your goal of eating the best you can, being active and staying in school.

Parents: Managing type 2 diabetes does take a toll on your child. You may feel that at certain times, or on certain days, it helps to give them a break from their diabetes. It's not the occasional excursions that are most critical, it's the overall blood sugar level. Your child's 3-month A1C will give you a good picture of how he or she is doing.

As your child becomes a teenager, you can expect struggles when it comes to dealing with their diabetes. Remember when you were a teenager...this is normal. These struggles are a sign of growing up but may also be a sign of boredom, or a loss of direction or hope, or the opposite, being over-programmed. Diabetes is one more challenge for a struggling teenager. This doesn't make it easier for you as a parent(s), grandparent or caregiver. If there is anger, this is very hard for you, and your child.

In adolescence, teens begin to establish their independence. Also, many teenagers feel immortal. It might not make sense to them to keep up good preventative care habits on a daily basis to avoid long term illness. It's hard for them to imagine themselves as adults! Even while struggling, your teenager will still need your daily support and guidance.

As caregivers, you need to be calm and strong, and be there for them. As tough as it is, this means you need to keep providing rules and setting limits. Rules should be age appropriate and have a purpose. These rules and limits can help show your love and care for your children. It makes them feel safe and secure. For children with diabetes, this support and guidance can also help them live longer, healthier lives.

Pregnancy and Gestational Diabetes

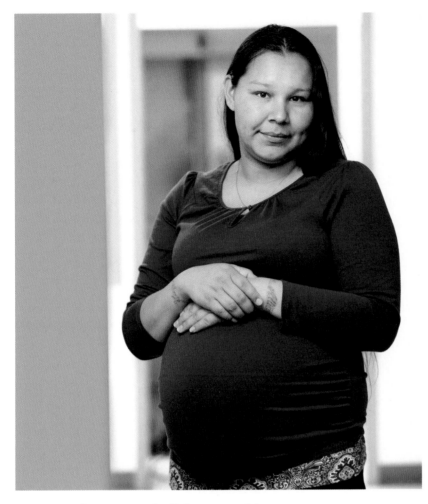

> ### *Avoid Problems*
> You can have a healthy pregnancy, a healthy baby and a healthy you! Follow the steps outlined on pages 383–390.

You may have type 2 diabetes and be pregnant, or your doctor may have told you that you have gestational diabetes. Gestational diabetes means you developed the diabetes during your pregnancy (see page 15).

At 24–28 weeks, your doctor will do a test to see if you have gestational diabetes. If you do, or if you have type 2 diabetes, you may be referred to a specialist – often an obstetrician.

A special test called an amniocentesis will often be done at about 36 weeks. This determines the health of your fetus (fetus is the medical term for your unborn baby). She may order other tests, for example, one or several ultrasounds. An ultrasound is sound waves that take a "picture" of your fetus. Looking at this picture, your doctor can estimate the size of your fetus. This information is useful in determining if you need to start on insulin.

Problems that may occur

If your blood sugar is consistently high and you gain too much weight during your pregnancy:

- Your blood pressure could go up during your pregnancy. This extra stress can also affect your kidneys, eyes and heart.

- Your baby could grow too large. It is harder to deliver a large baby. You may need a Caesarean-section (C-section).

- If any tests show that your baby is not healthy, you may need to deliver early. Then your baby is more likely to have breathing problems or jaundice.

- You are more at risk of losing your baby in your third trimester if your blood sugars are poorly controlled. This risk is lowered with good blood sugar control.

After birth, your baby may have:

Breathing problems
When a baby is large or premature, his or her lungs may not have developed fully. Your baby is likely to need oxygen, and in some cases, may need resuscitation.

Jaundice
Jaundice is yellowed eyes and skin. It occurs when a normal body chemical called bilirubin builds up. Normally, the liver removes excess bilirubin from the blood. However, when a baby is born premature, the liver is not fully developed and so can't work properly. Putting the baby under special lights easily treats the jaundice.

Low blood sugar
If your blood sugar was high before delivery, your baby gets some of this extra sugar. Then your baby's pancreas makes extra insulin in the womb. This continues for a while after birth, and causes your baby's blood sugar to go low when first born. A newborn with low blood sugar will be jittery and crying. He may be given numerous blood tests in the first two days of life. The hospital may separate the baby from you to give him formula or sugar by intravenous. As a new mom, it's hard to see your baby unhappy and taken away from you. Prevent or reduce these problems by taking care early on.

Breast milk is ideal to bring up your baby's blood sugar

Starting breastfeeding as soon as possible after your baby is born is the best way to bring your baby's blood sugar back to normal. See pages 387-389.

Optometrist appointment

When you have diabetes, pregnancy can affect your eyes. See your optometrist before your third month of pregnancy.

Once you have your baby, the diabetes normally goes away. However, you are at risk of getting it again with your next pregnancy. You, and your baby, also run the risk of developing type 2 diabetes later in life. Fortunately, you can reduce these risks by following the steps in this section.

Seven steps to having a healthy baby

1. Keep active

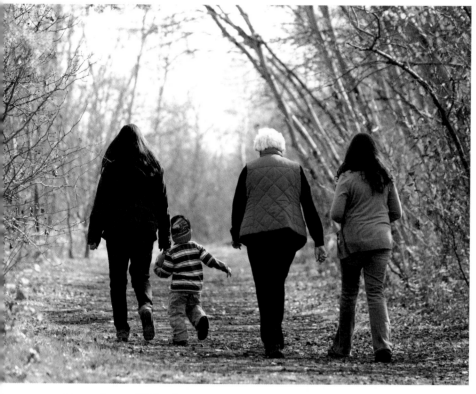

If your blood sugar is higher in the morning, this is an especially good time to go for a walk.

Exercise will help you:

- Prevent too much weight gain during your pregnancy.
- Use insulin more effectively and improve your blood sugar.
- Prevent back pain and constipation.
- Get in good shape for your labor and delivery.

Walking, using an exercise bike or low-impact aerobics are good exercises when you are pregnant. Swimming is also very relaxing, especially in the last trimester. Aim for an hour of walking – split this into a few walks, especially after meals. Use common sense. Sports or exercises that increase the chance of jolts or falling are risky.

When shouldn't you exercise?
Your doctor will tell you if you need to reduce your exercise or be on bed rest. Common reasons for bed rest are persistent vaginal bleeding or if your doctor thinks you may go into labor too early.

2. Gain a healthy weight

Just because you are pregnant does not mean you should eat whatever you want. Keep your portions controlled and aim for a slow gradual weight gain during your pregnancy. The amount of weight you should gain depends on your weight just before you got pregnant. See guidelines below.

Overweight by more than 30 lbs/14 kg (BMI* of 30 or more):	Overweight by up to 30 lbs/14 kg (BMI of 25–29.9):
Gain 11–20 lbs (5–9 kg). Your doctor may recommend you gain even less than 11 lbs.	Gain 15–25 lbs (7–11 kg).

Normal weight (BMI of 18.5–24.9):
Gain 25–35 lbs (11–16 kg)

Underweight (BMI of under 18.5), a teenager or expecting twins: Doctors recommend a larger weight gain than those with normal weight.

*See page 340 to learn about BMI, or Body Mass Index.

The faster and the more weight you gain during pregnancy, the larger your baby will grow. During the first three months you only need to gain a couple of pounds (1 kg) in total. After that, your weight should gradually go up, and you should gain most of your weight in the last trimester (month 6–9). If you are overweight, your average weight gain should be about half a pound (0.25 kg) a week averaged over the last two trimesters.

Weigh yourself once a week or at your doctor appointments. Adjust your food portions or exercise, as needed. It is a good idea to spread your food out throughout the day by including three meals and three snacks. The size of your snacks and whether you choose the small or large meals (see page 151) will depend on your appetite and weight gain.

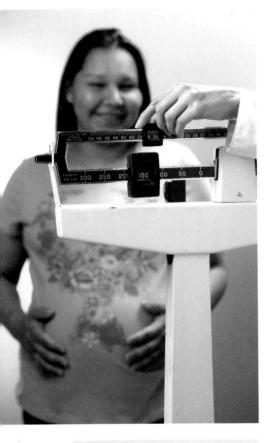

Talk to your doctor or dietitian about the right weight gain for you.

3. Make wise nutrition and health choices

- **Use the meal plans in this book as a guide.**
  You may need to choose the large or small
  meal plans, depending on your weight gain.

- **Choose foods rich in iron, folic acid, vitamin C,
  calcium and vitamin D.** See pages 132–133.

- **Take a prenatal multivitamin and mineral pill every
  day during your pregnancy.** Ideally, start three
  months before you get pregnant. It is wise to
  continue the supplement during the first 6–12
  months of breastfeeding.

- **Choose high fiber foods** (see page 58 and 91–93),
  **drink water and walk every day to lessen or avoid
  constipation.**

- **Do not smoke, drink alcohol or take street drugs.
  These go directly to your baby, there is no safe
  amount.** Talk to an addiction counselor if needed.

- **Limit caffeine:** Limit caffeine to no more than 300 mg
  a day. This would equal about 2 cups (500 mL) of coffee
  (270 mg of caffeine). A cup (250 mL) of tea or can of cola
  each have about 45 mg.

- **Limit some fish:** If you eat fish almost daily, talk to your
  doctor or dietitian about portions. Some fish are high
  in mercury and should be limited during pregnancy.

- **Avoid some low calorie sweeteners:**
  cyclamates or saccharin.

4. Take insulin if needed

If you are not on insulin, your doctor may prescribe some for
you during your pregnancy, especially in the third trimester.
This is when blood sugar usually goes up the most. *Insulin is
safe for your baby.* It does not cross the placenta to your baby.
Taking the insulin will allow you to manage your blood sugar
and still eat enough for proper weight gain. The doctor will
usually stop the insulin when you go into labor. If you have
type 2 diabetes and took insulin before you got pregnant,
you may need less, or none, while breastfeeding.

Diabetes pills: Doctors say you should stop taking diabetes
pills, some blood pressure and cholesterol pills, and most
other pills while you are pregnant or breastfeeding. The
doctor may recommend other pills instead, such as for your
blood pressure. *Talk to your doctor about all your medications
before you get pregnant or as soon as you know you're pregnant.*

*If you are nauseous
or vomiting, try some
of the meal suggestions
on page 148. It may
help to eat a few soda
crackers (kept at your
bedside) before you
get up in the morning.*

*Caffeine: Research
is unclear whether
high amounts of
caffeine could cause
miscarriage. You may
choose to consume
only small amounts
of caffeine or avoid
all caffeine during
pregnancy. Try a
decaf coffee or decaf
tea or chicory root
coffee substitute
(such as Caf-Lib).*

*Doctors commonly
prescribe these
kinds of insulin
during pregnancy:*

- *An evening dose of
  intermediate insulin.
  If needed, you'll take
  short or rapid insulin
  during the day.
  Short insulin allows
  you to eat snacks
  in between doses.*

- *If you are vomiting,
  rapid insulin is
  often the best choice.
  You can take it after
  you feel you will be
  able to hold down
  the meal.*

Ask your doctor or diabetes educator how often you should test.

5. Test your blood sugar

Your doctor will likely ask you to test your blood sugar during your pregnancy, especially if you are taking insulin. See pages 345–349 for guidelines on testing. Your doctor may recommend testing one hour after a meal, as well as at two hours. If you are taking rapid insulin, you will need to also test before meals.

To help protect your growing fetus, doctors recommend that your blood sugar levels be a bit lower than at other times. See usual targets below; these may be increased if you are having low blood sugars.

Recommended blood sugar levels during pregnancy	
Before meals	less than 5.3 mmol/L (95 mg/dL)
One hour after a meal	less than 7.8 mmol/L (140 mg/dL)
Two hours after a meal	less than 6.7 mmol/L (120 mg/dL)

Your doctor may recommend you take insulin
if your blood sugar stays above these levels.

To avoid a low	stay above 4 mmol/L (70 mg/dL)

Feeling down?

Pregnancy and the birth of a baby bring many changes and emotions. Some women feel upset, blue or stressed during pregnancy or after their baby is born. For suggestions on managing stress, please see pages 354–364. Talk to your doctor if your feelings are difficult to manage or you feel depressed (see page 365). It is often helpful to be referred to a counsellor specializing in post-partum depression.

6. See your doctor regularly

During pregnancy
Your doctor will check your blood pressure, and order lab and urine tests. She will check the growth and health of your fetus. She/He will order special tests, see page 381.

After your baby is born
About 2–6 months after your baby is born, have your doctor check your blood sugar. Then have it checked annually, or as recommended by your doctor. This is to see if you have any early signs of type 2 diabetes.

It is also a good idea to get your thyroid checked about one month after your baby is born. This is especially important if you feel tired, sad, or are having a hard time losing weight.

7. *Breastfeed to protect against future diabetes*

Breastfeeding reduces your risk of developing type 2 diabetes later in life. This is mostly because breastfeeding helps you lose weight. Breastfeeding also reduces your baby's risk of getting type 2 diabetes as a teenager or adult. This is because, on average, breastfed babies gain less body fat than bottle-fed babies. Rapid weight gain during the first six months of life may cause your child to gain too much weight by the time they are three or four years old. This fat then tends to stay with children into their teenage and adult years. Research recommends breast milk as the baby's only food or drink for the first six months. After this point, you can introduce table foods, and breastfeeding should continue. Some babies will wean themselves towards the end of their first year, others breastfeed longer.

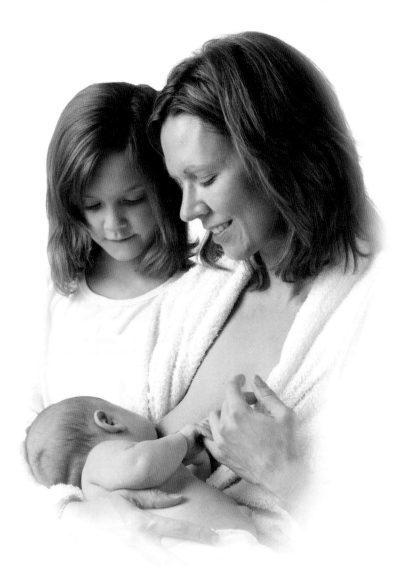

Breast milk benefits your baby. It:

- *Is good for your baby's brain.*
- *Protects your baby from ear and lung infections, diarrhea, gum and tooth decay, asthma, allergies and childhood cancers.*
- *Saves you money.*
- *Can help you bond with your baby.*

Other benefits to the breastfeeding mother:

- *It reduces your risk for breast and ovarian cancer, high blood pressure, high cholesterol and heart disease.*

The longer you breastfeed in your lifetime, the lower your risk for all these conditions.

Breastfeeding is healthier for you and your baby. However, your family or those in your community may be most familiar with bottle feeding. You may have to fight some resistance among your family and friends when you make this important health choice for yourself and your newborn.

Breastfeeding support persons

Your doctor
Talk to your doctor or obstetrician about breastfeeding.

Lactation Consultant
This is a health care professional that specializes in helping mothers to breastfeed. This even includes breastfeeding a premature baby.

Doulas
A doula doesn't provide medical care or deliver babies. She gives you support during labor and after your baby is born. She can help with breastfeeding and help you at home and with the care of your baby.

Midwives
This is a health care professional who works with pregnant women and helps in childbirth. She can work independently or with your doctor to assist you during labor and birth, and breastfeeding.

Supporting breastfeeding

Breastfeeding is wonderful for your health and your baby's health. However, two things can work against breastfeeding. First, if your husband, partner or family is not supportive, this may make you less likely to breastfeed. Second, many women may not receive proper support in hospitals for successful breastfeeding.

Breastfeeding needs to start early. Most women need help in learning to breastfeed. In some busy hospital maternity wards, you may not receive this help. You may go home without establishing good breastfeeding skills. This may be very upsetting for you as a mother, and can even trigger a blue mood. Once home, with a crying baby in hand, it is hard to cope with this on your own, although many make a courageous effort. If breastfeeding didn't work for you, remember you are still a good mother. There are many things you can do for your baby. See page 390 for tips on bottle feeding.

Here are some things that you can do to increase your chances of successfully breastfeeding:

1) Before you deliver, seek help and support.

- Find a friend, family member, diabetes educator or La Leche League member who has successfully breastfed. She can help you learn about breastfeeding before and after you deliver your baby. However, for special challenges such as breastfeeding a premature baby, consult a professional.

- Hire a doula to work with you.

- Your lactation consultant or midwife, if you have one, can be a wonderful help for you.

These support people can help your husband, partner or family to learn about the benefits of breastfeeding.

Ask your doctor or public health nurse, a La Leche League leader, or new mothers to recommend a midwife, doula or lactation consultant where you live. You can also search for them on the internet.

2) Try to choose birthing and hospital options that encourage and support breastfeeding:

- **Find a "Breastfeeding Friendly" hospital.** This means the hospital has policies in place that support breastfeeding. Well-trained nurses help you learn how to breastfeed so your baby latches on properly and feeds well. Lactation consultants work on some larger maternity wards. A birth team or doctor that supports you is very important.

- **Early breastfeeding helps.** Try to bring your baby to your breast to feed within 30 minutes of birth. This is when your baby has a strong instinct to suck. It's not always in your control to have your baby right away. The medical staff wants to ensure that your baby is safe and healthy. Don't worry; just try as soon as you can.

  If you have had a C-section it is also important to begin breastfeeding as soon as possible. A regional anesthetic (epidural) is a good choice, if possible, as you will be either fully awake or mildly sedated. You will see your baby being born, and be able to breastfeed sooner. With a general anesthetic, there will be some delay, but you can breastfeed once you are awake and able to hold your baby.

- **Take minimal or no medications, if possible.** If you have medications with labor, this medication also goes to your baby. Your baby may be sleepy and slow to suck when born. This is why it is so helpful to have a midwife or doula assist you through labor. This support can help you get through the pain of labor without medication or with less medication. If you had pain medication (or had a C-section), your baby will be more alert and ready to breastfeed once the drugs wear off.

- **Keep the baby with you and maintain skin-to-skin contact.** Most hospitals allow your baby to stay with you, if your baby is well enough to do so. This helps you know when your baby is hungry and that it's time to try feeding. The more you feed, and the more skin-to-skin contact you have with your baby, the more milk you make!

- **Avoid bottles, especially in early days.** Sometimes doctors recommend supplemental feeding with formula or expressed breast milk. Your baby sucks differently from a bottle than your breast. If you offer a bottle in the days and weeks before breastfeeding is well established, this may interfere with successful breastfeeding.

Colostrum is the thicker breast milk that a new mother makes in the first couple of days after her baby is born. It has lots of nutrients and antibodies to fight infection. It is very important for your baby.

Ahead of time ask a family member, friend or professional to advocate for you in the hospital after either a C-section or vaginal birth. They can speak out to get your baby to you as soon as possible, and encourage both you and your baby to be kept awake for those early feedings.

Labor medications include if your labor is induced, or you receive pain medication such as an epidural or Demerol.

If your baby needs supplemental feeding, a bottle is not the only way to do this. A newborn can feed with a spoon, cup or through a tiny tube taped to the mother's breast. If you or your baby is ill, a feeding tube may provide intravenous nutrition.

389

Tips for bottle feeding moms

There are times when a woman cannot breastfeed. For example, certain adult medications can interfere with the health of her baby by passing through her breast milk. In this case, for the woman's personal health and well-being she must continue to take her medications and bottle feed her baby formula.

Other times, a mother has not been properly supported to breastfeed, by health providers, family and friends, as discussed on page 388.

Once you have decided you are going to bottle feed your baby, still talk to your public health nurse about:

- borrowing a breast pump
- the type and amount of formula you should feed your baby, and
- a healthy baby's weight gain.

It is possible to learn to express milk from your breasts by hand or using a breast pump. Then your baby can be fed expressed breast milk or formula, or a combination of the two.

Bottle Feeding Time:
This is your time to pay special attention to your baby. Hold your baby close to your body so your baby feels secure and can see your face. Your baby feels loved when you look at him or her, and learns language when you talk and sing during the feeding. This is bonding time that you give only to your baby. This time also boosts your "happy hormones." Dad and other family members can bottle feed baby now and again too. These are all bonding times that will last a lifetime.

Caution

Feeding your baby canned milk, juices or soft drinks can be harmful to your baby's growing body and brain.

Being a Mom

Mothering begins the day you find out you are pregnant. Being a new mother can be wonderful – but is also challenging. The early years with your first child, including feeding your baby, can be the toughest because you are learning so much about yourself and being a mom.

Don't be shy – ask for help from all sources, public health nurse, doctor, community nutritionist, infant program leaders at your community resource centre.

All mothers know that you will do your very best and you will continue for the rest of your life; loving, comforting, teaching and caring for your child.

How many children do you want?

If you would like to have another baby, start planning early. The good news is that if you make lifestyle changes now, you may be able to prevent or delay getting gestational diabetes in your next pregnancy.

Once you've had gestational diabetes, you are at high risk of getting gestational diabetes again or getting type 2 diabetes. With multiple pregnancies, your risk can increase. This is because you may be at a higher weight at the beginning of your next pregnancy, and you will be older.

You can reduce this risk after your baby is born:

- Eat well, but eat less, so you can gradually lose weight. Try to get back to your pre-pregnancy weight or a lower weight if you are overweight.

- Continue daily walking and other exercise as soon as you recover from your birthing or C-section.

If you have type 2 diabetes and want to get pregnant:

It is best to have your blood sugar under control at the time of conception. The first trimester is when the fetus' organs are developing. Good blood sugar in this period reduces your baby's risk of health problems.

Birth control

You may want to wait a few years between one pregnancy and the next. Alternately, you may not want any more children, especially if you have developed some diabetes complications. Please discuss birth control with your doctor or public health nurse, as well as any side effects and their effectiveness. On the internet search "birth control hotline."

Having your tubes tied (tubal ligation) or vasectomy for your partner

This is a permanent choice. Although sometimes a doctor can reverse a vasectomy, a woman's tubes can rarely be untied.

Temporary birth control

Recommended options for women with diabetes include low-dose oral contraceptive pills and the IUD (intrauterine device) inserted by your doctor. The diaphragm or cervical cap combined with spermicidal foams or jellies, and condoms with spermicidal foams are other options. These are all safe during breastfeeding. Discuss other birth control options with your doctor or public health nurse.

Emergency birth control

Women with diabetes can take emergency oral contraceptives ("the morning after pill") after unprotected sex. It's not a good idea to use this for regular contraceptive use.

Caution

Certain diabetes pills can increase your fertility, especially for pre-menopausal women. See pages 317 and 321. Make sure you protect yourself from pregnancy if you do not want to risk further health concerns at this stage of your life.

Remember, the only thing that keeps you safe from sexually transmitted diseases (other than abstinence) is a properly used condom.

Sexuality and Diabetes

Caution

This section is for adults who are on your own, or who as a couple, both want to have sex with each other.

See page 391 for information about birth control.

To protect against unwanted sexually transmitted infections (STIs) use a condom. A condom is also necessary for those who are with a new sex partner. Oral or genital contact can pass sexual infections (such as HIV, or herpes from cold sores) from one person to another. If you are unsure of the risk of your partner's health, please talk to an STI nurse (at a confidential toll-free phone line). She can also help you and your partner to take precautions for intercourse, oral sex or other sexual activity to protect yourself from STIs.

To find a toll-free phone number search "STI hotline" and the area that you live. STIs are sometimes called STDs (sexually transmitted diseases) so you could also search "STD hotline."

Lovemaking offers the following benefits:

- It is a wonderful way to be intimate.
- It increases your circulation.
- It tightens and then relaxes muscles.
- It releases hormones that relax you.
- It can help you sleep.
- It decreases blood sugar if your session is active or long lasting.

Good solutions for sexual changes and diabetes

The Diabetes Complications section, on pages 49–50, covered information about the types and causes of sexual changes. This explained how high blood sugar over many years can lead to blood vessel and nerve damage to your sexual organs. Men can have difficulty getting an erection (called erectile dysfunction), to different degrees. Vaginal dryness and sensitivity changes can occur in women. Diabetes can also make you tired or contribute to depression, so you may be less interested in sex.

Some gradual sexual changes are a natural part of aging. A man's penis may not get as firm as quickly as when he was younger, and a woman's sexual response may be slower than when she was younger. This is normal and shouldn't be confused with not being able to have sex. If sex takes longer and is softer, this still leaves room for fun and pleasure.

Just because you have diabetes, or are getting older, does not mean you will develop sexual changes. You can stop or reduce problems with an open mind, regular exercise and eating well. Exercise stimulates blood vessels throughout your body, including to your sexual organs! Try to keep your blood sugar, cholesterol and blood pressure at healthy levels.

Today's society bombards us with sexual images, yet sex still remains one of the hardest things to talk about. You are not alone if you find it embarrassing to talk about sex to your wife or husband or partner, even if you've shared a bed for five or fifty years. If it is also difficult to talk to your health care provider about sex, please gather the courage to do so. Your doctor is busy and may not ask you about sex – but that doesn't mean he/she can't help you. Please don't suffer in silence.

If you are a man who enjoyed sex in your relationship, and then began to have a slower or softer erection, you may decide it is easier to stop having sex. If you are a woman with dryness or lack of desire, you may turn away from your partner and lose an important part of your relationship. These changes might lead to frustration, and even resentment. Consider talking with your partner about what is important to you as individuals and as a couple.

It's worth it to look for solutions if you or your partner struggle with sexual changes. Hopefully, after you read through this section, it will be easier to start the conversation. Along with talking to each other, try talking to your doctor or another health professional. If possible, see a sexual therapist with your partner.

Sexuality and sexual intimacy

Much of our sexuality is between our ears, rather than between our legs. Sexuality is how you feel about yourself, your body and your gender. It's the way you express yourself in how you dress, hold yourself and smile. It's the friends you have and the compliments you give each other. Talking, laughing, sharing and touching are all part of sexuality. It is about others appreciating you, just for who you are. You may not have a sexual partner, but you are still sexual. This is part of all of us.

Sexual intimacy is something you share with one person only, that you do with no one else. It is the knowledge that you have of how your body, and your partner's body, functions. Pleasure and fun are key – even as you get older and your body changes.

What's a sex therapist?

This is a counselor who specializes in loving relationships. A sex therapist understands the importance of sex in your partnership. He or she also has suggestions for how to cope with physical and emotional issues that may come up. To find one near you; search "sexual therapist" on the internet or go to www.aasect.org

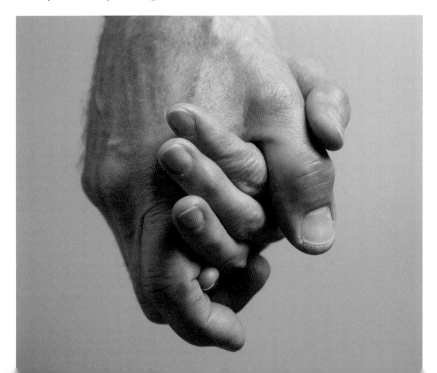

Sexuality is also about the way others treated you as a child, teenager or adult. If there is hurt or abuse in your past, this affects how you feel about yourself and sex. It may be difficult for you to get close to another through sexual intimacy. As a result, you may not choose sex to be part of your life. Other things may fill your life instead. You may have had an unhappy sexual relationship in the past, and be struggling to be comfortable with sex from a caring person who is now part of your life. If you feel at any time that you need support from a counselor, please seek it.

A couple's sexual life can vary like different kinds of car rides. Everyone likes a different kind of ride: fast, slow, smooth or rough, frequent, just occasional, or not at all. Some couples have the same or opposite sexual appetite. It might be high, or low. Some feel sex is a disappointment or chore. Perhaps it's an invigorating and important part of life, especially as you get older, and have more time. Many men and women come into their peak sensuality in their forties or fifties, and beyond.

Six approaches to sexual changes

The first approach is to take steps to make yourself a healthier person so that your blood flow and nerve stimulation to your sexual organs improves. Exercise and eating well are very important. The second and third approach is to allow yourself self-fulfillment and if needed, the use of lubricants, whether you are on your own or part of a couple.

The last three approaches are primarily for couples, although if you are single, some of the information is suitable for you also. In the fourth approach you'll find ideas for romance and intimacy, and different positions for more comfortable sex. The fifth approach is to use medications (to enhance erections or sex drive) or an erection device (such as a penis ring or vacuum pump). Whether you choose medications or a device may depend on how much sexual change you experience, costs, and the possible side effects of the treatments. The last, but not least thing is that you may not want to take more pills or rely on erection devices. Instead explore other ways to enhance the totality of your sexual experience (Approach 4, pages 397–399) and bedroom alternatives (Approach 6, page 407–411).

> Whichever way you choose, these six approaches offer a potential to make your sex life *better*.

1) Boost your circulation and nerves

- **Keep your blood sugar in good control.** Improved blood sugar can, in some cases, actually reverse some of the damage to your blood vessels and nerves. Then erectile dysfunction or vaginal sensitivity can improve. When your blood sugar is in good control, you are energized and ready for sex.

- **Keep your blood pressure and blood cholesterol in good control, and try to quit smoking.** These changes also improve the health of your blood vessels – now more blood flows to the penis or vagina.

If you are a man who smokes, you are more likely to have difficulty with erections than someone who doesn't smoke. This is because smoking narrows your blood vessels. It also reduces how much nitric oxide you make (see below, under Exercise). If you are a smoker, please think of this as one more important reason to quit. See "Becoming a Non Smoker" on pages 263–280.

- **Eat a healthy diet.** Nutrition that is good for your heart is also good for your sexual organs (see pages 119–121). Antioxidants and nutrients help keep blood vessels and nerves in your genitals healthy.

- **Exercise regularly.** Exercise helps increase the flow of blood and oxygen to your sexual organs. Exercise stimulates your blood vessels to produce something called nitric oxide. This helps arouse a man's or woman's sexual organs.

Do you take pills for depression or high blood pressure? Some men find these pills affect their ability to have a firm erection. The good news is that regular exercise can help improve your blood pressure as well as your mood. Then your doctor may be able to change or reduce your medication.

Being active also helps both men and women feel up to having sex. Whether you have a large or small body, you can keep fit by regular walking and a proper diet. When you are fit, you will have more flexibility and stamina for sex.

Toning up can help you, as a man or woman, feel sexier.

- **Limit or avoid alcohol.** While the first drink can relax you, the second drink or more can slow or stop a man's erection.

Schedule a doctor's appointment for a complete physical.

- *Your doctor can rule out other causes (besides diabetes) for erection changes, vaginal dryness, or decreased sex drive for men or women. Medications such as some blood pressure pills and anti-depressants can cause a lower sex drive or other problems. If you are on these pills, ask if there are other options.*

- *If you have had a recent heart attack or surgery talk to your doctor about when it is safe for you to have sex. Generally sex is safe if you can tolerate light – moderate exercise.*

- *Your doctor may refer you to a urologist or gynecologist. With this doctor, you can discuss concerns about your sex drive, arousal or genital functioning.*

- *Ask about going to a diabetes education center. There, you can get advice on how to improve your blood sugar, cholesterol and blood pressure.*

2) Self-fulfillment

You may be widowed, divorced or single, and do not currently have a sexual partner. You may be married or with a partner but not be in a sexual relationship. You are still a sexual person. You can still do things that are sexually and/or emotionally fulfilling. Whether or not you are in a sexual relationship, the first step in nurturing the sexual part of yourself is to look after "you." Sometimes we are so busy looking after others or working that we forget to nurture ourselves. This means taking time to relax and do things that we enjoy (see Step 6, Staying Upbeat pages 354–364).

Non-sexual physical closeness

- companionship with a special friend
- visit with grandchildren
- touch (as outlined on page 362) – from a hair cut to a foot massage
- talk to, and pet and play with your dog or cat
- keep your treasured memories of loved ones close to your heart by looking at photo albums and mementos, and listening to music.

Sexual self-fulfillment

Masturbation helps your body make "happy hormones" (endorphins). It can help you relieve tension and sleep better at night. It also helps keep your erectile tissue (in a man's penis or woman's clitoris) elastic and healthy. Some men or women use a lubricant or vibrator (page 397 and 411), and find this enhances their experience.

- **Women:** Some women say that as they got older they became more comfortable with their own body. They now know what feels good, and what visual stimulation or thoughts they need to orgasm. Masturbating may be more natural.

- **Men:** Are you a man without a sexual partner, and with a low sex drive or erectile dysfunction? You may be interested to know that erection enhancement medications or devices used by couples, can be used by a man alone to either enhance or enable masturbation. This would include erection pills, vacuum devices, penis rings or local therapies (creams, pellets or injections) used on the penis itself to get or maintain an erection. All of these will be discussed on pages 402–406.

Walking and keeping physically active helps keep your body fit. This gives you energy and drive to do things – including masturbation.

3) Lubricants

If you feel dry during sex or masturbation you may want to consider buying some "personal lubricant." You can buy it off-the-shelf at your local pharmacy. It can be used by men or women. If you put it on your genitals, it helps them feel smooth so sexual activity is easier. For women with diabetes who are dry during sex, using a lubricant can help reduce the risk of a yeast infection (see pages 301–304 for more information).

- Start with a water-based lubricant such as K-Y, Astroglide, Wet or Sliquid, or less expensive store brands.

- If you find the water-based lubricant dries out too quickly, you may want to try a silicone-based lubricant. However, this type is difficult to wash off yourself and your sheets, and should not be used with silicone sex toys.

- Lubricants are sold in drugstores in single packets, tubes or small bottles.

- Avoid "warming" lubricants or those with flavors or colors which can irritate your skin. Flavored lubricants may also have sugar added which might make you more likely to get a vaginal or urinary tract infection.

Caution

Don't use oil-based creams or Vaseline as a lubricant! These can break a condom. These are also more difficult to wash off your body after sex, and may stain your clothes or sheets.

Check the best-before date to make sure the lubricant you are using is not expired. Apply lubricant with clean hands to prevent bacteria getting into the lubricant, or use single-packet lubricants only.

Vaginal Moisturizers

*Vaginal moisturizers are **not** the same thing as lubricants. This is a product used by women to keep their vagina feeling moist for several days in a row. It's a good idea to try lubricants first. Then, if you are still having pain with vaginal dryness you could try a vaginal moisturizer to see if it helps. Common brands are Replens, Gyne-Moistrin, Hylafem and K-Y Liquibeads. You have to use an applicator to insert the moisturizer up into your vagina. Usually you put it in every day for a week, and then 2–3 times a week for ongoing moisturizing. Some of them can cause a harmless white discharge to later leak out of your vagina.*

Joyce's story:

I started having problems with dryness, and intercourse was painful. After a while I started finding reasons to not do it. I knew it was affecting my relationship with my husband, but I didn't know what to do about it. When I went to see the diabetes nurse for my six-month appointment, I decided to talk to her about this.

She asked me if I had ever tried a lubricant. I didn't really even know what this was. She explained that you could buy a little tube for about five bucks in the pharmacy. She suggested a water-based lubricant. This may seem funny to you, but I had to ask her where do I put it? She told me that just before intercourse to squeeze out a blob of lubricant (about the size of the tip of my pinky finger to begin with). Then, to open my legs and use my fingers to spread it over my clitoris, labia, around my vagina and even a little bit inside my vagina.

I tried it, and you have no idea what a difference this made. It removed the dryness, and sex was comfortable again. When I think back how simple the solution was, and yet it took me so long to discover it.

4) Build intimacy

Nurture yourself and your relationship outside of your normal household activities. It is important to make time for yourself, and for each other. Spending time together gives you a chance to talk, have fun, renew your friendship and build intimacy. Then you will be more comfortable talking about and considering new approaches to managing sexual changes. It may mean that as a couple you will decide to try an erection medication or erection device (Approach 5). You may also want to explore new bedroom techniques (Approach 6).

Improve your sexual relationship through good communication. Talk about what's important to you.

Nurture your relationship and celebrate each other
Eat meals together so you have time to talk.

Every day, do something with your partner, even if it is something small. Give each other compliments. Say thank you. Turn off the TV and computer, and go for a walk together. Hold hands. A touch, kiss and hug are all very good too. Be gentle and kind; make your partner feel good, and you will feel good too.

Plan a regular date night – and stick to it. Watch a romantic movie or enjoy a meal, just the two of you. You're never too old for romance.

In your relationship with your partner, focus on each other as individuals with unique feelings. You each have your own bodies – bodies that aren't perfect, but that can be sensual and sexy. No matter your size or shape, what makes you sexy is what is inside – your desire to give and receive.

Put more intimacy into your relationship
Think about things that you could do as a couple that will help you focus more on increasing touch, fun and pleasure in the time you spend with each other. Consider:

Accepting sexual change is difficult, but it doesn't mean giving up sexual intimacy.

- **A sensual massage:** Rub in body cream or body oil. For some, a back massage or foot massage is a satisfying experience. It doesn't have to lead to further activity.

- **A sexual massage:** You may take the massage one step further and massage sexual parts of your partner's body. This could lead to one of you masturbating (or both of you together), or one of you helping the other. If you aren't sure how to do this as a couple, ask your partner how he/she normally does it when alone. Ask him/her to show you how. A lubricant helps to relieve dryness and enhance pleasure for both of you (see page 397).

Accommodate your special needs when having sex

You may have aches and pains or you may have a disability. Small changes in your sexual pattern can help enhance or bring back sex and intimacy into your life.

A short session or a long one?

Sometimes you may be up to just a short session. Maybe only one of you needs relief at that moment. It's okay to make it a quickie and move on. Other times it's nice to stretch out lovemaking in the afternoon or early evening. Don't always leave sex until later. At bedtime, you may have no energy left.

Comfortable positions

Do you have arthritis, back pain or a disability that makes sexual activity difficult or painful? Sometimes a simple change like a pillow to support a man or woman's back or under a woman's hips can make a difference. Consider trying new sex positions than your "usual." You may want to talk, laugh about it and experiment with positions that feel comfortable for you both. There are no rules for positioning that work for everyone. Discuss different positions with your partner – just talking about this can itself help build excitement and intimacy.

Helpful tips prior to sexual activity:

- *Be well rested.*
- *Relax and try not to think about your worries.*
- *Don't drink excess alcohol or take street drugs.*
- *Don't eat a heavy meal.*
- *Choose a room that is warm (not cold or hot).*
- *Men, you may find erections are more likely at certain times of the day or evening. This will depend on when you take your pills, and how you and your partner feel.*

Sex is as individual as each of our personalities. Remember, good communication is essential to building intimacy.

Here are some ideas for male/female couples:

If fatigue or reduced erection hardness makes intercourse too strenuous or difficult, consider alternatives. This might include using a vibrator or other adult toy (see page 411). It also might include oral sex. If this isn't something you have done before but you want to try it, please read pages 407–410.

- If her back, knees or hips hurts: With the man on top in "missionary" position, place a small pillow beneath her lower back or a wedge pillow behind her knees for support. To take pressure off her hips, he can try putting his legs outside her legs. Placing a pillow under her buttocks can be helpful if both couples are large.

- If his back, hips or knees hurt (or he is quite large): Try sex with the woman on top, then the man doesn't have to support his own weight. This is often also a very pleasurable position for a woman. A small pillow or towel under the man's back may also help.

- If you both have sore knees: 1) Try lying or standing in spoon position (man behind woman, with his chest to her back, with both of you facing the same direction). 2) If lying down, a pillow between your knees can help too. 3) If standing, the woman can lean on a table or high bed for support (to take weight off her knees) and the man enters from behind. This rear-entry position can work for some larger couples, especially if the woman leans forward (or moves closer to the edge of the bed and the man stands).

- Books or DVDs on sex can give you lovemaking ideas. You may find ideas for new sex positions that are more stimulating and comfortable for you. Look for resources that present sexual options for self-stimulation or for adult couples in a respectful way for both of you. Just because you see it on TV or the internet, don't feel pressured to use anything or do anything you are not comfortable with.

Do you have a fear of urinary incontinence during sexual activity?
It helps to empty your bladder and shower just prior to sexual activity. Taking other steps long before intercourse also help. Drink water to keep your urine clear, pee regularly, and limit coffee, tea, alcohol and smoking. This helps reduce bladder irritation so you are less likely to have leakage. Constipation can contribute to incontinence so exercise daily, eat lots of fiber and drink water. Regularly doing easy exercises (kegels) to keep your pelvic muscles strong is important (on the internet, search "kegel exercises for women" or "kegel exercises for men").

If you have a physical disability such as a spinal cord injury or are fully dependent on a wheelchair: Consider reading "pleasureABLE: Sexual Device Manual for Persons with Disabilities." Search for "DHRN sex manual" on the internet.

5) Medications and erection devices

If getting or maintaining an erection is a concern, talk to your doctor. Your doctor may suggest and prescribe either medications or erection devices, or both. In some cases your doctor may refer you to a urologist. This section explains these medications and devices and how they work.

Doctors most commonly recommend erection drugs, such as Viagra-like drugs (called PDE5's). If your hormones are low, the doctor may recommend taking testosterone for men or estrogen for women. Rather than medications, your doctor might recommend a penis pump (a device shaped like a cylinder, that creates a vacuum to make the penis go hard, and then is removed). Another option is an erection medication called prostaglandin, that can be applied on or into the penis.

Some couples wish to explore sexual options that don't involve medication or the use of erection devices. These "bedroom alternatives" takes longer to discuss in the doctor's office. Some doctors don't take the time to mention these options. If you wish to learn more, please see pages 407–411.

Surgically placing inflatable rods into the penis would be the last resort for the treatment of advanced erectile dysfunction when other methods have not worked. This is surgery done by a specialized urologist and is not covered in this book. For more information about this surgery you can search "penis implants" on the internet.

Talk to your doctor

Different medications and devices have varying levels of effectiveness and safety. If one option isn't appropriate for you (due to your health or other medications you are taking), your doctor will likely be able to suggest something else. Likewise, if you try a treatment and it doesn't work, your doctor can recommend another option. It's important to know how to take a medication and how much, and how to safely use an erection device. Each treatment has both benefits and side effects. Do not order devices or drugs over mail order or the internet, unless your doctor has recommended it and you know it is government approved as safe.

Herbal products or other over-the counter products

Prior to the use of Viagra and the other PDE5s, doctors sometimes prescribed the herb yohimbine hydrochloride to help with erections. Today, doctors rarely prescribe it as the PDE5s are more effective. Yohimbine has risks, and only mild and inconsistent benefits.

There are a variety of drugs sold over-the-counter and on the internet that say they will improve an erection. These drug advertisements and lower prices may be tempting, but beware they are often counterfeit. They are virtually useless except in the mildest cases of erectile dysfunction. Researchers have not done proper scientific trials on these drugs. Some of these products have been found to have no medication, while others have a dangerous amount of medication or additives. **Do not take them!**

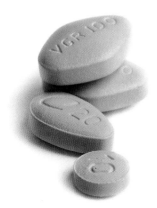

If one type of PDE5 pill does not work for you, it's worthwhile to try one of the other ones. Talk to your doctor.

Caution

Doctors don't prescribe Viagra or the other PDE5 inhibitors if you take nitroglycerine. They also may not recommend them if you have:

- decreased liver or kidney function.
- very low or high blood pressure.
- recently had a heart attack or stroke, or other heart conditions
- certain eye disorders.

It is wise to learn about the risks as well as the highly advertised benefits. **Talk to your doctor.**

Viagra and other PDE5 inhibitors

These pills help fill the penis with blood. *They will not increase your sex drive, per se.* To make this kind of drug work, you need to combine it with foreplay so you will feel excited and get hard.

The medical name for these pills is phosphodiesterase type 5 inhibitors, or PDE5s. They include:

- sildenafil (Viagra)
- vardenafil (Levitra)
- avanafil (Stendra) – approved for sale in the USA, but not Canada
- tadalafil (Cialis) – long acting

Sildenafil, vardenafil and avanafil work over a 4-6 hour period. Tadalafil lasts in your system for up to 36 hours, which means you could consider having sex anywhere in that 1½-2 day period. Whichever PDE5 drug you use, you should wait about one hour after taking it before you have sex.

High fat meals affect your body's absorption of the short-acting PDE5's including Viagra, Levitra and Stendra. Don't eat a greasy, heavy meal, or you may find these pills won't work as well. What you eat does not affect Cialis as it is longer acting than the other two. Some people wonder if drinking alcohol will affect how these pills work. The answer is that you can drink alcohol with these pills, but drinking too much alcohol affects anyone's sexual abilities, so avoid alcohol or drink only in moderation.

If you use PDE5's regularly, it can get costly, and they are not covered under most drug plans. Fortunately, some of these pills are now available as generics (non-brand names), which are cheaper, and you may also be able to buy brand name PDE5's at the same lower price. Call a pharmacist to get a price.

Although PDE5's are a great option for many men with diabetes, they may not be right for you. Talk to your doctor about other options listed on pages 403–406.

Side Effects of PDE5 inhibitors

You may get a headache, stuffy nose, flushed face, mild vision changes, or indigestion after taking one of these pills. Go back to your doctor after you have tried it. If this happens, discuss dosage and any effects you've noticed. Also, although very rare, if an erection lasts longer than four hours, see an Emergency doctor right away. If you experience a loss of vision or hearing, which is also very rare, stop use of the pills. Go see a doctor or specialist right away.

Hormones for men or women

If blood tests indicate an imbalance of your sex hormones, your doctor may recommend taking hormones. Testosterone for men, and estrogen for women.

Testosterone: Both men and women have testosterone in their bodies, but men have a much larger amount. It has an important role in a man's sex drive. Men typically have a steady decrease in their testosterone levels as a natural part of aging. Men with diabetes are more likely to have low testosterone levels. Bringing the testosterone level back to a normal level can help a man's sex drive, and help him ejaculate or reach orgasm easier. It may or may not help erections. To help with erections, men usually need in addition to take PDE5 pills or use an erection device. The PDE5s work better with a normal level of testosterone. A doctor may prescribe testosterone as a pill, a gel or cream, or by injection.

Taking testosterone may not improve your erection, but it usually helps improve your sexual desire and energy.

Estrogen: Both women and men have estrogen in their bodies, but women have a much larger amount. As a woman gets older, estrogen continues to have benefits including keeping her bones strong. Estrogen helps with natural vaginal lubrication and comfort. Estrogen decreases in women after menopause. To enhance a woman's sex drive or decrease vaginal dryness, a doctor may prescribe estrogen. This can be prescribed as a pill, skin gel (that you rub on your arm) or as a patch (that you stick on your skin). Alternately, an estrogen cream can be put around the vagina, or a tablet, cream or ring containing estrogen can be placed inside the vagina.

Estrogen can increase blood sugar. Women often find they have blood sugar swings during their period. Their blood sugar usually increases before and during menstruation. When estrogen levels change during menopause, this can cause blood sugar swings.

While estrogen has many benefits in the body, post-menopausal women may be cautioned by their doctor against taking an estrogen supplement as it may increase the risk for breast cancer, heart disease and stroke for certain women. It also increases blood sugar. However, in many cases, the benefits of taking estrogen may be greater than the risks. Fortunately, lower doses of hormones (both estrogen and testosterone) carry less risk. Low doses still have benefits.

Please discuss with your doctor the benefits and risks of taking hormones, whether it's testosterone or estrogen.

Caution

If you have a bleeding condition or are on blood thinners such as Warfarin, penis rings and pumps can increase your chance of bruising.

Hinge effect

The vacuum pump helps the small tubes in the outer part of your penis become erect, but not the inner tubes of your penis that attach to your pelvic bone (so there is no strut, or brace, for the erection). This means the erection you get with a vacuum device and held by a ring, may pivot at the base (called the "hinge effect"). During sex, some men find it helpful to adjust their angle to avoid slipping out of their partner, especially for missionary position. Some couples who use the pump find that female-on-top position works well.

Penis rings and vacuum pumps

When used properly, a penis ring or a penis vacuum pump can be a very good non-medicinal option for men with erection problems. You can buy them without a prescription, however beware, there are many cheap, poor quality, or used products sold on the internet. So you don't harm your penis, buy good quality and **always follow the manufacturer's directions** (see box on page 405).

A penis ring: If you are able to get an erection but can't hold it as long as you'd like, a penis ring is an inexpensive, effective option for you. It is a special rubber ring that you can stretch and place at the base of your penis once you start getting hard. Some find that just a little lubrication at the base of the penis or on the ring, can help ease the ring on. The ring then helps keep you firm. Do not leave the ring on longer than 30 minutes. Never use a regular rubber band, this could cause serious harm.

Some men buy a device especially designed to help put on the penis ring, or use a hard plastic pipe fitting from a hardware store called a "coupling" (that looks like a napkin ring) and comes in different sizes. It should fit over your erection, but not be too big – so you can stretch the ring over it. Slip the device (with the attached ring) over your penis as far as it will go. Then carefully slide the ring off to the base of your penis.

A penis vacuum pump: This uses a specially designed pump *and* a penis ring. The vacuum pump is a hard plastic tube (or cylinder). You manually pump out the air around your penis creating a vacuum and the ring will hold the erection. See diagram below. If your hand strength is poor, consider buying a pump that is battery-operated. Using the pump takes a bit of practice, but can be an effective solution with few side effects. This makes it a good alternative to medications.

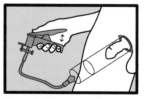

Step 1. Place sterile lubricant on the base of your penis to allow for a good seal. Then, place the plastic tube around your penis.

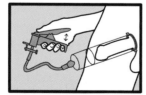

Step 2. Using a stop-and-go action, pump out the air around your penis using the hand-held pump. This creates a vacuum and helps draw blood into your penis. An erection will be created within a few to ten minutes.

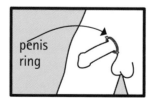

Step 3. There is a penis ring attached to the base of the plastic tube. Once your penis enlarges, you slip the ring off the tube and over the base of your penis. This holds the erection. Then you remove the plastic tube. If you use a condom, have it all ready, and put it on at this time.

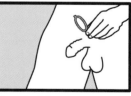

Step 4. After sex, you remove the penis ring and the erection will go down. The ring should not be left on longer than 30 minutes.

(You can watch an instructional video online at youtube.com search "Osbon ErecAid").

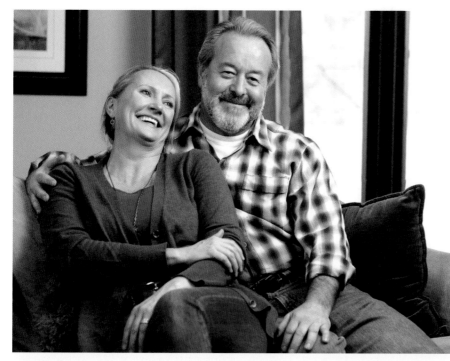

Ron's Story:

My wife and I have enjoyed a loving sex life together. But about a year ago I noticed changes in me. I couldn't get as hard as I used to or I'd lose it quickly. I thought this was just because I was getting older. Then I was reading that diabetes could cause this, and I have had diabetes for 11 years.

We talked about Viagra, but I didn't want to take any more medications with my diabetes. We looked into other options and decided to order a vacuum erection device (a pump).

When we got the pump, it made us laugh, as it was kind of bigger than we expected! The instructions said that if you haven't had erections for a while, that it is important to take your time learning to use the pump. The first time I used it, I pumped slowly, and released the vacuum, and pumped slowly again, and repeated this a few times over 10 minutes. I felt a pulling, but I didn't get an erection. I felt disappointed, but then I realized that it wasn't going to work the first time. So like the instructions said, over the next two weeks I practiced on my own. After about a week of practice I was able to get an erection. I held the pump on and kept my erection for about a minute, then released the vacuum, and repeated it once or twice. Soon I felt comfortable to pump at the right speed and pressure to create an erection. The second week I also practiced a couple of times putting the ring on to keep the erection. Now I can get an erection in about 2-3 minutes using the pump.

Then it was time to try it together! I got ready for bed as usual, and brushed my teeth, then I pumped myself erect and slipped on the ring to keep me erect. I came to bed and we started with intimate touch and foreplay. When we were ready, my wife went on top and she helped insert my penis. Without telling you more of our private details, I can say we got it to work! My wife did mention that my penis felt less warm than normal, but otherwise she said I felt hard – and we had fun again.

That was about six months ago. I feel happier and I have a reason to be healthy and fit, so I've started walking more. I'm even thinking about quitting smoking. Now that my wife and I have tried this, we both feel a bit more open to talk about these things. Sometimes we can have intercourse using just the penis ring, without the pump, but more often we need them both. The vacuum pump is probably not for everyone, but it's been really good for us both.

If you feel comfortable to talk to your doctor or urologist, ask him to recommend a brand of vacuum pump or penis ring. The doctor, or doctor's nurse, can explain how to use them.

Where to buy a pump: 1) at a medical supply store, 2) ask a pharmacist to order one in for you, or 3) purchase at an online store such as Amazon.com, or search brand names: for example, a top-of-the line quality pump is about $500 from Osbon, and lower cost acceptable versions are available from Encore or Augusta for $150–$250. The penis rings bought on their own usually cost under $20. Some drug plans cover these costs. After a year or two, the one-time cost of a vacuum pump is for many people a cheaper option than erection medications that cost $10 or more for *each time.*

Applying erection drugs on or in the penis

Prostaglandin EI, also called alprostadil, is a prescription erection drug that can boost blood flow into the penis. It can be delivered in three ways: 1) injected into the penis (ICI), 2) put into the end of the penis as a small pill (MUSE), or 3) dispensed on the head of the penis as a cream (Vitaros).

ICI – a penis injection

The medical name for this is IntraCavernosal Injection or ICI. Alprostadil often works better in combination with another two drugs called papaverine and phentolamine, called trimix (or "Triple P"). Another combination is called bimix and doesn't have the alprostadil. You would inject the drug(s) into the side of your penis. You give the injection about ten minutes before intercourse (or masturbation). It can last up to an hour. These drugs create an erection by increasing the blood flow to the penis. They work best when you are relaxed, and aroused and stimulated. Although not effective in all men with diabetes, for some it can be effective. Some men find ICI produces a more firm erection than PDE5 inhibitors.

MUSE – a penis pill

MUSE is short for "Medicated Urethral System for Erection." Instead of an injection, a small dose of alprostadil (as a tiny pellet) is gently put in the end of your penis. This is done about ten minutes before intercourse. It stimulates an erection, but is not as effective as ICI in men with diabetes, and is expensive. However, if you don't like the idea of using an injection this might be worth a try.

Vitaros – a penis cream

This is an alprostadil cream that you drip into your urethral opening and rub on the head of your penis. It is quickly absorbed and can work in five minutes. This new application looks promising for men without severe erectile dysfunction.

Ask your doctor or urologist, or the doctor's nurse, to show you (or you and your partner) how to use ICI, MUSE or Vitaros.

Intimacy grows from partnership when using an erection medication or device.

Before you buy or use an erection medication or erection device, talk to your partner. If you think you might both be interested in trying one of these new things, then go together to see your doctor or urologist. This can help you both be more comfortable to talk more about it with each other. To increase intimacy and fun, incorporate your use of the erection medication or device into your overall sexual experience with your partner. For example, your wife or partner can place the "blue pill" or vacuum pump on your bedside table as a seductive suggestion for the evening. As part of your sexual foreplay, your partner, might do the ICI injection for you, or help you pump up your penis. This involvement can enhance sexual desire and intimacy.

Side Effects

Alprostadil can cause aching in the penis for some men. If this is a problem for you, bimix (which doesn't have alprostadil), might be an alternative for you. If you give yourself an ICI injection regularly, there is a very small risk of scarring at the injection site. In an occasional case your erection may stay hard (and hurt) so try ejaculating or an ice pack to reduce the erection. Although rare, if your erection does not go down after four hours, see your doctor right away (or go to Emergency). This problem can be prevented with proper technique and dose of medication. Discuss this with your doctor ahead of time.

6) *Bedroom alternatives*

Some couples decide they don't find medical therapies effective or that the pills and devices are too expensive, or just don't fit their lifestyles. Some are looking for more "natural" alternatives to try in their bedroom. If the male partner is unable to have or maintain a hard erection you may be looking for alternatives to intercourse.

Perhaps you would like to consider new ways of lovemaking? It's okay if you feel a bit embarrassed about it. Don't let this stop you from trying to make each other feel good! If you have physical limitations to intercourse, or are a man having some erection changes, or a woman having a decrease in sensation or desire, your sexual life may be different – but it doesn't have to end. In the past, your sex may have included a small amount of foreplay, followed by intercourse. Now, consider having more touch and foreplay, with or without the penetration. Sometimes changes require creative solutions. If the old way that you always did something isn't working any more, then try something different.

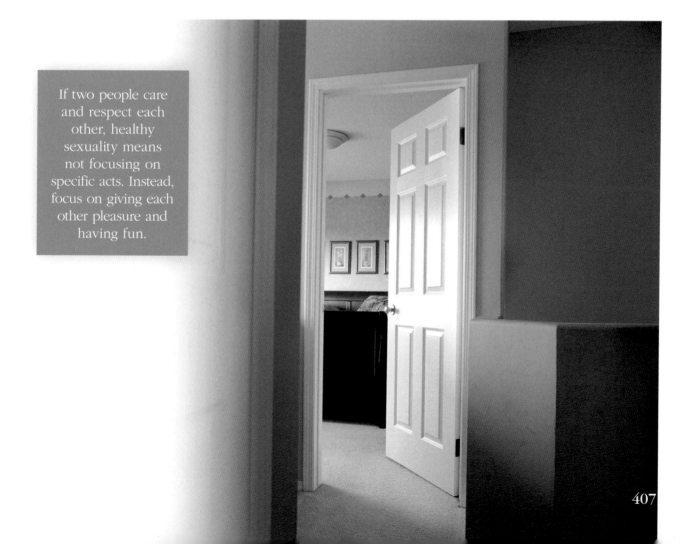

If two people care and respect each other, healthy sexuality means not focusing on specific acts. Instead, focus on giving each other pleasure and having fun.

Ideas to give pleasure to your woman
with vaginal dryness, decreased sensation or desire.

Gentle lips and hands, and kind and encouraging words make you a great lover. Say every word that you can think of that means she is beautiful and sexy. She needs to hear this – over and over. She needs to know you want her. She needs to be touched in her special places and in ways that only you know.

One of the most exciting things for many people is seeing your partner aroused. If you are not sure what feels arousing for your wife or partner, then ask her. Even if you've been married for 40 years, it's never too late to ask! Every person is different in what feels good.

Kiss her, and touch her love spots – perhaps her neck, back, ear lobes, lips, fingertips, nipples and vagina area. Keep asking her, "Where does it feel good?" Her clitoris is tiny compared to a penis but you might be surprised to know it has all the same parts: a covering like a foreskin, a shaft, and a head. Save touching her sensitive clitoris for last. She will tell you if she wants less or more touch.

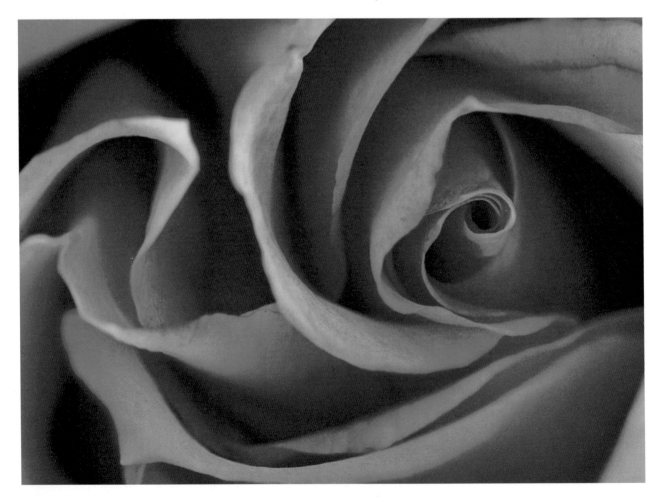

Women can enjoy orgasms from direct genital stimulation without intercourse. For example, she may be able to orgasm by rubbing her clitoris on your leg or penis (soft or erect). Ask her if you may put a generous dab of lubricant on her genitals. Gently touch her there. Some women also want direct stimulation to the vagina. Stroke the inside of her thighs. If she opens her legs for you, you know she is ready for more. For men who don't want to attempt penetration, she may invite you to enter her slowly with your finger. Make sure your nails are short, smooth and clean. You may also want to try using a vibrator or dildo (see page 411). If you can get her excited, and sometimes bring her to orgasm, this is awesome! You may feel yourself moving in that direction too. Most women do not have orgasms every time they have sexual intimacy (and some never do) but they can still enjoy being with their partner and being intimate.

For information on over-the-counter lubricants or moisturizers for dryness, see page 397.

If she would like, would you be comfortable giving her oral sex? If so, this would mean using your lips and tongue to stimulate her genitals. If this is new, it may be embarrassing to her. If you are respectful and loving, you can help her relax. She may want to try this intimate experience. If she has vaginal dryness, then your mouth will keep her wet and comfortable.

Sexual experiences that don't focus mostly on penal-vaginal intercourse are different, but can still be intimate and arousing for you both. The key is to add in something else for each of you. The sensual attention that you give your woman, she can give back to you (see next page) for a joint erotic experience.

Never try to force or coerce each other. Sexual activities should be comfortable for you both.

Preventing urinary tract infections (UTIs)

Showering together, or separately if you prefer, is a good way to start off a love making session. This helps you both relax, and leaves you both fresh and clean. To prevent vaginal or urinary tract infections, the partner needs to then avoid anal contact (where germs lie). Also avoid giving a woman oral sex if you yourself have diabetes and have a gum, mouth or tongue infection. It is also really important that the woman's genitals are well lubricated. Without lubrication, friction can cause tiny cuts and can lead to a yeast infection.

For information on preventing UTIs see pages 301–304. For information on sexually transmitted infections, see page 392.

Ideas to give pleasure to your man
with erectile dysfunction or decreased desire.

When you care about your partner and your relationship, and want intimacy, it is sometimes helpful to take a more active role in the bedroom. One of the things that turns your man on the most is seeing you excited. If in the past, you tended to lay back and let him take charge, then think about a change. At first, trying new things in the bedroom can be intimidating, and feel awkward. But over time it becomes more natural. Giving pleasure with your mouth (oral sex) is something you may wish to consider. In some cases, this can be a stepping stone back to intercourse. If you have never tried it with your man, or want a bit more practice, then read on. These three easy steps will get you started.

Step one. When you have a few spare moments on your own, wash your hands and give your fingers a relaxing massage. Sip on some water so your mouth is moist. Then gently suck on each of your fingertips. Imagine you have just dipped them into melted chocolate! Tighten your mouth so your finger presses against your lips, but don't bite with your teeth.

Step two. One evening while you are sitting on the couch, maybe watching TV with your husband or partner, ask him if you can wash and massage his hands with a warm washcloth. Then ask him if you can kiss his fingers. At first he may wonder what you are doing, but he may be interested. If he is shy, tell him you don't want sex, you just want to touch him. Once he's comfortable, slowly move his finger in and out of your mouth. He may not be able to take his eyes off you!

Step three. If this has been nice for you both so far, when you feel ready, you may want to go a bit further. Both take a shower and climb into bed. This is your turn to please him – later he can please you. Hold him. Let him know you want intimacy. Touch his back, ears and face, and kiss him gently. As he relaxes, kiss his fingers and let him watch so he will know you want to be with him. Move your hand to touch his penis and scrotum while kissing his fingers. You can start moving down his body kissing his nipples and belly area and still touching his penis with your hand. Take your time with your tongue and lips. Take his penis into your mouth and gently move it in and out of your mouth. Ask him "what feels best?" Watch and you may feel him get a bit firm. He may not become firm if his nerves are unable to give his genitals the signals, but he will still be aroused.

This will be an intimate sharing for you both.

Intimate touch is a very personal thing. What is comfortable for one person may not feel comfortable and safe for you. Holding on to intimacy with the one you care for is important, so help each other discover your own way to be together.

This technique is so stimulating that some men can experience an orgasm without an erection, although it may be less intense.

Adult toys for couples or if you are single

Do you like to use something for fun in your bedroom – such as lingerie, a tie or romantic lighting? Then, you are already using a type of adult toy! Do you have a "personal massager" at home for your back or arms? This is useful for stimulating other parts of your own or your partner's body, either directly or through the vibrations that go to your fingertips. At some point you may even be curious and experiment with a vibrator or dildo.

Vibrators or dildos

Vibrators or dildos come in a variety of shapes and colors. Some are hard (acrylic) or soft (silicone). Vibrators are electrical or battery operated (and can be set on rechargeable pads, like cell phones). Dildos are typically shaped like an erect penis. Dildos are not electrical. A vibrator or dildo can stimulate a man or a woman. These are best used with a water-based lubricant (see page 397). With a little humor and adventure, a vibrator or dildo can become an erotic part of your sexual life.

Strap-on dildo

If you are a man with full or partial erectile dysfunction, you may want to consider a strap-on dildo. This can be a fun way to have intimate relations with your partner without having to worry about getting an erection. You strap a penis-shaped dildo onto your body, just above your own penis. Once firmly attached you can enter your partner the same way you would have with regular sex. While you are wearing the dildo, you and your partner have full body contact with each other. You can have the natural and familiar hip movements of intercourse. Your partner can lubricate and then stimulate your genitals. If you would like to read a story about this, go to this internet link: http://wassersug.medicine.dal.ca/story.pdf

Adult toys as part of your sex life

If this is new, you might feel uncomfortable with having or using, an adult toy. You may wonder if these take the romance out of your lovemaking. If you are on your own, you may wonder if this is too sexual. These are normal thoughts, but adults can have fun with these. If your energy level is low, these can help you have a longer session. If you have a sore back or knees, these can allow for pleasure without stressing your joints. If you or your partner has erectile dysfunction, these can bring back pleasure, without stress and worry about erections. Used in private, these toys may enhance your experience.

Caution

Only buy good quality adult toys. Always ensure they are in good condition and clean before each use. There is some concern about chemicals in soft rubber toys. Covering these with a condom before use is advisable. If you have any allergies, such as to latex, avoid toys made with these.

To avoid causing injury or irritating tender tissues, don't insert a toy too deeply, nor use it roughly, nor too frequently. Using a lubricant is recommended. Women with diabetes may have reduced feeling in their vagina (due to neuropathy) so be careful to avoid injury.

Where to buy adult toys

You can buy adult toys privately on-line or by phone (and have them mailed to you). However, if possible, it's always better to actually see the product. Most of us, perhaps you included, have never been in an adult toy store. Even the thought of it is embarrassing. Consider going with your partner. You will find the store clerks are not embarrassed, and will be helpful.

Diabetes Glossary

A1C   A blood test that measures your average blood sugar over the past three months.

ABC's   Three important diabetes blood tests: **A**1C, **B**lood pressure and blood **C**holesterol.

albumin creatinine ratio (ACR)   A urine test that measures the amount of albumin (a type of protein) in your blood; a sign of kidney damage.

atherosclerosis   Hardening and narrowing of blood vessels.

carbohydrates   Starches, natural sugar from fruits, vegetables and milk, and table sugars.

dialysis   A machine that works like a kidney to filter and clean your blood.

dilated eye exam   A special test done by an optometrist or ophthalmologist to make your pupil go larger so the back of your eye can be examined.

erectile dysfunction   For a man, difficulty getting hard or maintaining an erection.

gastroparesis   Nerve and blood vessel damage in your gut that causes poor digestion.

gestational diabetes   Diabetes that develops during your pregnancy.

GI   See Glycemic index.

glomerulus   Part of the kidney that helps filter and clean your blood.

glycemic index   A rating of how quickly a carbohydrate food raises your blood sugar.

gum disease   A serious bacterial infection of your gums and jaw bone.

infection   A growth of disease-causing germs in your skin or body.

inflammation   Swelling and redness of your tissues.

insulin   A hormone made by your pancreas that moves sugar from your blood to your brain, muscles, tissues and organs.

insulin receptor   These are areas on your body cells that allow insulin to work properly.

low blood sugar   When your blood sugar is under 4 mmol/L (70 mg/dL).

low-calorie sweeteners   Products that taste sweet but are not sugar; they have few calories.

macroalbuminuria   Advanced kidney damage with loss of large amounts of protein (albumin) in your urine.

microalbuminuria   Early kidney damage with loss of small amounts of protein (albumin) in your urine.

nephron   Part of the kidney that helps filter and clean your blood.

neuropathy   Nerve damage that can cause a variety of problems such as skin pain or numbness in your feet.

non-proliferative retinopathy   Early diabetes eye damage.

pancreas   The organ in your body, behind your stomach, that makes insulin.

pre-diabetes   Your blood sugar levels are higher than normal but lower than what is diagnosed as true diabetes.

proliferative retinopathy   Advanced diabetes eye damage.

retinopathy   Diabetes eye damage to the back of the eye.

type 1 diabetes   This is generally diagnosed in children or teenagers, and insulin must be taken as the body does not make insulin.

type 2 diabetes   This type of diabetes most often occurs in adults and is related to being overweight, inactive and genetics.

ulcer   An open wound (sore) with severe skin breakdown.

urinary tract infection   Infection that affect the kidney, bladder or urethra (urine tube).

Index

A

A1C, 14, 315, 340, 343, 344, 349
ABCs, 297, 341
acarbose, 319, 334
ACE inhibitors, 322
acids in foods, 92
    and tooth decay, 107, 297, 298
Actos, 321
acupuncture, 273
addictions, 135, 271, 354, 385
aerobics, 232-33
albumin creatinine ratio (ACR), 341
alcohol, 59, 134-37, 148, 402
    benefits, 136
    limiting, 74, 76, 121, 307, 395
    mixed with energy drinks, 136, 279
    and preventing low blood sugar, 336, 338
    risks, 135-36, 140, 256, 332, 385
Aloe vera, 128
aerobic exercise. *See* exercise
alpha-glucosidase inhibitors, 319
alprostadil, 406
Amaryl, 318
ankle rotations, 81, 239
anti-depressants, 49, 52, 366, 395
antioxidants, 120, 122, 123, 132-33, 156
Apidra, 329
apnea, 53, 362
appetite, poor, 143, 147-48
appointments, 310-14
Aquafit, 230
ARBs, 322
arm chair pushup, 242
arm roll, 242
arthritis, 237, 246, 247-49, 314, 399
aspart, 329
aspartame. *See* low-calorie sweeteners
atherosclerosis, 25
Avandia, 321

B

back health, 244-45
beans, peas and lentils, 193
belief, 358-59
biceps curl, 242
bicycling, 223, 228-29, 234, 237
biguanides, 317
bimix, 406
birth control, 302, 378, 391
bitter melon, 128
blood glucose meters, 300, 331, 345-49
blood pressure, 119-121
    and exercise, 221, 236, 241, 255
    and healthy feet, 283, 286
    improving, 109
    lab tests, 340, 343, 344
    and mouth care, 297
    pills, 322, 332, 385, 395
    and sex, 395
    and sodium, 109
    testing at home, 350

blood sugar, 16-17. *See also* high blood
    sugar; low blood sugar
    and exercise, 221
    and healthy feet, 283
    during illness, 139
    lab tests, 340, 343
    and mouth care, 297
    normal level, 16
    random and fasting, 340, 343, 344
    target, 343, 344, 346
    testing at home, 140, 277, 332, 334, 337,
        340, 345-49, 374, 386
blood vessel damage, 24-25, 38, 44, 51, 342.
    See also high blood sugar
blurring of vision, 38
BMI, 143, 340, 384
bottle feeding, 20, 44, 389, 390
bowel problems, 51, 314
brain food, 360
bread and bagels, 97, 158, 204, 205
breakfasts, 152-58, 202-4
breastfeeding, 44, 382, 387-89
    and alcohol, 135
    and caffeine, 201
    and medications, 316, 322
    protection against diabetes, 15, 20
burgers, 208
Byetta/Bydureon, 320

C

caffeine
    limiting, 121, 140, 201, 279, 362, 285
    mixed with alcohol, 136, 379
calcium-rich foods, 57, 109, 120, 133, 297
calf stretch, 239
calorie counter, 64-66
calories, 96, 134, 135, 158
    apps, 63
    boosting, 143-46
    in meals and snacks, 71, 151, 20
carbohydrate choices, 150
carbohydrates, 85-93, 158, 201, 329, 332, 335
    available, 97, 150, 196-200
cardiologist, 314
cataracts, 38
Cell "Insulin Helpers," 316, 321
cereals, dry, 97, 156, 202
chair exercises, 248-49
chicken, 172, 176, 188, 207
children with diabetes, 368-80
cholesterol, 24, 96, 144, 221, 283, 297, 395
    good and bad, 322, 341
    lab tests, 341, 343, 344
    lowering, 92, 118-21, 127, 152
    pills, 322, 385
Cialis, 402
cinnamon, 127, 152
circulation
    and healthy feet, 283
    and high blood sugar, 24-25
    improving, 81, 221, 232, 238, 264, 362, 395

    measuring, 286
    poor, 27, 30, 224
clothing tips, 231, 303, 361
clutter, reducing, 360
coffee, 78, 92, 121, 278. *See also* caffeine
colds, preventing, 306-7
colesevelam hydrochloride, 319
constipation, 51, 279, 385, 400
cotton wool spots, 40, 41
cranberries and cranberry juice, 152, 304,
    305
cravings, managing, 69, 101, 275-76, 278
Crestor, 322

D

dairy products, 98, 105, 213
dancing, 223, 232-33
dehydration, 136, 138, 140, 307, 379
dental hygienist or dentist, 43, 44, 280, 300,
    314
dentures, 299
depression, 52, 360, 365-66, 386, 392
dermatologist, 296, 314
desserts, 100-108, 215. *See also* recipes
detemir, 326, 331
Diabeta, 318, 331
diabetes. *See also* type 2 diabetes
    common questions, 10-12
    types, 14-15
diabetes education center, 23, 311, 312, 323,
    395
diabetes educator. *See* health care team
diabetes medications, 315-21. *See also*
        insulin; *specific diabetes medications*
    during illness, 139
    and infection, 295, 301
    and low blood sugar, 136, 331, 332, 336,
        337
    during pregnancy, 385
    for teenagers, 378
    and testing blood sugar, 347, 348
    and weight gain, 143
dialysis, 37
Diamicron, 318
diarrhea, 51, 139, 140, 308, 337
dietitian, 36, 51, 63, 277, 312, 314, 329
dilated eye exam, 342, 343, 344
dinners, 168-93
doctor appointments, 310-14, 386, 395
doctors. *See* health care team; *specific types
    of doctors*
driving safety, 338

E

eating out. *See* restaurant meals
ECG (electrocardiogram), 257
elliptical machines, 224, 234, 235, 237
endocrinologist, 310
energy drinks, 136, 373, 379
erectile dysfunction, 50, 392, 395, 396,
    401-6, 410, 411

estimated Glomerular Filtration Rate (eGFR), 341
estrogen, 49, 50, 403
exanatide, 320
exercise, 218-62
    aerobic, 82, 223-237
    benefits of, 121, 148, 221-22, 277, 307, 363, 395
    classes, 233
    flexibility, 238-39, 245
    getting started, 219-220
    and heart problems, 255-58
    high-impact, 31, 219, 255, 260
    on holidays, 77, 81
    and low blood sugar, 136, 256, 262, 337
    low-impact, 223-237, 246-254, 260
    managing setbacks, 254
    precautions, 254-62
    during pregnancy, 383
    recommended amount, 223, 241, 374
    strengthening, 240-45
    and sunlight, 360
    youth, 369, 372, 373, 374-77
eye problems, 38-41, 135
eyes and exercise, 236, 259
eye exam. See dilated eye exam

F
family planning, 391
fats in foods, 95, 96, 99, 105, 119, 145-46, 201
    healthy, 58, 152, 360
    unhealthy, 59, 108
feet and lower legs
    avoiding burns and cuts, 289
    daily foot check, 284-86, 341
    distorted shape, 31, 286
    doctor visit, 286
    dry, cracked skin, 30
    and exercise, 260-61, 283
    foot exam, 341, 343, 344
    hygiene and maintenance, 287-89
    infections, 29-31, 282-93
    managing small problems, 294
    socks and shoes, 290-93
    urgent foot problems, 282, 341
fiber
    high-fiber diet, 51, 97, 193, 201, 336, 385
    soluble, 119, 128, 152
    types, 92
Fitness Plan 1 (least active), 247-49
Fitness Plan 2 (active), 250
Fitness Plan 3 (most active), 252
flavorings, 104, 110, 120, 148
flu, preventing, 306-7
fluids, sugar-free, 140, 141
Food Guide, Hands-On, 55-59
food labels, 94-99, 101-3, 111
food poisoning, 308
food record, 62-63
fruits, 56, 98

G
gastroenterologist, 314
gastroparesis, 51, 308

genital problems, 49-50
gestational diabetes, 15, 381-86, 391. See also pregnancy
gifts, healthy, 372
ginkgo biloba, 126, 127
ginseng, 126, 127
glargine, 326, 331
glaucoma, 38
glibenclamide, 318
gliclazide, 318, 331
glimepiride, 318, 331
glitazones, 321
glomeruli, 34-36
Glucobay, 319, 334
GlucoNorm, 318
Glucophage, 317
glucose tablets, 262, 334, 335, 336
glulisine, 329
Glumetza, 317
glyburide, 126, 318, 331
glycemic index (GI), 91-93, 123, 336
Glycet, 319, 334
grains and starches, 56
grocery shopping, 68, 94-99, 101-3, 156
gum disease, 43-45, 300, 409
gymnema sylvestre, 128

H
hair growth, loss of, 29, 286
hamstring stretch, seated, 239
hand washing, 306, 308
Hands-On Food Guide, 55-59
health care team, 9, 84, 310-14, 324, 337, 354, 380
health claims, 96
healthy eaters, 83
healthy food choices, making, 201-16
heart attack, 27-28, 258, 322, 395
heart rate, 255-56
hemochromatosis, 20, 130
hemodialysis, 37
herbs and herbal supplements, 89, 122-27, 276, 277, 278, 401. See also flavorings
high blood sugar
    and blood vessels, 24-25
    emergency, 138
    improving, 90
    and infections, 29, 30, 44, 46, 306
    and nerves, 26
    symptoms, 18
    and weight loss, 143
    when exercising, 262
holiday eating, 75-77
hormones. See also insulin; estrogen; testosterone
    gut or appetite, 17, 53, 316, 320
    "happy," 121, 222, 279, 358, 360, 362, 390, 395, 396
    pregnancy, 15
    sodium excretion, 109
    stress, 46, 53, 139, 307, 332, 349
Humalog, 329
HumalogMix 75/25, 330
Humulin 30/70, 330
Humulin N, 327

Humulin R, 328
hypnosis, 273
hypoglycemia. See low blood sugar
hypoglycemic unawareness, 332, 348

I
ICI (IntraCavernosal Injection), 406
identification bracelet, 338
illness, 138-42, 337
immune system, 30, 46, 295, 306, 307, 308
incontinence, 46, 303, 305, 400
incretin therapies, 320
infections, 282-308. See also feet and lower legs; gum disease; urinary tract infections
insomnia. See sleep
insulin (as medication), 315, 323-30. See also specific insulins
    adjusting, 337
    and infection, 295, 300, 301
    intermediate, 325, 327, 330, 385
    long, 325, 326, 330, 331
    and low blood sugar, 136, 300, 332, 336
    patterns, 350
    during pregnancy, 385
    premixed, 330
    rapid, 75, 325, 329, 330, 336, 348, 385, 386
    short, 325, 328, 330, 385
    side effects, 324
    sick days, 139, 140
    and skin problems, 42
    starting on, 323
    syringe or pen, 325
    for teenagers, 378, 379
    and testing blood sugar, 345, 347, 349
    and weight gain, 143, 324
insulin resistance, 17, 20, 53
insulin secretagogues, 318
insulin sensitizers, 321
Intestine "Sugar Blockers," 316, 319
Intestine "Insulin Boosters," 316, 320
inulin, 92
iodine, 109, 110

J
Januvia, 320
juice, 88-89, 98, 370, 373

K
kidney damage, 27, 33-37, 109, 126, 308. See also urinary tract infections
kidneys, 33-34, 314
    lab tests, 341, 343, 344

L
lab tests, 339-44
Lantus, 326
laser therapy
    for eyes, 259, 314
    for quitting smoking, 273
laughter, 357-58
legs. See feet and lower legs
leg walk, 248
Levemir, 326
Levitra, 402

lifting, proper technique, 244
linagliptin, 320
Lipitor, 322
liraglutide, 320
lispro, 329
Liver "Sugar Blockers," 316, 317, 348
Lodalis, 319
low blood sugar, 127, 138, 140, 300, 324, 331-38
  causes, 332
  and exercise, 136, 256, 262, 337
  in newborns, 382
  over-treating, 336
  preventing, 336
  safety guidelines, 338
  symptoms, 333
  in teenagers, 379
  treating, 334-35
low-calorie sweeteners, 101, 103, 105, 106-8, 334, 385
lubricants, 302, 397, 398, 409
lunches, 160-66, 205

M

macroalbuminuria, 36-37
massage, 42, 244, 258, 276, 283, 362, 398
medications. *See also* diabetes medications
  for associated conditions, 295, 301, 322, 401-2, 406
  during illness, 139
  interactions, 126-28
  for quitting smoking, 273
medication side effects. *See specific medications*
meditation, 359, 364
menopause, 50, 403
menstruation, 403
mental health professional, 279, 314, 354, 365, 366
metformin, 317, 378
microalbuminuria, 35, 341
miglitol, 319
milk, 57, 98, 105
mini exerciser, 229, 234
mouth care, 297-300
MUSE (medicated urethral system for erection), 406
music, 361

N

nateglinide, 318, 331
nature, 359
nausea, 51, 140, 148, 385
neck stretch, 239
nephrologist, 314
nephrons, 34-36
nerve damage
  and bowel problems, 51
  and eye problems, 38
  and healthy feet, 286, 287, 341
  and high blood sugar, 26
  and infections, 29, 44, 46
  neuropathic pain, 42
  reversing, 295
neurologist, 314

nicotine replacement products, 270, 271-72, 278, 279
nitroglycerine, 257, 402
noodles, 210
Nordic walking poles, 225, 251
Novolin N, 327
Novolin ge Toronto/Novolin R, 328
NovoMix 30, 330
NovoRapid, 329
NPH insulin, 327
nurse, 312. *See also* health care team
nutrient analysis of meals, 150

O

oatmeal, 152
obstetrician, 314, 381
Onglyza, 320
ophthalmologist, 313, 314, 342
optometrist, 313, 342, 382
orlistat, 322
orthotics, 293, 295
overeating, 63, 75

P

pain, managing, 42
Pancreas "Insulin Boosters," 316, 318, 331, 345, 347, 378, 379
PDE5 inhibitors, 401, 402, 403
pedometer, 220
pedorthist, 293, 314
penis implants, 401
penis injection (ICI), 406
penis pumps, 401, 404-5
penis rings, 404-5
Peripheral Arterial Disease (PAD), 30, 224
peritoneal dialysis, 37
pharmacist, 126, 143, 268, 312, 316, 325
physiotherapist, 235, 237, 246, 314
pills. *See* diabetes medications; medications
pioglitazone, 321
pizza, 166, 209
plaque
  blood vessels, 25
  teeth, 44, 300
podiatrist, 288, 289, 293, 314
portion control, 55-59, 67-91, 119
potassium, 120, 126, 128, 133
potatoes, 211
pramlintide, 320
Prandase, 319, 334
Prandin, 318
Pravachol, 322
prayer, 359
Precose, 319, 334
pre-diabetes, 14, 61
pregnancy, 15, 135, 201, 230, 322, 326, 378, 381-86
prepared foods, 99, 110, 112-17
preschoolers with diabetes, 369-72
prickly pear cactus, 128
propranolol, 332
prostaglandin, 401, 406
prostate, enlarged, 48, 301
protein, 57, 145, 146, 158, 193
  in urine, 27, 35

R

recipes
  Cauliflower and Broccoli Slaw, 181
  Cinnamon Apple, 177
  Crepes, 154
  Deluxe Sandwich, 160
  Easy Chicken Curry, 188
  Garlic Bread, 177
  Homemade Chicken Strips, 176
  Hot Chicken Salad, 176
  Lady Vivian's English Trifle, 169
  Lemon Zinger Pudding, 185
  Luncheon Wrap, 164
  Mayo Parmesan Salad Dressing, 181
  Minute Steak, 168
  Nuts and Bolts Stir Fry, 172
  Peach Cobbler, 173
  Pizza Bun, 166
  Seafood Chowder, 184
  Taco Soup, 162
  Vegetable Omelet, 192
  Vegetarian Sauce (for pasta), 180
recipe substitutions, 104-5
record keeping, 355
  blood sugar, 348, 349
  exercise, 254
  food, 62-63
  lab tests, 343-44
regular insulin, 328
regular meals, 67, 76, 147, 277, 324, 336, 370
relaxation techniques, 363-64
repaglinide, 318, 331
restaurant meals, 59, 67, 70-74, 110, 116-17, 164, 307
retinopathy, 38-41, 135, 223, 236, 241, 259, 314
risks for diabetes, 19-20
rosiglitazone, 321
rowing machine, 236

S

salads, 176, 181, 212
saliva, 44, 297
salt. *See* sodium
salts, in the body, 33, 36
sandwiches, 160, 164, 205
saxagliptin, 320
screen time, limiting, 67, 219, 226, 369, 374
seasonings. *See* flavorings
self blood glucose monitoring. *See* blood sugar, testing at home
sex, 392-411
  adult toys, 409, 411
  benefits of, 392
  bedroom alternatives, 407-11
  erection devices, 401
  as exercise, 240
  and genital problems, 49-50
  intimacy/romance, 393-94, 398-400, 406, 410
  medications, 401-3
  self-fulfillment, 396
  sexual changes with diabetes, 392-94
  special needs and positioning, 399-400
  as stress relief, 362

sex (*continued*)
  and teenagers, 378
  therapist, 393, 394
  urologist, 314, 395
  and UTIs, 46-47, 301, 302, 305, 409
sexual organs, 49-50
sexually transmitted infections (STIs), 302, 378, 391, 392
sick days. *See* illness
sitagliptin, 320
skin care, 296. *See also* feet and lower legs
skin problems, 42
sleep, 53, 222, 244, 279, 307, 362-63, 371
smoking
  effects on body, 44, 121, 264-65, 283, 297, 307, 385
  quitting, 263-80, 395
snacks, 78-79, 196-200, 214, 216, 278, 334, 336, 363
sodium, 109-17, 140, 201
  reducing, 59, 98, 105, 110, 120, 162
  effect on body, 109, 324
sodium charts, 112-17
soft drinks, 87-88, 373
sorbitol. *See* sugar alcohols
soups, 98, 162, 184, 206
special occasions, 75-77
spices, 122, 278. *See also* flavorings
Splenda. *See* low-calorie sweeteners
stair stepper, 235
starches, 56
Starlix, 318
statins, 322
Stendra, 402
stevia, 106
stomach problems, 51
stomach tucks, 240, 243
stress, 52, 121, 222, 349, 352-64
  determining yours, 352-53
  effect on diabetes, 353-54
  managing, 77, 267, 279, 354-64
stroke, 27-28
sugar, added, 85-89, 91, 96, 101, 103, 105, 373
sugar alcohols, 102, 103, 139
sugar-free fluids, 140, 141
sugary drinks, 59, 85-89, 121, 370, 373
sunlight, 130, 132, 148, 259, 296, 307, 360
support team, 84
sweeteners. *See* low-calorie sweeteners
swimming, 223, 230-31
Symlin, 320

symptoms
  of type 1 diabetes, 15
  of type 2 diabetes, 18
  of kidney disease, 36

T

target heart rates, 256
tea, benefits, 92, 123
teenagers with diabetes, 373-80
  and alcohol, 379
  diabetes team, 380
  getting active, 374-77
  low blood sugar, 379
  medications and insulin, 378, 379
  pregnancy, 378
  sex, 378
teeth, care of, 44, 297-99
television. *See* screen time, limiting
testosterone, 49, 50, 401, 403
thrush (yeast), 45, 300, 409
thyroid, 109, 386
tooth decay, 45
touch, 362, 398, 407-11
Tragenta/Tradjenta, 320
traveling, 80-81
treadmills, 223, 224, 227, 234
treat budget, 68
TriCor, 322
triglycerides, 24, 25, 118-21, 127, 135, 322, 341
type 1 diabetes, 15
type 2 diabetes. *See also* diabetes
  in children, 368-80
  definition, 14, 16-17
  in pregnancy, 381-86
  risks for, 19-20
  symptoms of, 18
TZDs, 321

U

ulcers, 295
urethra, 47, 48, 302, 305
urinary tract infections (UTIs), 46-48, 301-5, 409
urine, and blood sugar, 46-47
urologist, 314, 395

V

vaccines
  for flu and pneumonia, 306
  for quitting smoking, 273
vaginal dryness, 302, 392, 397, 403, 408-9

vaginal infections. *See* urinary tract infections
vaginal secretions and blood sugar, 47
vegetables, 56
vending machines, 373
Viagra, 401, 402
Victoza, 320
vision. *See* eye problems
vitamins and minerals, 95, 97, 119, 129-33, 295, 307, 360, 385
Vitaros, 406
volunteering, 359
vomiting, 138, 139, 140, 308, 332, 337, 385

W

waist circumference, 340
walking
  after meals, 74, 77, 90
  at work, 78, 79
  daily walks, 82, 219, 220, 374, 383
  as aerobic exercise, 223, 224-27
  with arthritis, 237
  when quitting smoking, 277
wall squat, 243
water, drinking
  to help with cravings, 69
  when ill, 140
  for mouth care, 298
  to prevent infections, 302, 305, 307
  when exercising, 256, 257, 262
weight gain
  with insulin, 324
  during pregnancy, 384
  preventing when quitting smoking, 277-78
  if underweight, 143-48
weight lifting, 223, 236, 240-42
weight loss, 61-84, 94, 95, 107, 118, 134, 283, 322
WelChol, 319
"winter blues," 360
workplace eating, 78-79

X

Xenical, 322

Y

yeast. *See* thrush; urinary tract infections
yohimbine hydrochloride, 126, 401

Z

Zocor, 322

Library and Archives Canada Cataloguing in Publication

Graham, Karen, 1959-, author
  The complete diabetes guide for type 2 diabetes /
Karen Graham, RD, CDE.

Includes index.
ISBN 978-0-7788-0458-1 (pbk.)

  1. Diabetes–Popular works. I. Title.

RC662.18.G734 2013   616.4'62   C2013-902249-X

Library and Archives Canada Cataloguing in Publication

Graham, Karen, 1959-, author
  Canada's complete diabetes guide for type 2 diabetes /
Karen Graham, RD, CDE.

Includes index.
ISBN 978-0-7788-0469-7 (pbk.)

  1. Diabetes–Popular works. I. Title.

RC662.18.G733 2013   616.4'62   C2013-902247-3